Gene Targeting Protocols

METHODS IN MOLECULAR BIOLOGY™

John M. Walker, SERIES EDITOR

METHODS IN MOLECULAR BIOLOGY™

Gene Targeting Protocols

Edited by

Eric B. Kmiec

University of Delaware, Newark, Delaware

Humana Press ✳ Totowa, New Jersey

Dedication

For my wife, Jennifer

Cover illustration: The cover depicts the presence of active Green Fluorescent Protein being expressed in Chinese Hamster Ovary (CHO) cells. The phenotypic change is a result of the activity of the chimeric oligonucleotide on CHO cells that have integrated copies of mutated (inactive) GFP genes. Cells that have not been targeted or corrected to wild-type appear in the background. The technique known as gene repair or chimeraplasty was pioneered by the editor who supplied this picture.
Cover design by Patricia F. Cleary

For additional copies, pricing for bulk purchases, and/or information about other Humana titles, contact Humana at the above address or at any of the following numbers: Tel: 973-256-1699; Fax: 973-256-8341; E-mail: humana@humanapr.com or visit our Website at www.humanapress.com

Gene targeting protocols / edited by Eric B. Kmiec.
    p. cm. -- (Methods in molecular biology ; v. 133
    Includes index
    ISBN 0-89603-360-0 (alk. paper)
    1. Gene targetting--Laboratory manuals. I. Kmiec, Eric.
    II. Series. III. Series: Methods in molecular biology (Clifton, N.J.) v. 133.
    [DNLM: 1. Gene Targeting laboratory manuals. W1 ME9616J v. 133
1999 / QH 442.3 G326 1999]
QH442.3.G46 1999
572.8'77--dc21
DNLM/DLC
For Library of Congress   99-10333
                                                                     CIP

Preface

The potential now exists in many experimental systems to transfer a cloned, modified gene back into the genome of the host organism. In the ideal situation, the cloned gene is returned to its homologous location in the genome and becomes inserted at the target locus. This process is a controlled means for the repair of DNA damage and ensures accurate chromosome disjunction during meiosis. The paradigm for thinking about the mechanism of this process has emerged primarily from two sources: (1) The principles of reaction mechanics have come from detailed biochemical analyses of the RecA protein purified from *Escherichia coli*; and (2) the principles of information transfer have been derived from genetic studies carried out in bacteriophage and fungi. A compelling picture of the process of homologous pairing and DNA strand exchange has been influential in directing investigators interested in gene targeting experiments.

The ability to find and pair homologous DNA molecules enables accurate gene targeting and is the central phenomenon underlying genetic recombination. Biochemically, the overall process can be thought of as a series of steps in a reaction pathway whereby DNA molecules are brought into homologous register, the four-stranded Holliday structure intermediate is formed, heteroduplex DNA is extended, and DNA strands are exchanged. Not much is known about the biochemical pathway leading to homologous recombination in eukaryotes. Nevertheless, in *Saccharomyces cerevisiae*, a great deal of information has accumulated about the genetic control of recombination and the molecular events leading to integration of plasmid DNA into homologous sequences within the genome during transformation. Substantial insight into the mechanism of recombination between plasmid DNA and the genome has come from studies using nonreplicating plasmids containing a cloned gene homologous to an endogenous genomic sequence. Transformation of *S. cerevisiae* at high frequency takes place when the plasmid DNA is cut within the cloned DNA sequence. Almost invariably, transformants contain plasmid DNA integrated into the yeast genome at the homologous site. Autonomously replicating plasmids containing gaps of several hundred nucleotide residues within the cloned gene also transform at high efficiency and are repaired by recombination using chromosomal information as a template.

What has emerged from these studies on transformation of *S. cerevisiae* is a body of observations that has helped shape strategies for gene targeting in higher organisms. Unfortunately, the limited biochemical data available from yeast, and the often confusing and sometimes contradictory results from the genetic studies, have not provided a thorough mechanistic foundation for experimentation. It is not completely clear from the transformation studies carried out that information on the genetic control of plasmid integration will be generally applicable to high eukaryotic systems under study by investigators interested in gene targeting. The significance of the functionally independent, yet structurally redundant, RecA-like *Rad51*, *Rad55*, *Rad57*, and *Dmc1* genes in *S. cerevisiae* is not clear. The virtual absence of the illegitimate integration events during plasmid transformation commonly observed in many other eukaryotic systems raises certain caveats about the generality of the recombination system in yeast. Nevertheless, structural homologs of *rad51* and/or *rad52* have been identified in several higher eukaryotes, providing some indication that fundamentally similar biological principles underlie the mechanism of homologous recombination from bacteria to higher animals and plants, as well as that rules of gene targeting learned from transformation analysis of lower eukaryotes will be widely applicable.

With respect to gene targeting in higher eukaryotes, the tantalizing carrot of gene replacement as gene therapy remains dangling. Though noble approaches are underway to incorporate this methodology in molecular medicine venues, it is unlikely that gene therapies will become elements of common practice in the near term. Hence, what we are left with is a powerful process and extension technique in which gene targeting protocols can be used to achieve equally important goals. That is what *Gene Targeting Protocols* is about—the use of gene targeting techniques to create experimental systems that help us understand biological processes at a genetic level.

We have requested chapter contributions from members of the scientific community who are at the forefront of those dealing with and/or overcoming many of the barriers caused by the low frequency of homologous recombination. Clearly, more techniques are under study than those represented here, but we have striven to present a wide range of approaches that may be intriguing and, we hope, useful to the reader.

One of the most important features of gene targeting is the delivery of the construct into the nucleus of the cell. Whereas viral vectors are naturally occurring delivery vehicles, naked DNA is taken up quite poorly by mammalian cells. To overcome this problem, a number of strategies have been employed, one of which is the use of cationic lipids. The field of liposome delivery is rapidly expanding and the literature is often misleading and confusing. In addition, the choice of a particular liposome transfer vehicle for delivery into a particular cell type is viewed as crucial. In the chapter by Natasha Caplen, the variety of liposomes available to investigators and the criteria for choosing one to fit the experimental purpose is discussed in detail. Caplen surveys commercially available liposomes and outlines the advantages and disadvantages of each.

Along the same lines, Barbara Demeneix and colleagues discuss the use of polyethylenimine (PEI) as a gene transfer vehicle. One of the most appealing aspects of PEI is its nontoxicity in vivo. Details regarding the importance of determining the optimal ratio of PEI to DNA are outlined and a specific case study using brain cells is provided. In contrast, Xi Zhao discusses a relatively new approach to gene delivery using electronic pulse delivery (EPD). The EPD system differs from traditional electroporation in the use of selected pulse waves and the ultralow current. This technique provides a transfer efficiency of over 80% with a viability index of EPD-treated cells approaching 90%. It may be the most efficient physical delivery protocol currently in use. In the chapter by Greg May and colleagues, electroporation conditions for transfer of oligonucleotides into plant cells are outlined. Though the focus of many gene transfer protocols is mammalian cells, the capacity to alter plant genomes is of utmost importance.

Since many of the protocols outlined above discuss the virtues and drawbacks of the transfer vehicle, it is also imperative to understand the cell itself. Clearly, the state of the cell in terms of metabolism and cell cycle position upon becoming manipulated affects the efficiency of transfer. Nancy Smyth Templeton discusses the various parameters that affect vector uptake. In addition, she discusses the design of the DNA vector itself in a protocol aimed at gene targeting in mammalian cells. What has become apparent is that the amount of vector introduced relative to the cell culture conditions is critical in improving gene targeting frequency. The method of transfer for this protocol is electroporation, which complements the May chapter on plant cell electroporation. The chapter contributed by David Strayer outlines an important use of the viral vector SV40. Strayer's group has developed an efficient delivery system to assess cellular uptake and extended expression of marker genes after integration. The use of this vector is novel and will likely overcome significant delivery problems.

The next group of chapters outlines a series of protocols commonly used for gene targeting. Among the most successful is Cre-lox, developed by Brian Sauer and colleagues. In his chapter, he outlines the strategy for creating cell lines that express specific transgenes using the Cre recombinase. This system has been widely used because of its remarkable versatility. Perhaps the most important aspect of Cre-lox is its reversibility. A transgene can be inserted, expressed, studied for cellular effects, and then removed. Kaarin Goncz and Dieter Gruenert outline a similar approach in which small fragments of DNA are used to alter the genome by site-directed insertion. Such a technique enables gene replacement strategies that can lead to molecular therapy or improve knockout events. The simplicity of the vector itself is a key feature in using this approach to disrupt mammalian cells.

Several viral-based systems are also described, including the use of a modified adenoviral vector by Ichizo Kobayashi and colleagues to create a cell line that is amenable to high levels of homologous recombination events. This work pulls together several aspects of this volume including cell culture manipulation and vector design. The adenoviral vectors can allow for nearly 100% of the cells to acquire the transfer without influencing viability. In the same vein, Jude Samulski and colleagues provide a protocol for using adeno-associated virus (AAV) to introduce transgenes at a specific site in chromosome 19. The objective of this strategy is somewhat different from the others reported herein, since the site of integration is determined by the viral vector, not by the transgene. AAV has a predilection for integrating at a specific site on chromosome 19, and if one wishes to introduce a transgene permanently into the chromosome for inheritable expression, this technique is optimal. Richard Bartlett and Jesica McCue provide an excellent background on AAV biology, detailing targeted integration and studies of rAAV-based gene therapy vectors. They also provide an introduction to the studies using an AAV-based plasmid vector to express human insulin in skeletal muscle of diabetic animals.

Two chapters in *Gene Targeting Protocols* take a fundamentally different approach to gene targeting. The first by Sun Song and Wayne Marasco utilizes a fusion protein, attached to a plasmid, to deliver the vector to a target, in this case a virus. Although many protocols are aimed at targeting host chromosomal genes, the field of gene targeting also includes virus targeting. These authors outline a protocol that can deliver a therapeutic gene to a specific cell in animals. The target cell may be one that has been infected with a virus and the expression of the gene once transferred into the correct cell may have a therapeutic effect. The chapter by Jovan Mirkovitch and colleagues provides an interesting system for overcoming a serious barrier to therapeutic gene targeting. This problem is centered on the regulation of transgene expression. In many cases, the chromatin structure covering the transgene heavily influences its expression and may subvert even heroic efforts used to introduce the gene into the chromosome. To avert this problem, these authors have designed an episomal-based Epstein-Barr viral vector that can modulate the chromatin assembly process. This contribution impacts the choices of integrative vectors and enables evaluation of gene therapy expression cassettes prior to introduction into mammalian cells.

The final section of *Gene Targeting Protocols* centers on the use of oligonucleotides in gene targeting. These types of molecules have been used in the antisense field for many years to block gene expression at the mRNA level. In most cases, the mechanism of inhibition involves the hybridization of the oligo with the complementary mRNA sequence and subsequent destruction of the hybrid by cellular enzymes. Clinical applications have received mixed reviews, but no one disputes the controlled environment in which synthetic molecules can be produced. The authors of these chapters are developing new strategies for the use of oligonucleotides in gene targeting. In all cases, the objective is to alter or manipulate the gene at the genomic level, in other words, within the coding region. Karen Vasquez and John Wilson employ specialized oligonucleotides capable of forming a third strand of the helix to block gene expression, while Howard Gamper and colleagues use modified single-stranded oligos to introduce an adduct at a specific site. Peter Kipp and colleagues use a novel chimeric RNA/DNA oligonucleotide to introduce a specific base mutation in the tobacco genome to render the target cells resistant to herbicide. Ryszard Kole and colleagues have developed an interesting strategy for altering the splice sites in pre-mRNA. Such changes are then translated into mRNA molecules that code for different proteins. The field of targeted gene manipulation by oligonucleotides is quite new and among all the areas of scientific endeavor, is likely to be one that revolutionizes the entire field. Even with such a promising future, the current targets are single bases only and larger conversions are likely to require futuristic designs.

In the past ten years, a number of genetic protocols aimed at improving the frequency of gene targeting have been developed. Some of them have been significantly limited in their applications, whereas others are still being evaluated. The scientific community is necessarily skeptical at the advent of new techniques until their validity can be irrevocably established. Clearly, politics often plays a role in the acceptance of new techniques, but even such opinions are ultimately rewritten by the accumulation of careful and rigorous scientific experimentation.

The authors who contributed to this volume, in our opinion, comprise a group of the most innovative and dedicated workers in the field. The majority of techniques presented here are described by the lab from which they originated. It is likely that many, if not all, of these protocols will become commonplace in future molecular genetics research. I wish to thank all of the authors for their contributions and their patience. I am indebted to Paul Dolgert from Humana Press and John Walker from the University of Hertfordshire for their continued support throughout this endeavor. Finally, I wish to thank my administrative assistant, Tony Rice, for his efforts on this project. He played a crucial role in organizing this volume and without his dedication it is unlikely this book would have been completed.

Eric B. Kmiec

Contents

Contributors

IRINA AFONINA • *Epoch Pharmaceuticals, Inc., Redmond, WA*

SUDHIR AGRAWAL • *Hybridon Inc., Worcester, MA*

RICHARD J. BARTLETT • *Diabetes Research Institute, Departments of Medicine and Neurology, University of Miami School of Medicine, Miami, FL*

M. CHIARA BASSI • *Swiss Institute for Experimental Cancer Research (ISREC), Epalinges, Switzerland*

PETER R. BEETHAM • *Kimeragen Inc., Newtown, PA*

EVGENIY BELOUSOV • *Epoch Pharmaceuticals Inc., Redmond, WA*

BRUCE D. BETHKE • *Department of Biology, St. Vincent College, Latrobe, PA*

NATASHA J. CAPLEN • *Clinical Gene Therapy Branch, National Human Genome Research Institute, Bethesda, MD*

BARBARA A. DEMENEIX • *Laboratiore de Physiologie Generale et Comparee, Museum National d'Histoire Naturelle, Paris, France*

JULIETTE FIVAZ • *Swiss Institute for Experimental Cancer Research (ISREC), Epalinges, Switzerland*

AYUMI FUJITA-KUSANO • *Department of Molecular Biology, Institute of Medical Science, University of Tokyo, Shiroganedai, Minato-ku, Tokyo, Japan*

HOWARD B. GAMPER • *Jefferson Center for Biomedical Research, Thomas Jefferson University, Doylestown, PA*

MOHAMED GHORBEL • *Laboratoire de Physiologie Generale et Comparee, Museum National d'Histoire Naturelle, Paris, France*

KAARIN K. GONCZ • *Cardiovascular Research Institute, Gene Therapy Care Center, and Cystic Fibrosis Research Center, University of California, San Francisco, CA*

DANIEL GOULA • *Laboratoire de Physiologie Generale et Comparee, Museum National d'Histoire Naturelle, Paris, France*

DIETER C. GRUENERT • *Cardiovascular Research Institute, Gene Therapy Core Center, and Cystic Fibrosis Research Center, Department of Laboratory Medicine, and Stomatology, University of California, San Francisco, CA*

PETER B. KIPP • *Boyce Thompson Institute for Plant Research Inc., Ithaca, NY*

ERIC B. KMIEC • *Department of Biological Sciences, University of Delaware, Newark, DE*

ICHIZO KOBAYASHI • *Department of Molecular Biology, Institute of Medical Science, University of Tokyo, Shiroganedai, Minato-ku, Tokyo, Japan*

RYSZARD KOLE • *Lineberger Comprehensive Cancer Center and Department of Pharmacology, School of Medicine, University of North Carolina at Chapel Hill, Chapel Hill, NC*

WAYNE A. MARASCO • *Dana Farber Cancer Institute, Harvard Medical School, Boston, MA*

GREGORY D. MAY • *Boyce Thompson Institute, Cornell University, Plant Research Inc., Ithaca, NY*

JESICA M. MCCUE • *Diabetes Research Institute, Department of Medicine, University of Miami School of Medicine, Miami, FL*

JOVAN MIRKOVITCH • *Swiss Institute for Experimental Cancer Research (ISREC), Epalinges, Switzerland*

YASUHIRO NAITO • *Department of Molecular Biology, Institute of Medical Science, University of Tokyo, Shiroganedai, Minato-ku, Tokyo, Japan*

STÉPHANE PINAUD • *Swiss Institute for Experimental Cancer Research (ISREC), Epalinges, Switzerland*

MIKHAIL A. PODYMINOGIN • *Epoch Pharmaceuticals Inc., Redmond, WA*

MELANIE PRICE • *Swiss Institute for Experimental Cancer Research (ISREC), Epalinges, Switzerland*

MICHAEL W. REED • *Epoch Pharmaceuticals Inc., Redmond, WA*

LARRY RICHMAN • *Swiss Institute for Experimental Cancer Research (ISREC), Epalinges, Switzerland*

IZUMU SAITO • *Department of Molecular Biology, Institute of Medical Science, University of Tokyo, Shiroganedai, Minato-ku, Tokyo, Japan*

RICHARD JUDE SAMULSKI • *Gene Therapy Center, University of North Carolina at Chapel Hill, Chapel Hill, NC*

BRIAN SAUER • *Developmental Biology Program, Oklahoma Medical Research Foundation, Oklahoma City, OK*

HALINA SIERAKOWSKA • *Institute of Biochemistry and Biophysics, Warsaw, Poland*

SUN U. SONG • *Department of Surgical Oncology, Massachusetts General Hospital, Boston, MA*

DAVID S. STRAYER • *Departments of Pathology, Anatomy, and Cell Biology, Jefferson Medical College, Philadelphia, PA*

NANCY SMYTH TEMPLETON • *Center for Cell and Gene Therapy, Baylor College of Medicine, Houston, TX*

JOYCE M. VAN ECK • *Boyce Thompson Institute, Ithaca, NY*

KAREN M. VASQUEZ • *Verna and Marrs McLean Department of Biochemistry, Baylor College of Medicine, Houston, TX*

JOHN H. WILSON • *Department of Biochemistry, Baylor College of Medicine, Houston, TX*

WEIDONG XIAO • *Department of MGB, University of Pittsburgh, Pittsburgh, PA*

SAMUEL M. YOUNG, JR. • *Gene Therapy Center, University of North Carolina at Chapel Hill, Chapel Hill, NC*

XI ZHAO • *InCell Inc., Santa Clara, CA*

1

Nucleic Acid Transfer Using Cationic Lipids

Natasha J. Caplen

1. Introduction

The use of cationic lipids or cationic polymers to mediate the transfer of nucleic acids into mammalian cells has become a widely applied technology in recent years. The principal reasons for this have been the ease with which the methodology can be applied to a wide range of cell types; the relatively low cytotoxicity compared to other techniques; the high efficiency of nucleic acid transfer in comparison with methods such as calcium phosphate or diethyl-aminoethyl-dextran-mediated transfection; and the potential application of these systems to human gene therapy. The use of positively charged lipid-based macromolecules to deliver nucleic acids makes use of the fact that DNA, RNA, and oligonucleotides carry a negative charge caused by the phosphate groups that form the backbone of these molecules. The electrostatic interaction between the negatively charged nucleic acid and the positively charged macro-molecule induces a range of structural changes that vary, depending on the macro-molecule used. In general, however, the process results in condensation or compaction of the nucleic acid and physical association of the nucleic acid with the lipid. The interaction generates a complex that is more amenable to cellular uptake, protects sufficient nucleic acid molecules to allow trafficking to the nucleus, and, in at least some cases, may also facilitate transfer into the nucleus.

Cationic lipid- and polymer-mediated nucleic acid transfer have been used mostly for the transfection of plasmid DNA in applications in which transient gene expression is sufficient or required, but nucleic acids in all forms, ranging from small oligonucleotides to artificial chromosomes, can be transferred using these systems (*1–5*). RNA has also been transfected using these techniques (*6,7*), and, recently, hybrid molecules containing RNA and DNA residues have been transfected using both lipid- and polymer-based delivery systems (*8,9*).

From: *Methods in Molecular Biology, vol. 133: Gene Targeting Protocols*
Edited by: E. Kmiec © Humana Press Inc., Totowa, NJ

Because of the rapid speed with which this technology has developed, the terms associated with it have at times been confusing. In an attempt to simplify at least some aspects of this evolving terminology, Felgner et al. *(10)* have recently described a consensus nomenclature. Accordingly, "lipoplex" refers to any cationic lipid–nucleic acid complex, and "polyplex" refers to any cationic polymer–nucleic acid complex. "Lipofection" should be used to describe nucleic acid delivery by cationic lipids, and "polyfection," nucleic acid delivery mediated by cationic polymers. This chapter will concentrate on the practical aspects of lipofection, although many of the technical points made can equally apply to polyfection.

1.1. Lipofection

The use of a positively charged lipid to deliver nucleic acids to mammalian cells was first reported in 1987 *(11)*. Cationic lipids are usually used in the form of liposomes (membranous lipid vesicles that enclose an aqueous volume), which are small (100–400 nm) and unilamellar, though the use of multilamellar cationic liposomes has also been reported. The lipids most commonly consist of a pair of fatty acids possessing a hydrophobic tail and a hydrophilic head group. In aqueous solutions, the hydrophobic tails self-associate to exclude water; the hydrophilic head group interacts with any aqueous liquid on the inside and outside of the vesicle. Cationic liposomes can be formed from double-chain cationic lipids, which form liposomes spontaneously; however, most positively charged liposomes produced for nucleic acid transfer contain a nonbilayer-forming cationic lipid and a neutral helper lipid, such as dioleoyl-phosphatidylethanolamine (DOPE), which stabilizes the liposome. The head group of the cationic lipid is responsible for interactions between the liposomes and DNA, and between lipoplexes and cell membranes or other components of the cell. The head group of most cationic lipids contains simple or multiple amine groups with different degrees of substitution. Other domains of the lipid are the spacer arm, the linker bond (which appears to be important in determining the chemical stability and the biodegradability of the cationic lipid, thus influencing the toxicity profile of the liposome), and the hydrophobic lipid anchor *(12,13)*. There are two forms of hydrophobic lipid anchors that have been used; anchors based on a cholesterol ring, such as DC-Chol *(14)*, and those based on a pair of aliphatic chains, such as DMRIE *(15)*. There have been several recent studies systematically assessing different combinations of these critical moieties and these should be referred to for further details *(15–17)*.

The interaction of the positively charged liposome with negatively charged DNA results in the spontaneous formation of a complex. Little is known about the interaction of the nucleic acid and the liposome; however, under optimal conditions, the association between the DNA and the lipid appears to be very tight, protecting DNA from DNase digestion *(18–20)*. Various models have been proposed that describe the DNA–lipid interaction *(18,19,21,22)*. One of the most recent models, using *in situ* optical microscopy and X-ray diffraction, visualized lipoplexes consisting of a higher-ordered multilamellar structure, with DNA sandwiched between cationic bilayers *(23,24)*. However, it is likely that different liposomes, particularly mono- vs multivalent cationic lipids, may interact with nucleic acids in different ways, and thus aspects of all the current models may be correct. It should also be noted that the lipoplexes formed have often been observed to be heterogeneous and dynamic; as yet, no model has fully taken this aspect into account. To facilitate delivery of the DNA to the cell, lipoplexes interact with mammalian cell membranes, but the mechanism is unknown. The initial interaction between the lipoplex and the cell membrane is electrostatic, as a result of the excess positive charge associated with the lipoplex and the net negative charge of the cell surface. Endocytosis, phagocytosis, pinocytosis, and direct fusion with the cell membrane may all play a role in lipoplex cell entry, depending on the cell type *(11,25–30)*. Different cationic lipids may produce lipoplexes that are taken up by cells in different ways, and different cell types, and even cells in various states of differentiation, may use alternative cell trafficking pathways. DNA probably needs to be released from lipoplexes prior to entry into the nucleus, because microinjection of lipoplexes directly into the nucleus results in poor transgene expression, in comparison with introduction of naked DNA *(29)*.

1.2. Formulation and Transfection Efficiency

The need to optimize the formulation of a lipoplex cannot be overstated. A significant number of biochemical, biophysical, and cellular variables can influence the final level of transgene expression mediated by any given lipoplex, by several orders of magnitude. The most critical, and thus most studied, variables are, the ratio of the nucleic acid and the cationic lipid, the concentration of these components, the total amount of nucleic acid and lipid, and the composition of the diluent in which the complexes are formed *(31–34)*. The ratio of nucleic acid to cationic lipid can be expressed in several ways, based on a weight:weight (w:w) formulation, on a ratio based on the molarity of the two components (mol:mol), or on the ratio of the positive to negative charge. The importance of the DNA and lipid ratio probably reflects the need to neutralize a critical amount of charge to form a complex of the DNA and lipid, and yet results in a net positive charge to the lipoplex, to facilitate interaction with the negatively charged cell surface. The initial concentration of DNA and lipid, when forming the lipoplex, appears to influence the interaction of the DNA and lipid and the degree of condensation. The final concentration of the lipoplex that comes into contact with cells is also important, because high concentrations of DNA and lipid can be cytotoxic. The absolute amount of DNA or lipid used appears to influence optimal interaction of the lipoplex with the cell, probably because insufficient DNA results in reduced transgene expression and excess lipid results in cytotoxicity. The composition of the diluent in which the complex is formed is critical, because this can modulate the available charge caused by the presence of chelating agents, salts, and the influence of pH; protein can also significantly interfere in the complexation process. In addition, the medium in which the lipofection is performed is important, given the need to balance conditions that favor gene transfer with conditions that maintain cell viability. Unfortunately, the determined amount for each variable often does not translate between cell lines, and, more important, from in vitro to in vivo applications.

The degree to which all these variables must be optimized will, to some extent, be dependent on the goal of the investigator. If lipofection is to be used to obtain transient transgene expression once (e.g., to simply confirm transgene expression from a new vector), then only minimal optimization is probably required. Often the use of standard conditions, as outlined in **Subheading 3.1.**, described by the manufacturer, or reported in previous literature, will be sufficient. However, if the ultimate goal requires relatively high levels of nucleic acid transfer (e.g., in the generation of replication-defective viral vectors), or if a comparative analysis of different plasmid constructs is the aim (e.g., assessment of the level of transgene expressione from different promoters), or if the methodology is to be related to gene therapy (e.g., assessment of a new cell target), then there must be due regard to the formulation used, as outlined in **Subheading 3.2.**

2. Materials

2.1. Lipofection

1. Many cationic lipids are available with proven transfection ability in multiple cell lines and cell types. **Table 1** lists some of the commercially available cationic lipids marketed for nucleic acid transfer, and **Table 2** lists several other cationic lipids reported in the literature. *See* **Note 1** for suggestions on the choice of lipid, and *see* **Note 2** for storage and preparation.
2. Cell lines (*see* **Note 3**).
3. Appropriate cell culture medium: Dulbecco's modified eagle medium (DMEM), minimum essential medium (MEM), or RPMI 1640; fetal bovine serum (FBS), and any additional growth factors and supplements, depending on the requirements of the particular cell line. Antibiotics, such as penicillin, streptomycin, or gentamicin, are optional. Trypsin-EDTA, or the appropriate trypsin for the cells or cell lines of interest.
4. Reduced-serum medium, such as OptiMEM, a modified eagle MEM (Life Technologies, Gaithersburg, MD).

Table 1
Examples of Commercially Available
Cationic Lipids Marketed for Nucleic Acid Transfer

Trade Name	Chemical	Composition	Company
Lipofectin®	DOTMA: DOPE (1:1 w/w)	N-[1-(2.3-Dioleyloxy)propyl]-N,N,N-trimethylammonium chloride and dioleoyl phosphatidylethanolamine	Life Technologies[a]
DMRIE-C	DMRIE:Cholesterol (1:1 mol/mol)	1,2-Dimyristyloxypropyl 1-3-dimethyl-hydroxylammonium bromide and cholesterol	Life Technologies[a]
Lipofect-Amine™	DOSPA: DOPE (3:1 w/w)	2,3-Dioleyloxy-N-[2(spermine-carboxamido)ethyl]-N,N-dimethyl-1-propanaminiumtrifluoroacetate and dioleoyl phosphatidylethanolamine	Life Technologies[a]
CellFectin™	TM-TPS: DOPE (1:1.5 mol/mol)	N,N^{I},N^{II},N^{III}-tetramethyl-N,N^{I},N^{II}, N^{III}-tetrapalmitylspermine and dioleoyl phosphatidylethanolamine	Life Technologies[a]
Lipofect-ACE™	DDAB: DOPE (1:2.5 w/w)	Dimethyl dioctadecylammonium bromide and dioleoyl phosphatidylethanolamine	Life Technologies[a]
DOTAP	DOTAP	N-[1-(2,3-Dioleoyloxy)propyl]-N,N,N-trimethylammonium methyl-sulfate[g]	Boehringer Mannheim[b]
DOSPER	DOSPER	1,3-Di-oleoyloxy-2-(6-carboxy-spermyl)-propylamid	Boehringer Mannheim[b]
LipoTaxi™	Not available	Not available	Stratagene[c]
Clonfectin™	–	N-t-butyl-N'-tetradecyl-3-tetra-decylaminopropion-amidine	Clontech[d]
Transfectam®	DOGS	Dioctadecylamidoglycyl spermine	Promega[e]
Tfx-10™, Tfx-20™, Tfx-50™	–	N,N,N^{I},N^{I}-tetramethyl-N,N^{I}-bis(2-hydroxyethyl)-2,3-dioleoyloxy-1,4-butanediammonium iodide and dioleoyl phosphatidylethanolamine	Promega[e]
TransFast™	–	(+)-N,N[bis(2-hydroxyethyl)-N-methyl-N-[2,3-di(tetradecanoyloxy)propyl]ammonium iodide and dioleoyl phosphatidylethanolamine	Promega[e]
PerFect Lipid™ transfection	pFx-1–8	Not available	Invitrogen[f]

[a]Life Technologies, Gaithersburg, MD; [b]Boehringer Mannheim, Indianapolis, IN; [c]Strategene, La Jolla, CA; [d]Clontech, Palo Alto, CA; [e]Promega, Madison, WI; [f]Invitrogen Corporation, Carlsbad,CA; [g]name derives from the nomenclature 1,2 -dioleoyloxy-3-(trimethylammonium) propane.

Table 2
Examples of Cationic Lipids used for Nucleic Acid Transfer

Name	Composition	Ref.
DC-Chol: DOPE	3β [*N-N',N'*-dimethylaminoethane) carbomoyl] cholesterol[a] and dioleoyl phosphatidylethanolamine (1:1 mol/mol)	*(14)*
DMRIE	1,2-Dimyristyloxypropyl 1-3-dimethyl-hydroxylammonium bromide	*(15)*
GL67	(3-amino-propyl) [4-(3-Amino-propylamino)-butyl]-carbamic acid 17-(1,5-dimethyl-hazyl)-10,13-dimethyl-2,3,4,7,8,9,10,11,12, 13,14,15,16,17-tetradecahydro-1H-cyclopenta[α]phenanthren-3yl ester and dioleoyl phosphatidylethanolamine (3:2 mol/mol)	*(16)*

[a]DC-Chol lipid can be obtained from Sigma, St. Louis, MO, (cat. no. C2832).

5. Phosphate-buffered saline (1X PBS): 137 mM NaCl, 2.7 mM KCl, 10 mM Na$_2$HPO$_4$, 1.8 mM KH$_2$PO$_4$.
6. Sterile, polystyrene, tissue culture plasticware. Most standard tissue culture treated plasticware is suitable for performing cationic lipid transfections; **Table 3** shows the plates and dishes most commonly used.
7. Hemocytometer or automatic cell counter (Coulter, Miami, FL).
8. Standard tissue culture facilities, including a flowhood suitable for sterile work, and CO$_2$ incubators.
9. Sterile polystyrene tubes. Typically, the author uses 6-mL (12 × 75 mm) or 14-mL (17 × 100 mm) Falcon tubes (Falcon no. 2058 or no. 2057; Becton and Dickinson, Lincoln Park, NJ).
10. Nucleic acid (*see* **Note 4** for preparation).
11. Pipet aids and pipetors for dispensing small and large volumes (1–20 mL). Sterile pipets and pipet tips for use with pipette aids and pipetors.
12. Means of analyzing transgene expression or other readouts of nucleic acid transfer (*see* **Note 5**).

2.2. Assessment of Formulation Variables

1. Materials 1–5 and 7–12 required for the standard transfection protocol listed above, are also required for assessment of formulation variables.
2. Sterile, polystyrene 24-well plates.
3. Assay of total protein content (*see* **Note 6**).

3. Methods

3.1. Transfection

The method described below was developed for transfection of plasmid DNA using DC-Chol:DOPE *(14)* or DOTMA:DOPE (Lipofectin®, Life Technologies). However, this protocol is equally applicable to many other cationic lipids, with

Table 3
Suggested Quantities of Some Reagents
Used for Cationic Lipid-Mediated DNA Transfection

Tissue culture plate/dish/flask	Number of cells: Adherent	Number of cells: Suspension	Amount of plasmid DNA	Final volume of lipoplex	Volume of OptiMEM medium
96-well plate	1×10^4	2×10^4	0.2–0.5 µg	10 µL	90 µL
24-well plate	1×10^5	2×10^5	1–2 µg	50 µL	450 µL
12-well plate	5×10^5	1×10^6	2–4 µg	100 µL	900 µLl
6-well plate	1×10^6	2×10^6	3–5 µg	200 µL	1800 µL
60-mm dish	5×10^6	1×10^7	5–10 µg	500 µL	4500 µL
100-mm dish	1×10^7	2×10^7	>7.5 µg	1000 µL	9000 µL

only minor modifications. Where space has allowed, some of these modifications have been noted, particularly with respect to the more widely used commercial cationic lipid preparations; adaptation to other nucleic acids is also relatively easy.

3.1.2. Cell Culture

3.1.2.1. ADHERENT CELLS

1. Routine cell culture should be followed using the appropriate subcultivation ratio when passing cells (*see* **Note 3**).
2. Seed cells to be between 50 and 70% confluent by the following day. The number of cells to be plated per well for most cell types are shown in **Table 3** (*see* **Note 3**).
3. Wash cells twice with PBS, and once with OptiMEM, prior to transfection to remove residual FBS. Add OptiMEM medium to the cells. **Table 3** shows the final volume of OptiMEM medium added to the well or dish of the most commonly used cell culture formats (*see* **Note 7**).

3.1.2.2. SUSPENSION CELLS

1. Routine cell culture should be followed, using the appropriate subcultivation ratio when passing cells (*see* **Note 3**).
2. Harvest cells by centrifugation, and wash cells twice with PBS, and once with OptiMEM, prior to transfection to remove residual FBS. Resuspend the cells in OptiMEM at a concentration of 1×10^6 cells/mL and transfer the numbers of cells per well, shown in **Table 3**, to the dish or plate of choice. Add further OptiMEM medium to bring the final volume up to that required in each well or dish, *see* **Table 3** for the final volumes needed for the most commonly used cell culture plates or dishes (*see* **Note 7**).

3.1.4. Formation of Lipoplexes

1. Plasmid DNA and liposomes must be diluted separately to reduce aggregation of the lipoplexes.

2. The amount of DNA transfected for a given number of cells is shown in **Table 3** (*see* **Note 8**). Dilute the DNA in OptiMEM medium, up to 50% of the final complex volume (*see* **Table 3**), in a sterile polystyrene tube. Add the DNA to prealiquoted OptiMEM. *See* **Note 9** for alternative diluents.

3. The amount of lipid to be used will be dependent on the optimum ratio (*see* **Subheading 3.2.**); however, for DC-Chol:DOPE and DOTMA:DOPE transfections of most cell types the most widely used ratio is 1:5 w:w (*see* **Notes 10** and **11**). The lipid is diluted in 50% of the final complex volume (*see* **Table 3**), in a sterile polystyrene tube. Add the lipid to prealiquoted OptiMEM (*see* **Note 12**). *See* **Note 13** for details of scale-up.

4. Lipoplexes are formed by mixing of the two separately diluted DNA and lipid solutions by addition of one solution to the other. Lipid can be added to DNA, or vice versa, with no obvious effect on transfection efficiency (*see* **Note 14**). Pipet one solution into the other, invert the tube once, or, if the volumes are small, gently tap the tube to ensure mixing (*see* **Note 15**). Allow the lipoplex to form for up to 15 min at room temperature; the solution should become turbid (*see* **Note 15**).

3.1.5. Addition of Lipoplex

3.1.5.1. ADHERENT CELLS

Add the lipoplex solution to the OptiMEM covered cells. Gently swirl the dish or plate to ensure equal distribution of the complex. Return cells to normal growth environment.

3.1.5.2. SUSPENSION CELLS

Add the lipoplex solution to the cells suspended in OptiMEM. Mix by gently aspirating the total volume up and down 2–3× with a pipet. Return cells to normal growth environment.

3.1.6. Posttransfection

For most cell types, exposure of cells to the complex for 8–18 h works most effectively (*see* **Note 16**). After exposure of the cells to the lipoplex, remove the OptiMEM medium plus complex from attached cells, and add normal growth medium. Harvest suspension cells by centrifugation, and resuspend in normal growth medium. Return cells to normal growth environment.

3.1.7. Assessment of Transfer

Peak transgene expression from most standard mammalian expression plasmids is usually detected 24–72 h after initiation of the lipofection process. *See* **Note 5** for potential assays of transgene expression. Transgene expression should be normalized in some way. This can be done by counting the total number of cells if it is possible to visualize transgene expression *in situ*, or by assessing the total amount of protein, if cells are lysed (*see* **Note 6**). For statistical validation, each experiment should be conducted at least in triplicate. Cells can be put under selection for the generation of stable clones 48–72 h after initiation of transfection. To do so, normal growth medium can be replaced by medium plus the selective agent, or cells can be passaged and plated in fresh growth medium containing the selective compound.

3.2. Formulation Assessment

3.2.1 Overview

The efficiency of gene transfer and the level of transgene expression can be increased by severalfold, if a lipoplex formulation is optimized for a particular application. Optimization of a lipoplex formulation is most critical when using a new cell line, cell type, or lipid. On the whole, once a lipoplex formulation has been determined for a particular nucleic acid, e.g., plasmid or oligonucleotide, this formulation should work for any other plasmid DNA or oligonucleotide of a similar size (up to approx 10 kb for plasmid DNA, and up to approx 50 nucleotides for an oligonucleotide) with the same lipid or cell line. The determination of an optimal formulation of a lipoplex can be difficult, because each of the key variables (DNA:lipid ratio, DNA and lipid dose, and DNA and lipid concentration) are interdependent. For example, variation of DNA-to-lipid ratio requires changes in either the quantity and concentration of lipid or the quantity and concentration of DNA. Furthermore, variation in the quantity of lipid necessitates a corresponding change in the quantity of DNA, if the DNA:lipid ratio is to remain constant (*see* **Note 17**). The following protocol has been designed to allow a relatively rapid screening of these variables, with the aim of determining the optimal lipoplex formulation for a particular application. The use of 24-well plates allows assessment of six different formulations, four wells per formulation, (*see* **Note 18**).

3.2.2. Assessment of Optimal DNA:Lipid Ratio

3.2.2.1. CELL CULTURE

1. Routine cell culture should be followed using the appropriate subcultivation ratio when passing cells (*see* **Note 3**).
2. Seed attached cells (1×10^5 cells/well) in a 24-well plate. Cells should be between 50 and 70% confluent by the following day (*see* **Note 3**). Wash cells twice with PBS and once with OptiMEM prior to transfection to remove residual FBS. Add 450 µL OptiMEM medium to each well.
3. Harvest suspension cells by centrifugation, and wash cells twice with PBS and once with OptiMEM prior to transfection to remove residual FBS. Resuspend the cells in OptiMEM at a concentration of 1×10^6 cells/mL, and transfer 2×10^5 cells (200 µL) per well. Add a further 250 µL OptiMEM.

Table 4
Scheme for Assessment of Lipoplex Formulation Variables

Assessment of lipoplex ratio						
DNA:Ratio	1:3	1:4	1:5	1:6	1:7	1:8
DNA μg	1	1	1	1	1	1
Lipid μg	3	4	5	6	7	8
Final DNA concentration μg/mL	2	2	2	2	2	2
Final Lipid concentration μg/mL	6	8	10	12	14	16
Final volume μL	500	500	500	500	500	500
Assessment of DNA and lipid dose						
DNA:Ratio	1:5	1:5	1:5	1:5	1:5	1:5
DNA μg	0.5	1.0	1.5	2.0	2.5	5
Lipid μg	2.5	1	7.5	10	12.5	25
Final DNA concentration μg/mL	1	2	3	4	5	10
Final Lipid concentration μg/mL	5	10	15	20	25	50
Final volume μL	500	500	500	500	500	500
Assessment of DNA and lipid concentration						
DNA:Ratio	1:5	1:5	1:5	1:5	1:5	1:5
DNA μg	1	1	1	1	1	1
Lipid μg	5	5	5	5	5	5
Final DNA concentration μg/mL	1	2	3	4	5	10
Final Lipid concentration μg/mL	5	10	15	20	25	50
Final volume μL	1000	500	333	250	200	100

3.2.2.2. FORMATION OF COMPLEXES

1. Set up six sterile polystyrene tubes with 4 μg DNA in up to 100 μL OptiMEM per tube. Add the DNA to prealiquoted OptiMEM.
2. Set up six sterile polystyrene tubes with increasing amounts of lipid. Testing ratios of 1:3, 1:4, 1:5, 1:6, 1:7, and 1:8 w/w represents a good range. This corresponds to 12, 16, 20, 24, 28, and 32 μg lipid, respectively (*see* **Table 4**). Dilute the lipid in OptiMEM, up to 100 μL per tube. Add the lipid to prealiquoted OptiMEM.
3. Add one 100-μL aliquot of diluted DNA to one 100-μL aliquot of diluted lipid. Repeat for all the aliquots of DNA and lipid. Allow lipoplexes to form at room temperature for up to 15 min; the solution should become turbid.
4. Add 50 μL lipoplex to each of the four wells per formulation under assessment. If adding to attached cells, gently swirl the dish or plate to ensure equal distribution of the complex. If adding to cells in suspension, mix by gently aspirating the total volume up and down 2–3× with a pipet. Return cells to normal growth environment.
5. For most cell types, exposure of cells to the complex for 12–18 h works most effectively (*see* **Note 16**). Remove the OptiMEM medium plus complex from attached cells, and add normal growth medium. Harvest suspension cells by centrifugation and resuspend in normal growth medium. Assay for gene expression 48 h after initiation of transfection (*see* **Note 5**).

6. An important assessment of an optimal lipoplex formulation is whether it is cytotoxic. To assess this, the total protein levels at the end of an experiment can be determined (*see* **Note 6**).

3.2.2.3. INTERPRETATION OF RESULTS

1. Determine the mean gene expression for each formulation, and plot against the different ratios tested. The data normally form a bell curve around a particular ratio. It is usually possible to chose immediately an optimum ratio from those tested, in which case, proceed to the next Methods Subheadings (**3.2.3.** and **3.2.4.**). However, if the curve seems particularly skewed or very flat, then it may be better to test additional ratios, investigating ratios at one extreme or the other, depending on the skew seen, or testing smaller increments in the amount of lipid.

3.2.3. Assessment of Optimal DNA and Lipid Dose (See **Note 19**)

3.2.3.1. CELL CULTURE

Follow the protocol described in **Subheading 3.2.1.1.**

3.2.3.2. FORMATION OF COMPLEXES

1. To assess DNA dose, set up six sterile polystyrene tubes, with increasing amounts of DNA: 0.5, 1.0, 1.5, 2.0, 2.5, and 5.0 µg DNA per well is a good range. Testing four wells per DNA dose corresponds to 2, 4, 6, 8, 10, and 20 µg DNA diluted in up to 100 µL OptiMEM in each tube. Add the DNA to prealiquoted OptiMEM.
2. To assess lipid dose, set up six sterile polystyrene tubes, with increasing amounts of lipid. The amount of lipid will be based on the choice of ratio determined by following the protocol described in **Subheading 3.2.2.** However, assuming a ratio of 1:5 (w:w) was found to be optimum, then this would use 2.5, 5, 7.5, 10, 12.5, and 25 µg lipid per well (*see* **Table 4**). Testing four wells per formulation corresponds to 10, 20, 30, 40, 50, and 100 µg lipid diluted in OptiMEM, up to 100 µL per tube. Add the lipid to prealiquoted OptiMEM.
3. Proceed as for **Subheading 3.2.2.2., steps 3–6**.

3.2.3.3. INTERPRETATION OF RESULTS

Determine the mean gene expression (and, if available, the amount of total protein or other measure of cytotoxicity) for each formulation, and plot against the dose of DNA and lipid tested. The plot usually shows a plateau at a particular dose of DNA, after which increasing the amounts of DNA and lipid do not increase the level of transgene expression. There may be some decline in transgene expression at relatively high doses of DNA and lipid, because of cytotoxicity. If the amount of DNA that is shown to be optimal is very different from that used in **Subheading 3.2.2.**, it may be desirable to repeat the initial analysis with this dose of DNA complexed with different ratios of lipid.

3.2.4. Assessment of Optimal DNA and Lipid Concentration (See *Note 19*)

3.2.4.1. CELL CULTURE

1. Routine cell culture should be followed, using the appropriate subcultivation ratio when passing cells (*see* **Note 3**).
2. Seed attached cells (1×10^5 cells/well) in a 24-well plate. Cells should be between 50 and 70% confluent by the following day (*see* **Note 3**). Wash cells twice with PBS, and once with OptiMEM, prior to transfection to remove residual FBS. To four wells add 950 µL OptiMEM per well, and then to each subsequent four wells, add 450, 283, 200, 150, and 50 µL OptiMEM per well.
3. Harvest suspension cells by centrifugation, and wash cells twice with PBS, and once with OptiMEM, prior to transfection to remove residual FBS. Resuspend the cells in OptiMEM at a concentration of 4×10^6 cells/mL, and transfer 2×10^5 cells (50 µL) per well. Add an additional 900 µL OptiMEM per well to four wells, and then to each subsequent four wells add 400, 233, 150, 100, and 0 µL OptiMEM per well (*see* **Table 4**).

3.2.4.2. FORMATION OF COMPLEXES

1. To assess DNA concentration, set up six sterile polystyrene tubes, each with the same amount of DNA. 1.0 µg DNA per well is usually an effective amount of DNA to start with. Dilute 4 µg DNA in up to 100 µL OptiMEM in each tube. Add the DNA to prealiquoted OptiMEM.
2. To assess lipid concentration, set up six sterile polystyrene tubes, each with the same amount of lipid. The amount of lipid will be based on the choice of ratio determined by following the protocol described in **Subheading 3.2.2.** However, assuming a ratio of 1:5 (w:w) was found to be optimum then this would use 5 µg lipid per well. Dilute 20 µg lipid in OptiMEM, up to 100 µL per tube. Add the lipid to prealiquoted OptiMEM.
3. Proceed as for **Subheading 3.2.2.2., steps 3–6**.

3.2.4.3. INTERPRETATION OF RESULTS

Determine the mean gene expression (and, if available, the amount of total protein or other measure of cytotoxicty) for each formulation, and plot against the DNA and lipid concentrations. The data normally form a bell curve around a particular concentration. It is usually possible to pick immediately an optimum concentration from those tested. Any subsequent assessment of a different DNA:lipid ratio, or of a different dose, should take this into account. Once this variable has been determined, particularly for a given cell line, this usually is applicable when the DNA:lipid ratio or the dose of DNA or lipid is changed.

3.2.4. Assessment of Additional Factors

Other variables that can be tested in this format include optimization of the complexation process by looking at time and temperature, the concentration of the DNA, and the lipid when the complex is formed and different diluents; the cell density of attached cells and the number of suspension cells; the medium in which the lipofection is conducted; and the time cells are exposed to the lipoplex.

4. Notes

1. The choice of lipid for any given application is likely to be determined by several factors including the stability of the lipid, the DNA binding and condensation capacity, the consistency of the lipoplex formed, the stability of the lipoplex, the biodegradability and toxicity of the lipid(s), and the resistance of the lipoplex to deactivation by serum. Unfortunately, no single cationic liposome is the one to use for a particular application, and testing different lipids is the only definitive means of making a final choice. However, a few generalizations are possible, and the following suggestions may be useful. Multivalent cationic lipids (for example, LipofectAmine™) are usually better than monovalent cationic lipids at transfecting larger nucleic acid molecules (e.g., plasmid DNA over 10 kb). If cells do poorly in the absence of serum, then use a lipid that is less susceptible to deactivation by protein, for example, DOTAP. If cytotoxicity is a particular problem, then lipids that contain biodegradable ester bonds may be better, for example, DC-Chol:DOPE. Some companies now supply several different lipids as kits, so a comparison, using the type of experimentation described in **Subheading 3.2.**, can be performed before committing to larger-scale experimentation.

2. Cationic lipids are usually supplied preformed as liposomes or as dried lipid films. Preformed liposomes must be stored at 4°C, and should be kept on ice during experimentation. Cationic lipids supplied as lipid films are usually stored at –20°C or –80°C. Sterile water is usually added to reconstitute dried lipids, which are allowed to rehydrate and form unilamellar liposomes, typically by vortexing. **Do not freeze liposomes** (TransFast™, Promega, Madison, WI, is one of the few exceptions to this rule, and is stored frozen once liposomes are formed).

3. The protocols described here are most suitable for the transfection of immortalized cell lines, however, once an optimum lipoplex formulation has been determined, this can usually be applied to primary cells of a similar lineage. Unfortunately, optimal in vitro formulations are not necessarily optimal for use in vivo, and additional optimization is required for animal experimentation. Cells allowed to become confluent, or that have undergone multiple passages prior to plating for transfection, often show a significant reduction in the efficiency of lipofection. To ensure consistency between experiments, it is essential to maintain cells in a healthy state and to minimize the number of passages prior to use. Ideally, frozen stocks of cells at similar passage numbers should be maintained which can be returned to when necessary. The numbers of cells to be plated per well, shown in **Table 3**, are a guide; cells with different growth rates may need to be plated at lower or higher densities to ensure a 50–70% confluency at transfection.

4. The nucleic acid should be as pure as possible (260:280 ratio of 1.8:1.9); aim for a plasmid DNA concentration of 1 mg/mL. Plasmid DNA can be prepared by

most standard purification methods, including alkaline lysis of the bacterial host, followed by centrifugation through cesium chloride. However, with the potential application of these methods to gene therapy, column purification, which eliminates the exposure of DNA to heavy metals and ethidium bromide, has been favored *(35)*. DNA purification columns from Qiagen (Valencia, CA) and Promega work well, though many others are also available. The presence of bacterial lipopolysacchrides (LPS) or endotoxin in DNA preparations can reduce the effectiveness of lipofection, and can be particularly toxic to primary cells *(36,37)*. Bacterial LPS can be removed using a detergent. At least one specific kit has been marketed for this purpose (Qiagen). The plasmid DNA is usually in the closed circular double-strand form; DNA may be linearized if the goal is stable transfection, but this is not required for transient transfections. Most standard RNA extraction methods or kits will purify RNA of sufficient quality for transfection; the RNA should be assessed by gel electrophoresis prior to use, to determine the degree of degradation, which should be minimal. Oligonucleotides can contain residual contaminants from the synthesis reactions, which may inhibit transfection; carefully check the quality control documentation supplied with commercially produced oligonucleotides; if necessary, oligonucleotides should be reprecipitated, washed, and resuspended. The nucleic acid should be resuspended in sterile water. Ideally, Tris-EDTA buffer should not be used, because the presence of even trace amounts of EDTA (a chelating agent) could effect the availability of the positive charge on the cationic lipid.

5. Any assay of nucleic acid transfer should be quantitative and easy to apply to multiple samples. Regarding assays of transient gene expression from plasmid DNA, several reporter genes are now available that can be used. In choosing a particular assay, it is important to decide whether determination of the total level of gene expression or the percentage efficiency is required. Usually, there is a correlation between higher gene expression and higher transfection efficiency on a per-cell basis, but it should be remembered that the same level of gene expression can be obtained from a few cells making a lot of protein, or from many cells making a small amount of protein. The most widely used reporter proteins for which there are quantitative assays are β-galactosidase (using 2-nitro-phenyl-β-D-galactopyranoside or chlorophenol red-β-D-galactopyranoside as soluble substrates), chloramphenicol acetyltransferase and luciferase. The genes encoding β-galactosidase (using 5-bromo-4-chloro-3-indolyl-β-D-galactopyranoside as an insoluble substrate) and green fluorescent protein have proven useful in assessing the number of cells transfected.

6. To determine total protein levels, use a protein assay such as that based on the color change of Coomassie blue (Bio-Rad, Hercules, CA, cat. no. 500-002) *(31)*. This assay can be conducted using a convenient 96-well-plate format, and can be used both to standardize gene expression and to assess the effect of different lipoplex formulations on the growth of cells. The amount of total protein appears to correlate well with the cytotoxicity of a lipoplex formulation, when compared to control cells that have been untreated *(32)*. An alternative means of assessing the

cytotoxicity of a given formulation would be to conduct cell proliferation or cell death assays on cells transfected in parallel with those being assessed for nucleic acid transfection.

7. Maximum nucleic acid transfer is usually obtained if the lipofection is conducted in serum free medium, because protein can interact with, or degrade, lipoplexes, making them unavailable for transfection. If cells cannot be grown in OptiMEM at all, or for only short periods of time (less than 4–6 h), then normal growth medium can be used, but it is recommended that the percentage of FCS be minimized (less than 5%). Also, try to avoid using enriched mediums such as RPMI 1640, though CD34[+] cells have been successfully transfected in this medium supplemented with FCS *(3)*. The final volume of medium in which the lipofection occurs is critical to maintaining the concentration of the lipoplex at a level tolerated by most cells. If significant toxicity is seen, this can be varied as described in **Subheading 3.2.4.** Do not add antibiotics or antifungal agents to the medium in which the transfection is performed. Antibiotics or antifungal agents can mask contamination of the reagents used in the lipofection. Also, some antibiotics or antifungal agents can make cells more susceptible to uptake of lipid containing macromolecules. Although this may sound advantageous, it can distort the evaluation of a particular lipofection, and can introduce a significant source of variation within and between experiments. All transfections should be conducted under sterile conditions.

8. The amount of plasmid DNA stated is for the total amount of DNA. Mixtures of plasmids expressing different transgenes can be used. It is unclear whether a mixture of nucleic acids (e.g., plasmid DNA and oligonucleotide) is either an advantage or a disadvantage. Plasmid DNA usually requires transport to the nucleus for expression, although most experiments using oligonucleotides have been antisense studies requiring only cytoplasmic uptake. Furthermore, these are two very different nucleic acid species, which probably form lipoplexes of different sizes and charge; thus, it is unlikely that one can act as a surrogate marker for the other.

9. The diluent in which the complex is formed must be serum-free, because protein interferes with the interaction of the DNA and the lipid. Alternative diluents that have been used include 20 mM HEPES-buffer, pH 7.4 (DOTAP, Boehringer Mannheim, Indianapolis, IN), HEPES-buffered saline (DOSPER, Boehringer Mannheim; Clonfectin™, Clontech, Palo Alto, CA), DMEM (LipoTaxi™, Stratagene, La Jolla, CA), 150 mM NaCl (for transfections using Transfectam® in the presence of serum [Promega]) and Krebs-buffered saline *(31)*.

10. It has been recommended that the ratio of DNA to lipid used to form a lipoplex be calculated and expressed as a charge ratio, because this best describes the electrostatic relationship between the nucleic acid and the cationic lipid *(10)*. The negative charge equivalents can be calculated from the concentration of the nucleic acid. For example, the average mol wt per nucleotide monomer is 330; thus, 1 mg/mL DNA is 1.6×10^{-3} M, or 1.6 mM in base pairs. Each base pair has two negative charges, so the concentration of negative charge is 3.2 mM. The positive charge equivalents will be dependent on the number of protonatable

nitrogen atoms and the pKa of each nitrogen atom, and must also take into account the presence of any counterions, such as chloride or bromide. For example, DOTMA, DOTAP, DC-Chol, and DMRIE have theoretical net positive charges of +1. GL67 has a net positive charge of +3, DOSPER +4, and DOSPA (Lipofectamine) +5. This information is not available for all lipids, particularly those marketed commercially in which restrictions have been placed on describing the exact composition of the lipids used. To allow easy application of the methods outlined here, the DNA:lipid ratio has been expressed on the basis of w:w, because this is probably the most widely used terminology at present. However, conversion to a charge:charge ratio may be phased in over the next few years.

11. The weight of lipid refers here to the total weight of lipid, cationic and neutral.

12. As a general rule, the stock of cationic liposomes should be kept on ice during experimentation, though it is recommended for a few cationic lipid formulations that the lipid be prewarmed to 37°C. Unless otherwise stated for a particular lipid, the diluted liposomes in OptiMEM can be maintained at room temperature, but the time prior to formation of lipoplexes should be kept to a minimum.

13. **Table 3** shows the amount of DNA to be added to lipid per well. Lipoplexes can be formed individually for each well, but scale-up to form lipoplexes for multiple wells can be done by simply multiplying the amount or volume of each component by the number of wells, and then adding the same volume of complex per well, as shown in **Table 3**. As long as the concentration of DNA and lipid remains constant there should be no theoretical limit to the scale-up that is possible. However, practically the total volume of lipoplex formed should be restricted to less than 10 mL. None of the volumes stated in the methods described here allow for pipeting error, and allowance should be made for this, as required.

14. If large volumes of lipoplexes (5–10 mL) are being formulated, aggregation and flocculation can be a significant problem, even if the DNA and lipid concentrations are consistent with smaller-scale experiments. Rapid addition of the diluted DNA to the diluted lipid can help to alleviate this problem.

15. Do not vortex or vigorously shake the mixture in any way. Allowing complexation to continue for more than 45 min usually results in a decrease in transfection as the complexes become aggregated.

16. Contact time in vitro between the lipoplex and the cell surface is critical, and is usually 4–8 h (29,31). Whether this time is required for sufficient lipoplexes to settle on the cells to obtain a meaningful amount of DNA transfer, and thus gene expression, or because this amount of time is required for the active uptake of lipoplexes, is unclear. If necessary, FBS (preferably 5% or less) containing medium can be added to cells 4–6 h after initiation of the transfection, with only a minimal effect on the overall level of transgene expression obtained.

17. The biological effect of these variables usually reflects a particular physicochemical interaction between the DNA and the lipid. Some of the literature cited discusses these issues (11,12,15–21,31–33,38), but additional details can be found in **ref. 39**.

18. A 24-well-plate format gives a high reproducibility within and between experiments, while minimizing the use of resources; six variables can be assessed per plate, with four wells per variable, allowing for a level of statistical validation.
19. It is best to run **Subheadings 3.2.3.** and **3.2.4.** side by side, because this enables an easier interpretation of the data from these two experiments.

References

1. Capaccioli, S., Pasquale, G. D., Mini, E., Mazzei, T., and Quattrone, A. (1993) Cationic lipids improve antisense oligonucleotide uptake and prevent degradation in cultured cells and in human serum. *Biochem. Biophys. Res. Comm.* **197,** 818–825.
2. Lewis, J. G., Lin, K.-Y., Kothavale, A., Flanagan, W. M., Matteucci, M. D., DePrince, R. B., et al. (1996) Serum-resistant cytofectin for delivery of antisense oligonucleotides and plasmid DNA. *Proc. Natl. Acad. Sci. USA* **93,** 3176–3181.
3. Kronenwett, R., Steidi, U., Kirsch, M., Sczakiel, G., and Haas, R. (1998) Oligodeoxyribonucleotide uptake in primary human hematopoietic cells is enhanced by cationic lipids and depends on the hematopoietic cell subset. *Blood* **91,** 852–862.
4. Chen, M., Compton, S. T., Coviello, V. F., Green, E. D., and Ashlock, M. A. (1997) Transient gene expression from yeast artificial chromosome DNA in mammalian cells is enhanced by adenovirus. *Nucleic Acids Res.* **25,** 4416–4418.
5. Ikeno, M., Grimes, B., Okazaki, T., Nakano, M., Saitoh, K., Hoshino, H., et al. (1998) Construction of YAC-based mammalian artificial chromosomes. *Nature Biotechnol.* **16,** 431–439.
6. Lu, D., Benjamin, R., Kim, M., Conry, R. M., and Curiel, D. T. (1994) Optimization of methods to achieve mRNA-mediated transfection of tumor cells *in vitro* and *in vivo* employing cationic liposome vectors. *Cancer Gene Ther.* **1,** 245–252.
7. Kariko, K., Kuo, A., Barnathan, E. S., and Langer, D. J. (1998) Phosphate-enhanced transfection of cationic lipid-complexed mRNA and plasmid DNA. *Biochim. Biophys. Acta* 1**369,** 320–334.
8. Cole-Strauss, A., Yoon, K., Xiang, Y., Byrne, B. C., Rice, M. C., Gryn, J., Holloman, W. K., and Kmiec, E. B. (1996) Correction of the mutation responsible for sickle cell anemia by an RNA-DNA oligonucleotide. *Science* **273,** 1386–1389.
9. Kren, B. T., Bandyopadhyay, P., and Steer, C. J. (1998) *In vivo* site-directed mutagenesis of the *factor IX* gene by chimeric RNA/DNA oligonucleotides. *Nature Med.* **4,** 285–290.
10. Felgner, P. L., Barenholz, Y., Behr, J. P., Cheng, S. H., Cullis, P., Huang, L., et al. (1997) Nomenclature for synthetic gene delivery systems. *Hum. Gene Ther.* **8,** 511–512.
11. Felgner, P. L., Gadek, T. R., Holm, M., Roman, R., Chan, H. W., Wenz, M., et al. (1987) Lipofection: a highly efficient, lipid-mediated DNA-transfection procedure. *Proc. Natl. Acad. Sci. USA* **84,** 7413–7417.
12. Gao, X. and Huang, L. (1995) Cationic liposome-mediated gene transfer. *Gene Ther.* **2,** 710–722.
13. Gao, X. (1997) Cationic lipid-based gene delivery: an update, in *Gene Therapy for Diseases of the Lung* (Brigham, K. L., ed.), Marcel Dekker, New York, pp. 99–112.

14. Gao, X. and Huang, L. (1991) Novel cationic liposome reagent for efficient transfection of mammalian cells. *Biochem. Biophys. Res. Comm.* **179**, 280–285.
15. Felgner, J. H., Kumar, R., Sridhar, C. N., Wheeler, C. J., Tsai, Y. J., Border, R., et al. (1994) Enhanced gene delivery and mechanism studies with a novel series of cationic lipid formulations. *J. Biol. Chem.* **269**, 2550–2561.
16. Lee, E. R., Marshall, J., Siegel, C. S., Jiang, C., Yew, N. S., Nichols, M. R., et al. (1996) Detailed analysis of structures and formulations of cationic lipids for efficient gene transfer to the lung. *Hum. Gene Ther.* **7**, 1701–1717.
17. Wheeler, C., Felgner, P. L., Tsai, Y. J., Marshall, J., Sukhu, L., Doh, S. G., et al. (1996) Novel cationic lipid greatly enhances plasmid DNA delivery and expression in mouse lung. *Proc. Natl. Acad. Sci. USA* **93**, 11,454–11,459.
18. Gershon, H., Ghirlando, R., Guttman, S. B., and Minsky, A. (1993) Mode of formation and structural features of DNA-cationic liposome complexes used for transfection. *Biochem.* **32**, 7143–7151.
19. Eastman, S., Siegel, C., Tousignant, J., Smith, A. E., Cheng, S. H., and Scheule, R. K. (1997) Biophysical characterization of cationic lipid: DNA complexes. *Biochim. Biophys. Acta* 1**325**, 41–62.
20. Ferrari, M. E., Nguyan, C. M., Zelphati, O., Tsai, Y., and Felgner, P. L. (1998) Analytical methods for the characterization of cationic lipid-nucleic acid complexes. *Hum. Gene Ther.* **9**, 341–351.
21. Felgner, P. L. and Rinegold, G. M. (1989) Cationic liposome mediated transfection. *Nature* **337**, 387–388.
22. Gustafsson, J., Arvidson, G., Karlsson, G., and Almgren, M. (1995) Complexes between cationic liposomes and DNA visualized by cryo-TEM. *Biochim. Biophys. Acta* **1235**, 305–312.
23. Rädler, J., Koltover, I., Salditt, T., and Safinya, C. R. (1997) Structure of DNA-cationic liposome complexes: DNA intercalation in multilamellar membranes in distinct interhelical packing regimes. *Science* **275**, 810–814.
24. Spector, M. S. and Schnur, J. M. (1997) DNA ordering on a lipid membrane. *Science* **275**, 791–792.
25. Smith, J. G., Walzem, R. L., and German, J. B. (1993) Liposomes as agents of DNA transfer. *Biochim. Biophys. Acta* **1154**, 327–340.
26. Legendre, J. Y. and Szoka, F. C. (1992) Delivery of plasmid DNA into mammalian cell lines using pH sensitive liposomes: comparison with cationic liposomes. *Pharm. Res.* **9**, 1235–1242.
27. Zhou, X. and Huang, L. (1994) DNA transfection mediated by cationic liposomes containing lipopolylysine: characterization and mechanism of action. *Biochim. Biophys. Acta* **1189**, 195–203.
28. Wrobel, I. and Collins, D. (1995) Fusion of cationic liposomes with mammalian cells occurs after endocytosis. *Biochim. Biophys. Acta* **1235**, 296–304.
29. Zabner, J., Fasbender, A. J., Moninger, T., Poellinger, K. A., and Welsh, M. J. (1995) Cellular and molecular barriers to gene transfer by a cationic lipid. *J. Biol. Chem.* **270**, 18,997–19,007.

30. Matsui, H., Johnson, L. G., Randell, S. H., and Boucher, R. C. (1997) Loss of binding and entry of liposome-DNA complexes decreases transfection efficiency in differentiated airway epithelial cells. *J. Biol. Chem.* **272,** 1117–1126.
31. Caplen, N. J., Kinrade, E., Sorgi, F., Gao, X., Gruenert, D., Geddes, D., et al. (1995) *In vitro* liposome-mediated DNA transfection of epithelial cell lines using the cationic liposome DC-Chol/DOPE. *Gene Ther.* **2,** 603–613.
32. Fasbender, A. J., Zabner, J., and Welsh, M. J. (1995) Optimization of cationic lipid-mediated gene transfer to airway epithelia. *Am. J. Physiol.* **269** *(Lung Cell. Mol. Physiol.),* L45–L51.
33. Eastman, S. J., Tousignant, J. D., Lukason, M. J., Murray, H., Siegel, C. S., Constantino, P., et al. (1997) Optimization of formulations and conditions for the aerosol delivery of functional cationic lipid:DNA complexes. *Hum. Gene Ther.* **8,** 313–322.
34. Liu, Y., Mounkes, L. C., Liggitt, H. D., Brown, C. S., Solodin, I., Heath, T. D., and Debs, R. J. (1997) Factors influencing the efficiency of cationic liposome-mediated intravenous gene delivery. *Nature Biotechnol.* **15,** 167–173.
35. Caplen, N. J., Gao, X., Hayes, P., Elaswarapu, R., Fisher, G., Kinrade, E., et al. (1994) Gene therapy for cystic fibrosis in humans by liposome-mediated DNA transfer: the production of resources and the regulatory process. *Gene Ther.* **1,** 139–147.
36. Cotten, M., Baker, A., Saltik, M., Wagner, E., and Buschle, M. (1994) Lipopolysaccharide is a frequent contaminant of plasmid DNA preparations and can be toxic to primary human cells in the presence of adenovirus. *Gene Ther.* **1,** 239–246.
37. Cotten, M. and Saltik, M. (1997) Intracellular delivery of lipopolysaccharide during DNA transfection activates a lipid A-dependent cell death response that can be prevented by polymyxin B. *Hum. Gene Ther.* **8,** 555–561.
38. Behr, J. P., Demeneix, B., Loeffler, J. P., and Mutul, J. P. (1989) Efficient gene transfer into mammalian primary endocrine cells with lipopolyamine-coated DNA. *Proc. Natl. Acad. Sci. USA* **86,** 6982–6986.
39. Lasic, D. D. (1997) *Liposomes in Gene Delivery*. CRC, Boca Raton, FL.

2

Optimizing Polyethylenimine-Based Gene Transfer into Mammalian Brain for Analysis of Promoter Regulation and Protein Function

Barbara A. Demeneix, Mohamed Ghorbel, and Daniel Goula

1. Introduction

The efficient and safe introduction of genes into the central nervous system (CNS) is a difficult, yet much sought after objective. Two broad classes of aims can be distinguished. On the one hand, there is therapy in which the ultimate target will be the modification of an endogenous gene by homologous recombination or the remedial addition of a gene coding for a deficient protein. On the other hand, there are analytical approaches in which the aim may be either to determine the physiological relevance of a given protein by blocking or by bolstering its expression, or to dissect the regulatory mechanisms impinging on promoter function in an integrated setting. Furthermore, analysis of promoter regulation will be a prerequisite for creating constructs with optimized regulatory sequences for expressing therapeutic proteins in physiologically appropriate conditions. Microinjection of different permutations of a specific promoter into defined brain regions is a rapid and inexpensive method for assessing function and for mapping transcriptional regulatory elements. Indeed, using somatic gene transfer can provide results that otherwise could only be obtained by labor-intensive germinal transgenosis, an approach that also requires a great deal of organizational prowess and expense for maintenance of the numerous lines created.

Gene transfer into the CNS can be based on cell grafting or direct delivery. For direct delivery, a variety of viral or nonviral methods are available. In mammalian systems, reports have appeared that describe the use of adenoviruses, lentiviruses, herpesvirus, and adeno-associated virus derived vectors. In amphibians, vaccinia virus has also been applied. However, besides their

From: *Methods in Molecular Biology, vol. 133: Gene Targeting Protocols*
Edited by: E. Kmiec © Humana Press Inc., Totowa, NJ

inherent safety problems in therapeutic settings, viral constructs are laborious to construct and verify. Moreover, their production in large quantities is often problematic. For these reasons, many groups have turned to synthetic, or nonviral, vectors to achieve gene transfer in the CNS. Two principal classes of synthetic vectors have been tested in the intact CNS: cationic lipids and cationic polymers. Here we describe the use of a cationic polymer, polyethylenimine (PEI). Indeed, of all the synthetic vectors so far tested in the mammalian CNS, low-molecular-weight PEIs (*see* **Note 1**) provide the most efficient gene delivery.

One of the most important features of PEI is its lack of toxicity in vivo. In the CNS the lesions inevitably created by microinjection into the brain tissue are no different following injection of carrier or injection of PEI/DNA complexes in carrier. This lack of toxicity with PEI is no doubt related to its high efficiency, which allows the use of very low amounts of DNA (in the nanogram range). The high efficiency of PEI is in turn related to its capacity for protonation *(1)*. In PEI, one in three atoms is an amino nitrogen that can be protonated, which makes PEI the cationic polymer having the highest charge density potential available. Moreover, the overall protonation level of PEI increases from 20 to 45% between pH 7 and 5 *(2)*.

PEI can be used for delivering plasmid DNA or oligonuclotides (*see* **Note 2**) to brains of adult and newborn mice *(3,4)*) and rats *(5)*. Moreover, it can be used in the CNS for intrathecal *(4,5)* or intraventricular delivery *(6)*, the latter route being one that could be particularly useful for delivery of therapeutic proteins, such as nerve growth factors. Work ongoing in the laboratory is showing that the method can be used for up and down modulation of protein production in defined brains regions and for analysis of neuron-specific promoter regulation (*7,8*; *see* **Note 3**).

When starting a gene transfer protocol in vivo, it is always preferable, whether one's aim is promoter analysis or production of protein, to optimize delivery by examining the quantitative aspects of transgene expression in the region targeted with luciferase, and then the spatial aspects with a β-galactosidase (β-gal) construct. Indeed, the authors have found that the optimal ratio of PEI amine to DNA phosphate can vary according to species and brain region targeted (*see* **Note 4**). Such preliminary work will also enable one to test which promoter will perform best in a given cell population/developmental stage. For these reasons, the authors detail methods for extracting and assaying firefly luciferase (from *Photinus pyralis*) in the brain, this luciferase being the best reporter gene available for setting up gene transfer protocols. It is three orders of magnitude more sensitive than β-gal (*see* **Note 5**), and the fact that it can be quantified with precision is an overriding factor for choosing it for optimization of PEI:DNA ratios, amounts of DNA to be used, time-course evaluation, and promoter analysis. Other reporter genes, such as chloramphenicol acetyl transferase (CAT) and β-gal can be quantitifed, but each has its drawbacks compared to luciferase. The chief problem with colorimetric quantification of β-gal expression in the CNS is excessive interference from endogenous enzymatic activity. Suppliers of kits for such methodology (such as Promega) recommend heat inactivation of endogenous enzymes. However, for the authors, such precautions have proven ineffective, and the extremely high background found throughout the mouse brain precludes precise quantification of expression of transgenes encoding β-gal. Similarly, when using histochemical procedures, it is vital to use appropriate fixation conditions to avoid interference from endogenous activity that can be high, particularly in the hippocampus. CAT is a good alternative for quantification, but, whichever method is chosen (usually enzyme-linked immunosorbent assay or the method of Seed and Sheen *[9]*), assay time is longer and the methodology laborious. Thus, the authors recommend starting off with luciferase, thereby determining, first, optimal PEI:DNA ratios, then kinetics and dose–response curves can be established (**Fig. 1**). Such experiments will also reveal the inherent variability of transfer efficiency in the target examined, and determine the need or not for normalization in experiments involving promoter regulation with luciferase.

However, β-gal remains one of the best markers for following spatial aspects of expression. Green fluorescent protein (GFP) is equally sensitive, but the fluorescent imaging, although esthetically pleasing, is not as satisfactory as standard light microscopy for anatomical detail. For this reason, the authors provide the methodology for β-gal relevation in whole brains. Indeed, histochemical analysis of β-gal expression on whole brains allows for rapid assessment of transfer efficiency and transgene distribution in small-sized samples (newborn mouse brains or regions of adult brains). The authors also provide a methodology for revealing β-gal expression on histological sections, a step that obviously permits more precise anatomical analysis, which is essential for determining brain regions and morphology of transfected neurons and glial cells. Furthermore, it is on such sections (prepared by vibratome or cryostat sectioning) that double labeling by immunocytochemistry can be performed to identify the cells expressing the transgenes. For instance, to identify neurons, one can use a neurofilament (NF) antibody or a Neuronal Nuclear Antigen (NeuN) antibody, and to identify astrocytes an antibody against glial acid fibrillary protein (GFAP) can be employed. Above all, one must remember that if one obtains just a few cells labeled with β-gal (a very insensitive method when dealing with transient expression in vivo), this level of efficiency will be more than sufficient to allow one either to proceed with promoter analysis using luciferase or to study the biological effects of a given gene of interest. Finally, the authors also suggest a very sensitive immunoautoradiographic method for measuring variation in expression of genes of interest at low levels (*see* **Note 5**).

Figure 1
Flow Chart for Optimizing PEI Transfection In Vivo

Step 1	Preparation of endotoxin-free plasmid and verification of the plasmid quality.
Step 2	Gel analysis of compaction with PEI.
Step 3	Establishment of optimal PEI/DNA ratios by microinjection and/or stereotaxic delivery of a luciferase construct.
	Use volumes of 0.5–5 µL (according to site of injection, intrathecal or intraventricular).
	The authors suggest testing N:P ratios from 2 to 10. Express plasmid for 24 to 48 h in these intitial tests.
Step 4	Time course (1 d to 3 wk).
	Dose–response (DNA concentration) test concentrations from 100 to 500 ng/µL.
Step 5	Spatial distribution.
	Different possibilities exist for assessing spatial distribution:
	a. β-galactosidase histochemisry on whole brains or sections or immunocytochemistry.
	b. immunoradiography.
Step 6	Expression gene of interest, if not used in **step 5**.

Fig. 1. Flow chart for optimizing PEI-based gene delivery into the intact CNS. The authors recommend setting up this method with a luciferase reporter gene under a CMV promoter.

2. Materials

2.1. PEI and DNA Preparation

1. PEI: Branched 25 kDa PEI is available from Aldrich (St. Quentin Fallavier, France) in anhydrous form. Linear 22 kDa PEI is available from Euromedex (Souffleweyersheim, France) at concentrations of 5 mM and 0.1 M. Both preparations should be stored at 4°C, having adjusted the pH to ≤4.0.
2. Plasmids: For setting up in vivo gene transfer with PEI, one can use commercially available plasmids, e.g., pCMV-luciferase from Promega; pCMV(nls)-Lac-Z from Clontech (Montigny-le-Bretonneux, France). For CAT, the most efficient construct the authors have tested is pcis-CMV-CAT, provided by R. Debs *(10)*.
3. Endotoxin-free plasmid DNA (*see* **Note 6**), prepared as in **Subheading 3.1., step 2**.
4. Appropriate restriction enzymes for verifying plasmids.
5. Agarose gels: 0.8% in 1X Tris Acetate EDTA (TAE) or Tris Borate EDTA (TBE) *(11)*.
6. Spectrophotometer for measurements of DNA concentrations (OD_{260}) and purity of DNA (OD_{260}/OD_{280} >1.8).

2.2. Condensation of DNA with PEI

1. Filtered (0.22 µm) 5% glucose solution.
2. Autoclaved 0.9% NaCl solution.
3. DNA resuspended in water at a final concentration of <0.5 µg/µL.
4. PEI solutions diluted extremporaneously to 0.1 *M*.
5. Sterile polypropylene tubes (1.5-mL).
6. Vortex.
7. Electrophoresis equipment for checking complexation (not required each time, but only for the first round of experiments).

2.4. Microinjections and Animal Care

1. Animals: adult and newborn OF-1 mice or Sprague-Dawley rats, both supplied by Iffa Credo (L'Arbresle, France).
2. Stereotaxic apparatus from David Kopf (Phymed, Paris, France). Stereotaxic coordinates for mice are determined according to Lehmann *(12)*.
3. Micromanipulator (Narishige, supplied by OSI, Maurepas, France) and microcapillaries (ext diam 1 mm, OSI). Capillaries are pulled to ext diam of 10–15 µm.
4. Capillary puller (Narishige).
5. Hamilton syringe (10 µL) with a 21-gage needle (ext diam of 460 µm; supplied by OSI).
6. Ice to anesthetize newborn mice (10 min on ice).
7. Sodium pentobarbital (Sanofi, France) diluted to 10% to anesthetize adult animals (70 mg/kg weight, ip).
8. Recovery chamber. Animals should be kept under an infra red lamp or a specially constructed heated cage until fully recovered from anesthesia and surgery.

2.5. Reporter Gene Revelation

2.5.1. Luciferase Activity in Brain Homogenates

1. Microdissection tools for dissecting out brain areas.
2. Ultra-Turrax (OSI) equipped with a small plunger to homogenize tissue samples directly in polyethylene tube.
3. Refrigerated benchtop centrifuge for Eppendorf tubes to pellet cell debris after homogenization, in order to recuperate supernatant for luciferase assay.
4. Luciferase assay kit from Promega. This system is based on the oxidation of luciferin by luciferase, in the presence of ATP and O_2, with photon production.
5. Luminometer (model ILA-911 from Tropix, Bedford, MA) to quantify light emitted.

2.5.2. β-Galactosidase Revelation

2.5.2.1. Detection with X-Gal Substrate

1. X-gal (Eurogentec, Seraing, Belgium) sold in powder form. Both the powder and stock solution (40 mg/mL), prepared in dimethyl sulfoxide (DMSO) must be kept at –20°C.

2. Phosphate-buffered saline (PBS) 0.1 M.
3. EGTA.
4. Paraformaldehyde (PFA, Sigma, St. Quentin Fallavier, France). Prepare a stock solution of 20% in PBS, and store at –20°C.
5. $MgCl_2$, 1 M.
6. Tween-20 (Sigma).
7. Heparin (10 U/L in 0.9% NaCl) for perfusion.
8. Peristaltic pump (Polylabo, Strasbourg, France) for perfusion of animals and fixation of tissues by perfusion.
9. Vibratome (Leica, Rueil-Malmaison, France) to section the tissues (20–40 µm thickness).
10. DMSO (Sigma) to make stock solutions of X-gal.
11. Small paintbrush to transfer tissue sections from one solution to another. Obtain from any art equipment supplier.
12. 25-mL sterile plastic vials (size no. 2) to collect sections
13. Potassium ferricyanide and potassium ferrocyanide (Sigma): Prepare 0.2 M stock solutions of each.
14. Alcohol series for dehydration (baths: 70, 95, 100% of ethanol).
15. Xylene, benzyl benzoate, and benzyl alcohol (all from Sigma) for delipidation of whole newborn brains or small blocks of tissue from adult brains.
16. Appropriate sized cover slips and glycerol (glycerol/PBS, 1V/3V) for mounting slides.
17. Plastic gloves. Benzyl benzoate and benzyl alcohol are irritants.
18. Glassware for delipidation solutions.

2.5.2.2. β-Galactosidase Detection using F-DG (Fluorescein-di-β-Galactoside) as Substrate

1. FDG (Molecular Probes, Leiden, The Netherlands): fluorescent substrate for β-gal.
2. PBS, 0.1 M.
3. DMSO (Sigma).
4. Small paint brush (*see* **Subheading 2.5.2.1.**).
5. Vibratome (Leica) for the same purpose as stated in **Subheading 2.5.2.1.**
6. Epifluorescence microscope equipped with activation/emission filters for fluorescein.

2.5.3. Double Immunocytochemical Revelation of β-Galactosidase and Neuron or glial Markers on Floating Sections

1. PBS, PBS–gelatin (0.2%).
2. Triton-X100 (Sigma).
3. Vibratome sections (40 µm).
4. Cromallun (Sigma).
5. Gelatinized slides prepared by dipping in a cromallun–gelatin solution (0.05/0.5% in distilled water) and dried overnight at 37°C.
6. Blocking solution: PBS–gelatin (0.2%).

7. Primary antibodies against β-gal and cell-specific markers (NF, NeuN, and GFAP) (Cappel, Organon Tetrika, Westchester, PA; Sigma; Dako, Glostrup, Denmark, respectively). To label neurons, NF can be replaced by NeuN antibody from Chemicon, Temecula, CA).
8. Coupling dye for labeling primary cell-marker antibodies (cy3.5; Fluorolink-AbTM). Labeling of the antibodies is carried out according to the manufacturer's instructions (Amersham, Les Ulis, France). The authors label the cell-specific antibodies (NF, NeuN, or GFAP), and use an antirabbit antibody coupled to fluorescein to reveal the β-gal immunoreactivity.
9. Mounting media: Vectashield (Biosys, Compiégne, France), or glycerol/PBS (1V/3V).
10. Fluorescent microscope (Olympus) equipped for visualizing fluorescein and Texas red emissions.
11. Small paintbrushes (*see* **Subheading 2.5.2.1.**)

2.5.4. CAT Assay

1. [^{14}C]chloramphenicol (Amersham CFA, 57 mCi/mmol). Aliquots stoked at –20°C.
2. Butyryl-CoA 10 mM (Sigma B1508, 100 mg). Aliquots stocked at –80°C.
3. Tris-HCl buffer, 250 mM, pH 7.5.
4. 2,6,10,14-tetramethylpentadecane/xylene (TMPD, 2:1; Aldrich).
5. Miniature polybrene vials for scintillation counter (Packard, Meriden, CT).

2.6. Immunoradiography

1. Appropriate primary polyclonal antibody raised in rabbit against gene of interest.
2. Cryostat (Leica)
3. Cryostat sections (15–20-µm thick) cut at –20°C.
4. Cromallun–gelatin coated slides (*see* **Subheading 2.5.3.**).
5. Desiccator.
6. PFA (as in **Subheading 2.5.2.**).
7. PBS.
8. Bovine serum albumin (BSA; Sigma).
9. Normal goat serum (Sigma).
10. Donkey antirabbit [^{35}S]IgG (200–2000 Ci/mmol, 100 µCi/mL). Amersham, Buckinghamshire, UK.
11. β-max films (Amersham).
12. Computerized image analysis system (Biocom, Les Ulis, France).

3. Methods
3.1. PEI and DNA Preparation

1. The stock solution (0.1 M) of PEI provided by Euromedex (22 kDa) is used as supplied. The 25 kDa obtained from Aldrich is prepared as follows: Weigh 4.5 mg of the solution, mix with 800 µL sterile water, thus obtaining a 0.1 M solution. Adjust the pH to ≤4.0 with 0.1 N HCl and the volume to 1 mL. Solutions are kept as aliquots at 4°C or at –20°C for long-term storage (>1 mo).

2. For plasmid DNA preparation and purification, the authors recommand use of Jetstar columns (Genomed, Research Triangle Park, NC, or Bad Oeynhausen, Germany). The system is based on anion exchange columns. According to the manufacturer's instructions and solutions supplied, bacteria resulting from maxiculture are lysed by alcali. Large membrane debris is eliminated using potassium acetate and centrifugation. The resulting supernatant is loaded on columns, and DNA is eluted with a solution containing ~2 M NaCl, then centrifuged after isopropanol precipitation. The pellet is washed with 70% ethanol (–20°C), and is resuspended in water or (TE) at high DNA concentration (≤5 µg/µL in TE). This is to ensure that when diluting DNA to its working concentration (≤0.5 µg/µL in 5% glucose) the final TE concentration is not greater than 1 mM Tris/0.1 mM EDTA (Standard TE/10). These plasmid preparations are endotoxin free (see **Note 6**).

3. One microliter of each DNA preparation is diluted in 1 mL sterile water, and analyzed at 260 nm and 280 nm. According to Sambrook *(10)*, 1 U DO$_{260}$ corresponds to 50 µg/mL double-strand DNA.

4. Agarose gel electrophoresis is used to verify that the plasmid DNA is not denatured, is free of RNA, and is mostly supercoiled. Restriction map analysis can be used to check constructions at this point. To this end, native and digested plasmids are analyzed using 0.8% agarose gel electrophoresis in TAE, with bromophenol blue and a DNA mol wt marker *(11)*. The gel is observed on a UV transilluminator (312 nm), and photographed with Sony video equipment from OSI (Maurepas, France).

3.2. Condensation of DNA with PEI and Analysis

1. Plasmid DNA is diluted in sterile (0.22 µm filtered) 5% glucose to the chosen concentration (usually 0.5–2 µg/µL). After vortexing, the appropriate amount of a 0.1 M PEI solution is added, and the solution revortexed. The required amount of PEI, according to DNA concentration and number of equivalents needed, is calculated by taking into account that 1 µg DNA is 3 nmol phosphate and that 1 µL 0.1 M PEI is 100 nmol amine nitrogen. Therefore, to complex 10 µg DNA (30 nmol phosphate) with an amine/phosphate (N:P) (see **Note 4**) ratio of 5 eq PEI, one needs 150 nmol PEI (1.5 µL of a 0.1 M solution). To minimize pipeting errors, it is best to dilute PEI to 50 or 10 mM, but this should be done extemporaneously. Dilute DNA to 10 µg (final concentration 0.5 µg/µL) in 20 µL final 5% glucose. Add the necessary volume of PEI to form the desired N:P ratio, and, water qsp 20 µL.

2. When using a plasmid preparation for the first time, the authors recommend analysis of complexes by agarose gel electrophoresis (**Fig. 2**), and comparing their migration to that of naked DNA (plasmid alone, N:P ratio = 0) after adding 1–2 µL of bromophenol blue. This gives a gel retardation profile in which DNA–PEI complexes formed at N:P <1 migrate similarly to naked DNA. At N:P >6, complexes are so positively charged that they migrate to the negative pole (see **Note 4**).

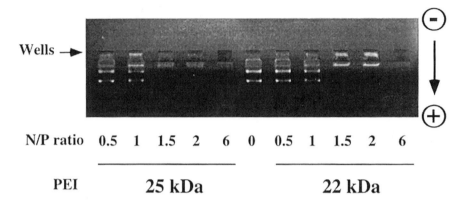

N/P ratio 0.5 1 1.5 2 6 0 0.5 1 1.5 2 6

PEI   **25 kDa**   **22 kDa**

Fig. 2. Verification of DNA compaction by linear 22 kDa and branched 25 kDa PEI. A pCMV-luc construct (1 μg) was mixed with PEI at various charge ratios, and DNA–PEI complexes were electrophoresed in 0.8% agarose gel stained with ethidium bromide. The position of wells and the direction of the electrophoretic migration are indicated on the right.

3.3. Injections

1. Obviously, all the procedures described herein that involve animals and their care must be conducted in conformity with appropriate institutional guidelines, that are in accordance with national and international laws and policies.
2. Adult (1–2-mo-old) mice are anesthetized using sodium pentobarbital (Sanofi, France) diluted to 10% in 0.9% NaCl. Animals are anesthetized by an ip injection (70 mg/kg). Adult mice or rats are placed in the stereotaxic apparatus. An incision is made to expose the cranial skull and a hole is made with a 21-gage needle at chosen stereotaxic coordinates. Between 0.5 and 5 μL of complexes in 5% glucose are injected slowly (<5 min) with a Hamilton syringe adapted to a stereotaxic apparatus, small volumes are used for intrathecal injection and larger volumes for intraventricular injection. The needle is left in place for 2 min postinjection, to limit backflow from the injection site.
3. Newborn mice are anesthetized by hypothermia on ice, and 1 μL of the complexes is injected with a microcapillary adapted to a micromanipulator. The head of the anesthetized pup is held manually for direct microinjection. Again, injections should be as slow as possible, and the capillary is left in place for at least a minute to limit backflow.
4. Animals are left in a recovery chamber until active. When optimizing PEI delivery, newborns are returned to the dam for 24 h before sacrifice; adults are kept for 72 h before sacrifice, because expression is usually maximal at these time points.

3.4. Sacrifice of Animals and Reporter Gene Detection

To quantify luciferase expression, animals are sacrificed by decapitation after anesthesia (**Fig. 3**). The dissected brains are separated into hemispheres, and

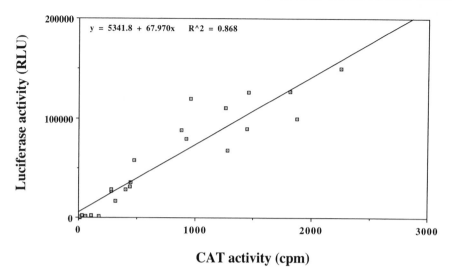

Fig. 3. Correlation between luciferase and CAT activities following PEI-based in vivo gene transfer in the newborn mouse brain. Plasmids (0.35 µg pCMV-luc and 0.15 µg pCMV-CAT in 2 µL 5% glucose) were complexed with PEI 22 kDa (4 Eq), and injected into the lateral ventricle. After 18 h, mice were anesthetized, decapitated, and brains removed for luciferase and CAT asssays.

homogenized using an Ultra-Turrax, in 2-mL Eppendorf tubes containing 200 µL (for the newborn) or 500 µL (for the adults) of luciferase lysis buffer. Homogenates are centrifuged, and 20 µL of each supernatant mixed with 100 µL luciferase assay substrate and vortexed. The light emitted is quantified (in Relative Light Units [RLU]), using a luminometer.

β-galactosidase can be revealed by several means:

1. Histochemical X-gal revelation, whether on sections or carried out *in toto*, requires intracardial perfusion of the anesthesized animals, using a peristaltic pump. First, tissues are fixed by perfusing 2% PFA (in PBS), then fixation is continued by leaving tissue blocks overnight in the same solution. Tissues are then vibratome-sectioned, and sections incubated in a 0.8–1 mg/mL X-gal solution for 2–4 h (30°C). It is important to precede the fixation by perfusion with saline containing 10 U of heparine, to help remove blood and blood cells from the vessels. The fixative (2% PFA) can contain 1.25 mM EGTA and 2 mM MgCl$_2$, which improves the X-gal reaction. To make the reaction mixture, the stock solution of X-gal (40 mg/mL in DMSO) is diluted to 0.8–1 mg/mL PBS containing: 0.1% Tween-20, 4 mM potassium ferricyanide, 4 mM potassium ferrocyanide, and 2 mM MgCl$_2$.

2. Immunocytochemical revelation also requires fixed vibratome sections, mounted on cromallun–gelatin-coated slides. Polyclonal anti-β-gal monoclonal anti-GFAP

and monoclonal anti-NeuN antobodies are used in the authors' experiments. Monoclonal and polyclonal antibodies can be labeled using appropriate labeling kits from Amersham. The authors used cy3.5 (Fluorolinf-abTM), according to the manufacturer's instructions, to label monoclonal antibodies. Primary antibodies are diluted to the concentrations recommended by each manufacturer, in 0.1 *M* PBS (containing 0.2% gelatin, 0.3% Triton X-100, and 3% normal goat serum). Anti β-gal is revealed using fluorescein coupled antirabbit antibody. Sections are protected from light to avoid fading of the fluorescence, and are mounted with glycerol/PBS (1V/3V) or Vectashield (Biosys) and examined under a fluorescence microscope. Luciferase antibodies can also be used to follow transgene expression in a double-labeling protocol. However, there are currently some problems with obtaining good luciferase antibodies for in vivo work (*see* **Note 7**).

3. Fluorescein-DI-β-Galactoside (FDG) is another substrate for β-gal. Hydrolysis of FDG by β-gal results in the liberation of both a monogalactoside and fluorescein. This second product is easily detectable, and theoretically makes this method very sensitive. Its chief limitation for the authors is that it is not suitable for fixed tissues, so that it is difficult to obtain good morphology in brain preparations. Moreover, on unfixed tissue, as cells die, the fluorescein product diffuses out. Thus, the revelation procedure must be very fast. Also, it is not possible to perform double staining to identify cell types. This method, which has the theoretical advantage of higher sensitivity than X-gal, is in fact rather limited for in vivo studies.

4. *In toto* X-gal revelation requires intracardial perfusion of the anesthetized animals, using a peristaltic pump. Fixation and postfixation are performed as for vibratome sections, but organs are treated as whole mounts. Incubate tissues in a 0.8–1 mg/mL X-gal solution for 2–4 h (30°C), rinse in 0.1 *M* PBS (2 × 5'), and transfer in series of ethyl alcohol under mild agitation: 70% (2 × 2 h), 95% (overnight, and another bath of 1 h), 100% (2 × 2 h). Dehydration times can be adapted, depending on the tissue size, to ensure thorough dehydration, one can leave the tissue in the second 100% alcohol bath overnight. Put dehydrated tissues into xylene (2 × 2 h in glass), then transfer them into benzyl benzoate/benzyl alcohol (2V/1V) in a glass container until clarification.

   N.B. Use gloves and glass containers at all steps involving benzyl benzoate and benzyl alcohol. These agents are irritants and also dissolve plastic.

3.5. Use of CAT Activity to Normalize Luciferase Expression

1. Before using a co-injected, ubiquitously expressed gene *(CMV-CAT)* to normalize for expression from a physiologically regulated transgene, it is appropriate to validate this approach by quantifying the correlation between the expression of two constitutively expressed genes co-injected into the same brain area. For this, two plasmids (0.35 µg pCMV-luc and 0.15 µg pCMV-CAT in 2 µL 5% glucose) are complexed with PEI 22 kDa (4 eq), and co-injected into the brain area targeted. After 18 h, mice are anesthetized, decapitated, and brains removed for luciferase and CAT assays.

2. For CAT assay, transfer a 50-µL supernatant aliquot to a 1.5-mL polypropylene tube, keep tube on ice before adding 40 µL 0.25 M Tris-HCl buffer, pH 7.5. Start reaction by adding 10 µL mixed solution of butyryl-CoA (0.53 mM; Sigma) and [^{14}C]chloramphenicol (0.01 mM, 1.85 kBq per tube; Amersham). After 3–5 s of vortexing, incubate 1 h at 37°C. Stop the reaction by adding 200 µL TMPD:xylene solution (2:1). Vortex 20 s and place tube on ice. To separate products, centrifuge 5 min at 4°C (11,000g), remove 150 µL supernatant, and quantify products in a scintillation counter (Wallac, Evry, France).
3. Assay luciferase on another sample of supernatant (*see* **Subheading 3.4.1.**).
4. Plot luciferase against CAT values from the same sample. Correlation should be significant.

3.6. Immunoradiography

This protocol is adapted from **ref. *13***.

1. The cryostat sections are desiccated at 4°C, and frozen at –80°C until used. After a 3-min fixation (4% PAF in PBS) at 4°C, sections are preincubated for 1 h in PBS supplemented with 3% BSA and 1% goat serum, then incubated overnight in an appropriate concentration of polyclonal primary antibody raised in rabbit.
2. After extensive washes in PBS, sections are incubated for 2 h at room temperature in donkey antirabbit [^{35}S] IgG.
3. After abundant washing, sections are air dried and apposed to β-max film for 1–2 d.
4. Optical density is measured by computerized image analysis.

4. Notes

1. A number of PEIs with different mean mol wt are available commercially. For example, preparations of branched PEI, synthetized to different degrees of polymerization, are available from Sigma or Aldrich (800, 50, or 25 kDa). Preparations of very low mol wt (0.7 and 2 kDa) are also available from Sigma, but do not complex DNA efficiently. The authors have found that the branched 25 kDa and linear 22 kDa (Euromedex) polymers work best in the CNS *(1,6)*.
2. When using either the 22 and 25 kDa preparations to deliver oligonucleotides, one should only use phosphodiesters, and not phosphorothioates. The authors have found (as has E. Saison Behmoaras, CNRS/MNHN, Paris) that complexes of PEI and phosphorothioates are of lower efficiency than PEI–phosphodiesters complexes in vitro and in vivo.
3. A major area of discussion in the field at the moment is the physiological regulation and relevance of transient transfection which relies on following transcription from episomally located plasmids. However, the authors have found that, despite lack of integration into the genome, remarkably tight, physiologically appropriate regulation of cell-specific promoters can be optained in vivo. One illustrative example is thyrotropin releasing hormone (TRH) promoter regulation in the hypothalamus. The authors have microinjected complexes containing 1 µg of construct containing 900 bp of the rat TRH promoter upstream of the luciferase-

coding sequence, complexed with 22 kDa PEI into the hypothalamus of newborn mice in different thyroid states. In hypothyroid animals, transcription is twice that in normal, euthyroid animals, and, in hyperthyroid animals, transcription is reduced to half that of the normal group *(7)*. This transcriptional regulation faithfully reflects the negative feedback effect of circulating thyroid hormone on hypothalamic TRH production. Another example of physiological regulation of transgenes introduced by somatic gene transfer includes Krox-24 gene in the newborn brain *(8)*.

4. The authors have found that the optimal ratio of PEI amine:DNA phosphate (N:P ratio) can vary according to species (and perhaps also to site of injection). In mouse and *Xenopus* tadpole brains, the authors have consistently found that the N:P ratio of 6 provides the best transfection conditions. In contrast, when injecting PEI–DNA complexes into adult rat substantia nigra, the optimal ratio was 3 *(5)*. It is important to note that increasing N:P ratio from 2 to 6 not only increases the overall charge of complexes, but also decreases complex size, complexes excluding ethidium bromide (BET) and becoming less visible in the gel. This greater condensation has been confirmed by ζ-sizing *(6)*.

5. When assessing efficiency of gene transfer, one must take into account the sensitivity of the method used. Histochemical β-gal assay with X-gal is rather insensitive. The authors find that it gives roughly the same image of transgene distribution and number of cells labeled as an equivalent amount of GFP plasmid. It has been estimated that revealing a good GFP signal requires 10^5–10^6 molecules per cell to show up over background *(14)*. For this reason, the authors have also tried immunocytochemistry with a polyclonal antibody against β-gal (Cappel), but this method is generally no more sensitive than histochemistry. However, it is important to note that one can obtain very good, and statistically significant, modulation of endogenous proteins with PEI-based gene transfer in systems in which transferring an equivalent amount of β-gal reveals no apparent transgene expression. This was the case for a recent series of experiments in which the authors transfected plasmids expressing either sense or antisense sequences of the dopamine transporter (DAT) into the rat substantia nigra *(11)*. In conditions in which no β-gal activity could be revealed (0.5 µg CMV-β-gal in 1 µL 5% glucose), use of plasmid encoding DAT significantly increased DAT content. This was shown by immunoautoradiography and by biological measurements of dopamine uptake *(11)*. For this reason, the authors recommend immunoautoradiography for following low levels of expression of genes of interest against which good antibodies have been raised.

6. Even though the authors own (unpublished) results show that the presence of small amounts (≤1 EU endotoxin/µg DNA) of endotoxins (also referred to as lipopolysaccharides [LPS]) have no deleterious effects on short-term <4 d) expression in the CNS, there is no available data on the possible effects of their presence in the longer term. For this reason, the authors always use endotoxin-free plasmid preparations. Jetstar columns (Genomed) are recommended. The resulting DNA has ≤0.1 EU endotoxins/µg DNA. This value is not statistically

different from the values found in plasmids prepared with Qiagen Endotoxin-free columns.

If other methods of plasmid preparation are used, the authors recommend measurement of endotoxin content by Limulus Amebocyte Lysate Assay (LAL, or Coatest™ Endotoxin) manufactured by Charles River Endosafe, Charleston, SC, and distributed in Europe by Chromogenix Mölndal, Sweden. If values are ≥4 EU/μg DNA, then endotoxins should be removed by chromatography through Affi-prep™ Polymysin Matrix (Bio-Rad, Hercules, CA), according to the manufacturer's instructions and endotoxin content reverified. After chromatography, values should be ≤0.05 EU/μg DNA.

7. To the authors' knowledge, the only reasonable luciferase antibody currently available is that from Cortex Biochem (San Leandro, CA, distributed by Europa Biochemistry in Europe). Variable results have been obtained with this polyclonal antibody, according to batch number. Promega commercialized a polyclonal antifirefly luciferase up until the end of 1997, but it has been withdrawn from circulation because of titer problems. However, the authors have obtained reasonable results with some batch numbers. Santa Cruz Biotechnology (Santa Cruz, CA) also produces a luciferase antibody, but the authors have not yet tested this antibody in vivo.

References

1. Behr, J. P. and Demeneix, B. A. (1998) Gene delivery with polycationic amphiphiles and polymers. *Curr. Res. Mol. Ther.* **1,** 5–12.
2. Suh, J., Paik, H.-J., and Hwang, B. K. (1994) Ionization of polyethylenimine and polyallylamine at various pHs. *Bioorg. Chem.* **22,** 318–327.
3. Boussif, O., Lezoualc'h, F., Zanta, M. A., Mergny, M., Scherman, D., Demeneix, B., and Behr, J.-P. (1995) Novel, versatile vector for gene and oligonucleotide transfer into cells in culture and in vivo: polyethylenimine. *Proc. Natl. Acad. Sci. USA* **92,** 7297–7303.
4. Abdallah, B., Hassan, A., Benoist, C., Goula, D., Behr, J. P., and Demeneix, B. A. (1996) Powerful nonviral vector for in vivo gene transfer into the adult mammalian brain: polyethylenimine. *Hum. Gene Ther.* **7,** 1947–1954.
5. Martres, M. P., Demeneix, B. A., Hanoun, N., Hamon, M., and Giros, B. (1998) Up- and down-expression of dopamine transporter by plasmid DNA transfer in the rat brain. *Eur. J. Neurosc.* **10,** 3607–3616.
6. Goula, D., Remy, J., Erbacher, P., Wasowicz, M., Levi, G., Abdallah, B., and Demeneix, B. (1998a) Size, diffusibility and transfection performance of linear PEI/DNA complexes in the mouse central nervous system. *Gene Ther.* **5,** 712–717.
7. Guissouma, H., Ghorbel, M. T., Seugnet, I., Ouatas, T., and Demeneix, B. A. (1998) Physiological regulation of hypothalamic TRH transcription *in vivo* is T3 receptor isoform-specific. *FASEB J.* **12,** 1755–1764.
8. Ghorbel, M. T., Seugnet, I., Hadj-Sahraoui, N., Topilko, P., Levi, G., and Demeneix, B. A. (1998) Thyroid hormone effects on *Krox-24* transcription in the post-natal mouse brain are developmentally regulated but are not correlated with mitosis. *Oncogene* **18,** 917–924.

9. Seed, B. and Sheen, J. Y. (1988) Simple phase extraction assay for chloramphenicol acetyl transferase. *Gene* **67,** 271–277.
10. Zhu, N., Liggitt, D., Liu, Y., and Debs, R. (1993) Systemic gene expression after intravenous DNA delivery into adult mice. *Science* **261,** 209–211.
11. Sambrook, J., Fritsch, E. F., and Maniatis, T. (1989) in N. Ford, C. Nolan and M. Ferguson (eds.) *Molecular Cloning: a Laboratory Manual.* Cold Spring Harbor Laboratory, Cold Spring Harbor, NY, pp. 1.1–1.52.
12. Lehmann, A. (1974) in *Atlas stéréotaxique du cerveau de la souris* (CNRS, ed.), Paris.
13. Gérard, C., Martres, M. P., Lefèvre, K., Miquel, M. C., Vergé, D., Lanfumey, L., et al. (1997) Immuno-localization of serotonin 5-HT$_6$ receptor-like material in the rat central nervous system. *Brain Res.* **146,** 207–219.
14. Zlokarnik, G., Negulescu, P. A., Knapp, T. E., Mere, L., Burres, N., Feng, L., et al. (1998) Quantitation of transcription and clonal selection of single living cells with β-lactamase as reporter. *Science* **279,** 84–88.

3

Gene Transfer and Drug Delivery by Electronic Pulse Delivery

A Nonviral Delivery Approach

Xi Zhao

1. Introduction

Tremendous progress has been made in the understanding of human diseases and medical problems at a molecular level. This has led to the development of molecular medicine, that is, gene therapy and intracellular immunization. Among the major steps involved in the modification of target cells for these applications, gene transfer and the delivery of molecular medicine has become more and more critical.

The clinical targets dictate not only the choice of an in vivo or ex vivo delivery strategy, but also the delivery systems used to transfer the expression transgene constructs or other functional therapeutic molecules. Various delivery systems have been developed, including vectors derived from retroviral virus, adenovirus, adeno-associated virus (AAV), and liposome complexes. Each of these approaches transfers the genes through different mechanisms, and has distinct advantages and disadvantages. The most commonly used approach for ex vivo delivery is retroviral vectors. Theoretically, the target cells can be permanently modified by inserting retroviral vectors, because retroviruses transfer their genetic information into the genome of the target cells. However, the use of this approach is limited by disadvantages of retroviral vectors, such as high risk of cancer, potential insertion mutagenesis, retroviral shutdown, requirement of proliferation of target cells, and production problems related to low titers, recombination, contamination, and so on *(1–3)*. Adenoviral vectors, however, have been used only in in vivo human trials. The transgene delivered by adenoviral vector remains epochromosomal. Therefore, adenoviral vectors will have to be readministered periodically to maintain their continuous expression. This limitation, together with the nonspecific

From: *Methods in Molecular Biology, vol. 133: Gene Targeting Protocols*
Edited by: E. Kmiec © Humana Press Inc., Totowa, NJ

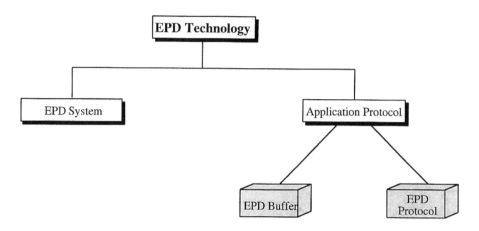

Fig. 1. EPD technology.

inflammation and antivector cellular immunity, restrict the application of adenoviral vectors *(4)*. AAV has been considered for use in delivering genes. Recent results suggest that AAV can be used for nonproliferating cells *(5)*. The drawbacks that AAV vectors present are several. They can only accept small DNA inserts; their lack of stable packaging systems leads to their limited delivery capability; and there is considerable difficulty in producing quantities of virus with consistent high titers and purity. The AAV transfer approach requires substantial improvement to be viable.

Vectors derived from different viruses face numerous challenges: to avoid the viral shutdown, and to express the transgene in a regulated pattern; to substantially reduce the risk of cancer, and active virulence; not to be recognized by the immune system, and not to induce any inflammation; and the ability to easily and reproducibly produce large quantities at high titers. Given the known limitations of viral vectors, the need for the development of a nonviral-mediated transfer methodology is obvious. Electronic pulse delivery (EPD) technology has been developed broadly in these applications, and refined to high transfer efficiency, with good survival rates of treated cells. EPD technology has demonstrated its nonviral, nontoxic and cost-effective advantages, as well as its potential in various clinical applications.

The EPD system and EPD application protocols for molecular delivery are two major portions of the EPD molecular delivery technology (**Fig. 1**).

The EPD system utilizes pulsed electronic effects to introduce exogenous molecules into a wide variety of living cells. The unique features of the EPD system include selected pulsed wave forms, ultralow current, precisely controlled instrument parameters of electronic pulses, well-defined sealed-operation environment, and selectable operation (batch operation or continuous process). Individual application protocols are critical for each specific delivery application. An application protocol includes the proprietary buffer for the delivery process and the EPD protocol, with the combination of various adjustable EPD instrument parameters. The application protocols have been optimized and established for transferring DNA, RNA, and/or protein into different types of target cells, including proliferating cells or nondividing cells. The optimized protocols permit the high molecule transfer efficiency (>80%) and good viability of EPD-treated cells (>90%).

The EPD system is significantly different from electroporation in apparatus, electrical parameters and the sophistication of the procedure. The EPD system subjects the target cells to electronic pulses in a computer-controlled transfer environment. Contrary to electroporation, EPD does not require contact of the electrodes to the mixture of target cells and molecules to be delivered. This significant feature not only permits a completely isolated operation environment, but also eliminates any possible contamination or electrocution, which are major problems caused by electroporators. With the unique patented electric circuit design, the EPD system delivers very low current, which permits the maintenance of the viability of the target cells. Conversely, electroporation often applies a significant current, resulting in the very poor survival rate of the electroporated cells. In addition, the optimized EPD protocols and test confirmed buffers increase the success of the delivery processes.

EPD technology has demonstrated the efficacy to efficiently delivery large molecules into target cells. The broad application of EPD technology has recently been focused on the delivery of molecular medicine, such as therapeutic genes and/or proteins, directly into the target cells. EPD delivery technology has not only been employed to various types of primary cells, culture cells, dividing cells, but also on nonproliferating cells, opening the door to modify different types of stem cells, as well as dendritic cells, whose therapeutic significance has been identified *(6,7)*. Further development of EPD applications will contribute significantly to molecular drug development and the realization of medical treatment with molecular medicine.

2. Materials

2.1. EPD System

1. EPD system controller (InCell, Santa Clara, CA).
2. EPD system monitor (InCell).
3. EPD reaction chamber for Petri dish (InCell).
4. EPD reaction chamber for receptacle container (InCell).
5. Petri dish (15, 60, or 100 mm).
6. Receptacle container (InCell).
7. EPD system software and Application Protocols™ (InCell).

2.2. Media

1. Phosphate-buffered saline: 8.5 g/L NaCl, 0.02 M phosphate buffer, pH 7.0.
2. EPD protein transfer buffer™ for protein delivery (InCell): Prewarm to 37°C prior to use.
3. EPD DNA transfer buffer™ for gene transfer (InCell): prewarm to 37°C prior to use.
4. Cell culture media: Select according to the target cells. For example, culture medium for NIH 3T3 cells: Dulbecco's modified Eagle medium (Gibco, Gaithersburg, MD), containing 10% bovine serum, 100 U/mL penicillin, and 100 μg/mL streptomycin; culture medium for human hematopoietic progenitor cells: Iscove's modified dulbecco's medium (Gibco), containing 10% fetal bovine serum, 50 ng/mL Interleukin (IL)-3, 500 μ/mL IL-6, 25 ng/mL Granulocyte monocyte colony stimulating factors (GMCSF) and 50 ng/mL stem cell factor (SCF); culture medium for CEM cells: RPMI 1640 (Gibco) containing 10% bovine serum, 100 U/mL penicillin, and 100 μg/mL streptomycin. Prewarm the culture media at 37°C prior to use.

3. Methods

3.1. Molecule Delivery into Cells in Suspension

1. Both primary cells and cultured cells that are in cell suspension can be treated by the EPD process directly. In a typical procedure, centrifuge the cell sample at 500g for 5 min, and discard the supernatant. Wash the cell pellet with a selected EPD DNA Transfer Buffer or EPD Protein Transfer Buffer for DNA delivery or protein transfer, respectively.
2. Discard the supernatant, and resuspend the cell pellets gently with the selected EPD DNA Transfer Buffer or EPD Protein Transfer Buffer. Adjust cell density to 10^6–10^8 cell/mL.
3. DNA constructs are prepared according to the standard procedure. After final precipitation with ethanol, the pallet is washed with 70% ethanol. The DNA sample is resuspended with DNA Transfer Buffer at the final concentration of 100 μg/mL.
4. If the delivery procedure is for protein transfer, the protein sample will be diluted to a final concentration of 1 mg/mL in EPD Protein Transfer Buffer.
5. Mix 10^5–10^7 recipient cells and the molecules to be transferred (100 μg/mL DNA or 1 mg/mL protein) in a Receptacle Container (InCell). Place the container into a reaction chamber **(Fig. 2)**.
6. Load selected EPD Protocols from the EPD system Controller **(Fig. 3)**, and follow the operating software step by step for the molecule transferring process. The selected EPD Protocols define all parameters concerning the EPD. The EPD process may take 10–40 s, depending on the chosen protocols.
7. After the EPD process is completed, the receptacle container is removed from the reaction chamber. The cells are transported to the appropriate media for further culture or analysis.

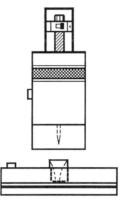

Fig. 2. EPD reaction chamber.

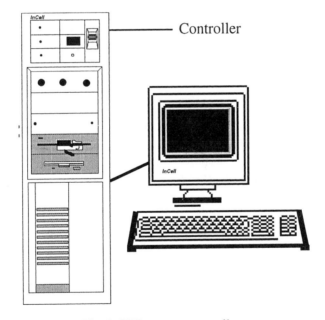

Fig. 3. EPD system controller.

3.2. Molecule Delivery into Cultured Monolayer Cells

1. The monolayer cultures can be subjected to EPD treatment either directly on the culture surface, for instance a Petri dish, or after the digestion by trypsin to prepare the cell suspension. The gene/protein delivery for suspended cells by trypsin should follow the procedure described in **Subheading 3.1.**
2. Discard the culture medium and rinse the culture with prewarmed PBS. Then aspirate the PBS from the Petri dish, wash the cultured cells with a selected EPD

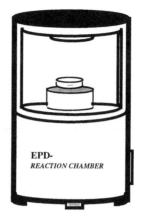

Fig. 4. EPD reaction chamber.

DNA Transfer Buffer or EPD Protein Transfer Buffer, for DNA delivery or protein transfer, respectively.

3. Discard the wash buffer, and add the selected EPD DNA Transfer Buffer or EPD Protein Transfer Buffer containing DNA (0.1 mg/mL) or protein (1 mg/mL) (cf. **Subheading 3.1., steps 3** and **4**) into the Petri dish.
4. Place the Petri dish into a reaction chamber shown, in **Fig. 4**.
5. Select the appropriate EPD Protocols from the EPD system software, and follow the operating instructions step by step for the molecule transferring process. Similar to the suspended cells, the EPD process for monolayer culture may take 10–40 s.
6. After the EPD process is completed, the Petri dish is removed from the reaction chamber, and the appropriate media will be added for further culture or analysis.

4. Notes

1. Cell preparation procedures are various, according to the cell types. When one isolates primary hematopoietic progenitors and matured blood cells from the mixed cell population, an immunoseparation process may be involved. Immunoaffinity columns, antibody-coated surfaces, magnetic beads coated with specific antibodies, and other methodologies are alternative approaches for the isolation of a specific cell population. When cells are isolated by immunomagnetic beads, the cells are often attached to the beads, and require a further separation for subsequent experiments. However, the EPD process does not require the separation of the cells from the magnetic beads. EPD delivery can be performed as described in **Subheading 3.1.**, and the beads have not been found to interrupt the EPD transfer process. If later assay or procedure requires detachment of the beads, the separation can either be done before or after EPD delivery.
2. It is important that the EPD delivery process has no serum contamination. When recipient cells are cultured in the medium-containing serum prior to EPD delivery, the culture medium should be removed completely. The selected EPD DNA Transfer Buffer or EPD Protein Transfer Buffer is used to replace the culture medium by washing the cells at least once or twice.

3. The combination of instrument parameters is very critical for producing high transfer efficiency and excellent cell viability *(8,9)*. The EPD system software and various EPD protocols are available for specific applications. These protocols defined the pulse parameters for each specific application.

4. EPD Transfer Buffer plays an important role in delivering the exogenous molecules into the target cells. Combined with appropriate EPD Protocols, high transfer efficiency can be achieved.

5. Besides the transferring of large molecules, DNA, and protein into the target cells, EPD can also be employed to deliver small molecules, such as peptides or oligonucleotides, into the cells. In addition, the EPD system has been used for cell fusion *(10)* and the production of transgenic animals *(11)*.

6. The EPD reaction chamber is a sealed device that integrates the concept of clinical applications with initial experimentation. Various formats of EPD reaction chamber can be further developed according to the specific clinical requirements.

References

1. Palmer, T. D., Rosman, G. J., Obsborne, W. R. A., and Miller, A. D. (1991) Genetically modified skin fibroblasts persist long after transplantation but gradually inactivate introduced genes. *Proc. Natl. Acad. Sci. USA* **88,** 1330–1334.

2. Dai, Y., Roman, M., Naviaux., R., and Verma, I. (1992) Gene therapy via primary myoblsts: longterm expression of factor IX protein following transplantation in vivo. *Proc. Natl. Acad. Sci. USA* **89,** 10,892–10,895.

3. Challita, P. M. and Kohn, D. B. (1994) Lack of expression from a retroviral vector after transduction of murine hematopoietic stem cells is associated with methylation. *Proc. Natl. Acad. Sci. USA* **91,** 2567–2571.

4. Marshall, E. (1995) Gene therapy's growing pains. *Science* **269,** 1050–1055.

5. Podsakoff, G., Wong, K., Jr., and Chatterjee, S. (1994) Efficient gene transfer into nondivinding cells by adeno associated virus-based vectors. *J. Virol* **68,** 5656–5666.

6. Kohn D. B. (1995) Current status of gene therapy using hematopoietic stem cells. *Curr. Opin. Pediatr.* **7,** 56–63.

7. Hsu, F., Benike, C., Fagnoni, F., Liles, T., Czerwinski, D., Taidi, B., Engleman, E., and Levy, R. (1996) Vaccination of patients with B-cell lymphoma using autologous antigen-pulsed dendritic cells. *Nature Med.e* **2,** 52–58.

8. Zhao, X. (1995) EPD, a novel technology for drug delivery. *Adv. Drug Deliv. Rev.* **17,** 257–262.

9. Zhao, X. (1996) Application of electronic pulse delivery in gene therapy: progress and perspectives, in *Artificial Self-Assembling Systems for Gene Delivery* (Felgner, P. L., ed.), American Chemical Society, Washington, DC, pp. 84–91.

10. Zhao, X. (1995) Use of electric-field-mediated cell fusion to produce hybridomas secreting monoclonal antibodies, in *Methods in Molecular Biology* (Davis, W. C., ed.), Humana, Totowa, NJ, pp. 61–67.

11. Zhao, X., Zhange, P. J., and Wong, T. K. (1993) Application of Baekonization: a new approach to produce transgenic fish. *Mol. Marine Biol. Biotechnol.* **2,** 63–69.

4

Strategies for Improving the Frequency and Assessment of Homologous Recombination

Nancy Smyth Templeton

1. Introduction

Gene therapy is a rapidly emerging field that holds much promise for the treatment of inherited disorders and acquired diseases. A major goal in most human clinical trials has been to produce long-term expression of therapeutic genes by integration of the DNA sequences encoding these genes into the chromosomes. Integration strategies include random, site-specific, and precise integration. To date, only random integration of retroviral vectors has been widely used in gene therapy clinical trials. However, there is concern that mutagenesis of essential genes or inactivation of tumor suppressor genes might occur as a result of random integration. Therefore, significant interest has emerged to develop site-specific integration and precise integration technologies for future gene therapy protocols.

Homologous recombination is the only method that can accomplish precise integration at endogenous chromosomal loci that have not been genetically engineered. Furthermore, precise integration is required to correct mutant sequences found within the genomic DNA of these chromosomal loci. The goal is to replace mutant sequences that produce aberrant gene products, or null mutations that prevent production of any gene product. In addition, it could be possible to eliminate harmful sequences, such as integrated HIV proviral DNA, by a knock-out strategy using homologous recombination. In vivo therapies based on precise integration require effective DNA delivery technology and efficient homologous recombination, in order to correct an adequate number of genomic DNA loci found within the target tissues and organs of interest. The low efficiencies of conventional in vivo DNA delivery and homologous

From: *Methods in Molecular Biology, vol. 133: Gene Targeting Protocols*
Edited by: E. Kmiec © Humana Press Inc., Totowa, NJ

recombination protocols have therefore limited application of precise integration to ex vivo applications, in which targeted alleles can be identified by selection.

Many publications have reported highly efficient homologous recombination in cultured cells and cell lines *(1–7)*. The efficiency of homologous recombination is assessed by two distinct frequencies, and both frequencies must be high, in order to achieve therapeutically useful levels of gene correction. One frequency is that for gene targeting which is an assessment of the amount of homologous recombination vs nonhomologous recombination. This frequency is calculated by dividing the number of homologous recombination events by the total number of integration events. Gene targeting frequencies as high as 80% have been reported *(7–9)*. The second frequency is called the absolute frequency of homologous recombination. This frequency is calculated by dividing the number of homologous recombination events by the total number of cells that are used for transfection. Typically, the number of homologous recombination events has been assessed by counting the number of colonies grown from single cells that have undergone precise integration of the targeting DNA. Recent reports from gene targeting experiments have shown that as many as 1 in 10 cells have been targeted by homologous recombination *(2,7)*. Therefore, the absolute frequency of homologous recombination can be at least 10^{-1}. If these high frequencies can be achieved in vivo, in animal models, homologous recombination could become a useful tool for gene therapy in humans.

Several factors influence the gene targeting frequency and the absolute frequency of homologous recombination in vitro. These factors include the design of the targeting DNA; the efficiency of DNA delivery; the culture conditions of the cells before, during, and after transfection; and the assessment of homologous recombination. This chapter will specifically address the use of replacement-type DNAs, as shown in Fig. 1. These DNAs can correct small genomic regions that contain insertions, deletions, and base substitutions (**Fig. 1,A–C**). In addition, large deletions can be corrected (**Fig. 1,D–F**), and large insertions can be removed (**Fig. 1,G–I**). Apparently, high gene targeting frequencies are obtained by using targeting DNAs that contain long lengths of homologies to the chromosomal allele. Regions that are 3.5–4 kb in length have produced high frequencies *(9)*. It is best if these regions contain few or no mismatches to sequences found in the chromosomal allele. Use of isogenic DNA has helped to increase the gene targeting frequency at certain chromosomal alleles *(8)*. For experimental purposes, a marker gene can be placed within the targeting DNA. The marker gene is placed between the regions of homology, so that production of the gene product encoded by the chromosomal allele is not disrupted. Marker genes can encode gene products used for positive selection, reporter genes, or cell surface markers. Ideally, targeting DNAs for use in human gene correction would not contain any marker genes.

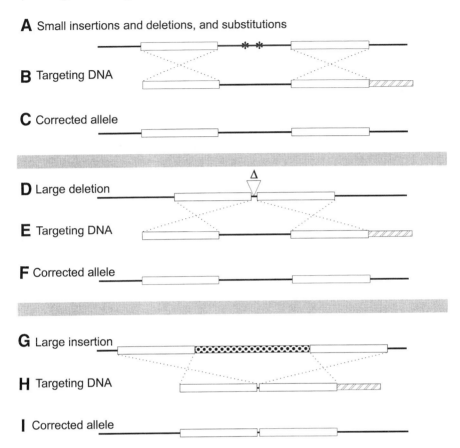

Fig. 1. Various schemes for DNA replacement. (**A–C**) Correction of small insertions and deletions, and base substitutions. Mutations in the chromosomal allele are indicated by asterisks in (**A**). The linearized targeting DNA shown in (**B**) contains the correct DNA fragment flanked by two regions homologous to the chromosomal allele (unfilled bars). The dotted lines indicate the regions where crossovers occur (between A and B; D and E; G and H). The cross-hatched bar indicates the vector backbone that does not insert into the chromosomal allele (B, E, H). (C) shows the corrected allele after homologous recombination between the targeting DNA and the mutant chromosomal allele at their regions of homology (unfilled bars). (**D–F**) Correction of a large deletion. The deletion is found between the two unfilled bars shown in (D). The targeting DNA shown in (E) contains DNA that corrects the allelic deletion found between two regions that are homologous to the chromosomal allele (unfilled bars). (F) shows the corrected allele after homologous recombination between the targeting DNA and the mutant chromosomal allele at their regions of homology (unfilled bars). (**G–I**) Elimination of inserted sequences (G, spotted bar) found in the mutant chromosomal allele. After homologous recombination occurs between the targeting DNA (H) and the mutant chromosomal allele (G) at their regions of homology (unfilled bars), the inserted DNA is eliminated, and the allele is corrected (I).

The absolute frequency of homologous recombination and the gene targeting frequency are influenced by the amount of DNA delivered into each cell. One major goal is to deliver the targeting DNA into the nuclei of as many cells as possible, thereby enabling a high absolute frequency. However, it is known that the frequency of non-homologous recombination increases when too many copies of DNA are delivered into the nucleus *(10)*. Therefore, transfection conditions should be optimized to deliver a limited number of DNA molecules into the nuclei of the greatest number of cells. Furthermore, these conditions will vary for different cell types and cell lines. Therefore, an approach to determining these optimized conditions is valuable. In addition, if transfections can be performed in small volumes, then several different conditions can be rapidly tested within a single experiment.

Electroporation is one method used for DNA delivery, and the conditions used for electroporation can easily be varied in order to modulate the DNA copy number that is delivered into the nucleus. This chapter will discuss the use of electroporation for efficient homologous recombination. It is also essential to know those conditions that produce high frequencies of nonhomologous recombination. The parameters that are most useful to vary include the amount of DNA, the voltage, the capacitance, and the temperature. The conditions used will also affect the survival of cells after electroporation. In order to test many different conditions quickly, microelectroporation chambers are used that hold a 25-µL volume. To test an entire battery of conditions would include the use of three different amounts of DNA, three different voltage settings, two different settings for the capacitance, and two different temperatures. This would require 36 different electroporations, which could reasonably be done using microelectroporation chambers, and then plating cells into wells of six-well tissue-culture clusters. Based on using these various conditions for electroporation of at least 10 different cell types and cell lines, the author and colleagues have developed guidelines to simplify optimizing the electroporation protocol. A guide for choosing a range of electroporation conditions for the most widely used applications is presented in Table 1, and the parameters listed should be applicable to almost all cell types and cell lines. This table covers work performed using the Cell-Porator™ Electroporation System (Life Technologies, Gaithersburg, MD). Therefore, to optimize conditions for homologous recombination in a given cell type or cell line, it would be necessary to try only two different amounts of DNA, one setting for capacitance, three different voltages, and two different temperatures. This would require performing only 12 different electroporations, and one can quickly assess the efficiency of homologous recombination in the cell pools soon after electroporation (*see* **Subheading 3.2.**). Specific conditions used to produce a high frequency of homologous recombination in mouse embryonic stem cells, E14TG2a, have been described

Table 1
Guide for Choosing Electroporation Conditions

Application	Cell death	T°	Amount of DNA	Capacitance[a] (μF)	Voltage[a] (V)
High transient transfection[b]	Low–moderate (<0.1–20%)	25°C	Moderate–high (50–110 nM)	Moderate (60)	Moderate (90–120v)
High-frequency nonhomologous recombination[c]	High (50–80%)	25°C	High (75–110 nM)	Moderate (60) High (330)	High (150v) Moderate (90–120v)
High-frequency homologous	Low (<0.01%)	4–25°C	Low (5 nM)	Moderate (60)	Moderate–high (90–150v)

[a]Capacitance and voltage settings listed are for use with microelectroporation chambers and the Cell-Porator Electroporation System (Life Technologies).

[b]These conditions produce the largest number of cells that express a reporter gene of interest, as detected by substrate staining, e.g., X-gal staining for β-galactosidase, or other visual methods.

[c]These conditions produce fewer live cells; however, all cells highly express a reporter gene of interest, as detected by enzymatic assays or ELISA performed on cell extracts. The amount of protein produced per μg cellular protein is about 10–20-fold greater than that produced using conditions listed for high transient transfection. In addition, many cells have integrated plasmid DNA. Therefore, these conditions can be used to create a large number of stable cell lines that have integrated a cDNA of interest.

[d]High frequency of homologous recombination is obtained using these conditions and linearized genomic DNA that has been optimized for targeting a particular chromosomal locus.

(7). As shown in Table 1, these conditions are not similar to those that produce high transient transfection or high levels of integration of cDNAs that do not contain long lengths of homology to genomic sequences.

The conditions used for cell culture greatly influence the frequencies and the assessment of homologous recombination *(7).* Specific details will be listed in the **Subheading 3.**, but some critical features will be briefly mentioned here. Cells used for gene targeting experiments should be grown to about 70% confluency prior to transfection. Cells and linearized targeting DNA should be mixed together and allowed to sit for about 20 min prior to electroporation; this mixture should remain undisturbed in the microelectroporation chamber for approx 15 min after electroporation. Cells should be plated at optimal density, so that these cells will grow to about 70% confluency the day after electroporation. Cells should be grown as pools for at least 60 h after electroporation. Ideally, it is best for cells to grow optimally for at least 1 wk after electroporation. The author has found that nonintegrated DNA persists in some nuclei for at least 1 wk after electroporation. Furthermore, DNA replication may be required for homologous recombination to occur *(11)*, although this hypothesis should be tested by performing gene targeting experiments in nonproliferating cells. Therefore, it is best to keep the cells growing optimally following transfection.

We have also shown that addition of selective media and plating cells at high dilutions after transfection can dramatically reduce the frequency of homologous recombination *(7)*. Several cell types and cell lines require specific extracellular matrix- and colony-stimulating factors that are only provided by neighboring cells of the same type. Many of these factors are not soluble, and, therefore, are not present in conditioned medium. For assessments of homologous recombination that involve formation of colonies, it is critical to optimize cell culture conditions, in order to produce high efficiencies of colony formation *(7)*. Therefore, for each cell type or cell line of interest, it is important to determine the efficiency of colony formation in nonselective media, and in appropriate selective media at various plating densities *(7)*. Furthermore, at high absolute frequencies of homologous recombination, large numbers of colonies will be obtained. Therefore, it is essential to use accurate methods for counting colonies *(7)*, and to use adequate methods for assessing homologous recombination in cell pools or in individual colonies (*see* **Subheading 3.2.**).

Electroporation may be useful for ex vivo applications of homologous recombination in gene therapy. To use homologous recombination in vivo, additional gene delivery methods are required. The author has interest in performing homologous recombination in vivo in adult animals using liposome-mediated DNA delivery. Initial experiments, involving intravenous injection of liposomes complexed with linearized targeting DNA, suggest that this is a feasible approach *(6)*. The goal is to create targeted liposome delivery that can modulate the DNA copy number introduced into the nuclei of cells in specific organs of interest. The author has assessed the frequencies of homologous recombination in total organ extracts. However, the author is also developing technologies to assess colonies grown from single cells of organs that have been transfected. These methods involve preparation of single-cell suspensions from dissociated organs: fluorescence-activated cell sorting (FACS) of targeted cells expressing an integrated reporter gene, such as β-galactosidase, after homologous recombination of a targeting DNA that contains the reporter gene; isolation of targeted cells that express an integrated cell surface marker after homologous recombination of a targeting DNA that contains the cell surface marker gene; and growth of these isolated single cells into colonies, in order to make adequate amounts of DNA for Southern blot analyses and polymerase chain reaction (PCR) analyses. Because all of the tools required for a thorough assessment of in vivo homologous recombination are available, it is now possible to optimize this technology for use in human gene therapy.

2. Materials
2.1. Gene Targeting Protocol

1. Cell-Porator Electroporation System (Life Technologies, cat. no. 11609-013): This system consists of the pulse control unit that delivers the electrical pulses and the chamber safe that holds the chambers during electroporation.
2. Disposable microelectroporation chambers (Life Technologies, cat. no. 11608-031). These chambers have two flat-topped electrode bosses that are separated by 0.15 cm **(Fig. 2B)**.
3. Several frozen stocks of the cells or cell lines of interest stored in liquid nitrogen. These stocks should be made from cells of the lowest passage number that is available (*see* **Note 1**).
4. Appropriate cell culture medium, including high-quality FCS, if required, and any necessary growth factors and supplements. HyClone Laboratories, Logan, Utah, is a good source for high quality fetal calf serum.
5. Cells grown to 70% confluency on 10 cm tissue culture dishes (*see* **Note 2**).
6. Hemacytometer.
7. Tissue culture hood.
8. Sterile, conical-bottomed microtube. The author prefers sterile Nunc CryoTubes (Nunc, Naperville, IL, cat. no. 377224; *see* **Note 3**).
9. Optimized gene targeting vector for replacement at the desired chromosomal locus (*see* **Note 4**).
10. Linearized targeting DNA that has been purified after restriction enzyme digestion (*see* **Note 5**). For gene targeting experiments, the final DNA concentration should be approx 1 µg/µL (*see* **Note 6**).
11. Spectrophotometer.
12. Trypan blue solution, 0.4% (Sigma, St. Louis, MO; cat. no. T 8154).
13. Gel electrophoresis equipment and reagents.
14. Appropriate restriction enzymes.
15. Inverted microscope.
16. Refrigerated tabletop centrifuge (Sorvall, Newtown, CT; model no. RT 7), or the equivalent.
17. Sterile, 15-mL disposable centrifuge tubes for use in the Sorvall centrifuge.
18. Trypsin-EDTA, or the appropriate trypsin for the cells or cell lines of interest.
19. Pipetors for dispensing small and large volumes. Sterile pipet tips for use with the pipetors.
20. Reagents required for proper cryopreservation of the cell types and cell lines of interest (*see* **Note 7**).
21. Distilled water chilled to 4°C.

2.2. Assessment of Homologous Recombination

1. Several materials required for the gene targeting protocol listed above are also required for assessment of homologous recombination (*see* **Note 8**).
2. Inverted microscope with a reticle or a dissection microscope with an eyepiece reticle.

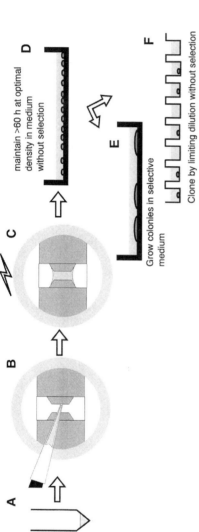

maintain >60 h at optimal density in medium without selection

Grow colonies in selective medium

Clone by limiting dilution without selection

Fig. 2. Gene targeting protocol. (**A**) Cells and linearized targeting DNA are mixed in a 25-μL vol consisting of at least 23 μL cell growth medium. A sterile, conical-bottomed tube is used, so that the mixture does not spread out over a large surface area. The tube containing this mixture of cells and DNA is placed at a specific temperature (on ice, at room temperature, or heated) for 20 min prior to electroporation. (**B**) The 25-μL mixture is placed into a microelectroporation chamber that is at a specific temperature (precooled, room temperature, or heated). The mixture is loaded into the microelectroporation chamber by using a pipetor to dispense the mixture onto one one of the electrode bosses. The mixture suspends between the two electrode bosses (C) by surface tension. (**C**) The loaded microelectroporation chamber is placed into a chamber safe that contains water at a specific temperature (chilled, room temperature, or heated). The chamber is inverted twice prior to electroporation, and electroporation is performed while the chamber is in the water that is in the chamber safe. After electroporation, the chamber containing the electroporated cells is placed at a specific temperature for 15 min (on ice, at room temperature, or heated). (**D**) Cells are plated into one well of a six-well tissue culture cluster, and are grown as pools for two passages. Isolation of colonies can be carried out by two different procedures, shown in E (using selection) or F (without using selection). (**E**) Isolation of colonies using selection. The author grows electroporated cells as pools for two passages. After cell pools no sooner than 60 hours after electroporation. The author grows electroporated cells as pools for two passages. After adequate growth in selection (approx 2 wk for each selective media), colonies will be formed. (**F**) Isolation of colonies by limiting dilution without the use of selection. After electroporated cells are grown as pools for growth from single cells, the cells are plated into 96-well dishes at limiting dilution. Wells are checked each day for growth from single cells, and all wells containing more than one colony are excluded. A colony is grown from each single cell, and is expanded in the well to approx 10^3–10^4 cells.

3. Multichannel pipetors for small volumes and for large volumes up to 200 μL.
4. Materials and reagents required for Southern blot analyses (*see* **Note 9**).
5. Materials and reagents required for PCR analyses.
6. Tissue culture dishes of various sizes, including 10-cm dishes, six-well tissue culture clusters, 12-well tissue culture clusters, 96-well dishes (*see* **Note 2**).
7. Wright-Giemsa stain (*see* **Note 10**).
8. Materials and reagents required for the preparation of genomic DNA.
9. Appropriate selective media, if selection is desired.

3. Methods (*see* Note 11)

3.1. Gene Targeting Protocol

3.1.1. Cell Culture

1. Routine cell culture procedures should be followed using the appropriate subcultivation ratio when passing the cells (*see* **Note 12**).
2. For gene targeting, grow cells to 70% confluency in 10 cm tissue culture dishes (*see* **Note 1**). Each dish provides enough cells for about six electroporations (*see* **Note 13**). Each 10-cm dish should be processed separately, and all six electroporations are performed before removing cells from the next 10-cm dish.
3. Remove the cells from the dish, following the appropriate procedure for the cells of interest. Most cells can be removed by trypsinization using trypsin-EDTA. However, trypsin cannot be used for some cells, and certain cells may require a special trypsin solution.
4. After removal from the dish, cells should be well suspended in a 10-mL final volume, using cell growth medium in a 15-mL disposable centrifuge tube.
5. Remove a small aliquot, about 20 μL, of the diluted cells, to view in a hemacytometer. Calculate the total number of cells in the 10-mL vol.
6. Centrifuge the cells in a tabletop centrifuge for 5 min at 1000 rpm. For some cells, it is best to spin at 4°C, and not at room temperature.
7. Decant the supernatant and resuspend the cell pellet in cell culture medium (*see* **Notes 13** and **14**). The cell pellet should provide enough cells to make six aliquots of about 2×10^6 cells (*see* **Note 13**). Each aliquot of cells for electroporation should be in at least 23 μL cell culture medium (*see* **Note 14**).
8. Place cells at the desired temperature on ice, at room temperature, or at 37°C (*see* **Note 15**).

3.1.2. Electroporation

1. Based on the guidelines in Table 1, set up several electroporations to test the range of variables as listed. For homologous recombination, use the following: voltage at 90, 120, or 150 V; capacitance at 60 μF; 4°C or room temperature; and 5 nM or 10 nM linearized targeting DNA. Therefore, 12 different electroporations will be performed using every possible combination of these variables.
2. Mix the cells (2×10^6, or one-sixth of the concentrated cell stock) and the DNA in a sterile, conical bottomed tube (**Fig. 2A**). The final volume of the mixture

should be 25 µL. Place the tube at the desired temperature for 20 min. Place the microelectroporation chambers at the same temperature as the cells + DNA mixture, and let sit for 20 min.

3. Place distilled water, at the desired temperature, into the chamber safe.
4. Load the DNA + cell mixture into the microelectroporation chamber by pipeting it onto one of the electrode bosses (**Fig. 2B**). The mixture will suspend between both electrode bosses by surface tension (**Fig. 2C**).
5. Invert the loaded microelectroporation chamber twice to suspend the cells well prior to electroporation. Place this chamber into the rack inside the chamber safe. Set the capacitance and the voltage on the pulse-control unit. Electroporate with an electrical pulse.
6. Let the chamber sit at the desired temperature for 15 min.
7. Repeat from step 2, until all electroporations are performed, using cells harvested from the same 10-cm dish. It is best to perform each electroporation immediately after the last, so that the aliquots of cells + DNA do not sit for more than 30 min prior to electroporation.

3.1.3. Plating of Cells After Electroporation

1. Invert the electroporated chamber once. For performing quantitative assays, remove 15 µL cell + DNA mixture from the microelectroporation chamber, and plate into one well of a six-well tissue culture cluster containing the appropriate cell growth medium (**Fig. 2D**). Approximately 1.2×10^6 cells are plated into a surface area of about 10 cm² (*see* **Note 16**) for electroporations that produce little cell death (*see* **Note 17**). It is difficult to remove 25 µL quantitatively from every chamber. For applications in which exact quantitation is not necessary, remove as much of the cell + DNA mixture as possible, and plate into cell growth medium (*see* **Note 18**).
2. Repeat all steps from **step 3** in **Subheading 3.1.1.**, until all electroporations have been performed.
3. Cells should be about 70% confluent the day after electroporation. Let cells grow as pools for more than 60 h in nonselective medium (**Fig. 2D**). If possible, let cells grow as pools beyond passage 1, and just prior to passage 2 after electroporation.

3.2. Assessment of Homologous Recombination

3.2.1. Assessment of Cell Pools

1. It is important to grow cells as pools after electroporation, to produce a high frequency of homologous recombination (*7*). If cells that are targeted by homologous recombination grow at the same rate as similar cells that have not been electroporated, then calculations of the frequency of homologous recombination within the cell pool, several days after transfection, will reflect the frequency of gene targeting events that occurred in the cells electroporated with the targeting DNA.
2. Southern blot analyses of genomic DNA from the electroporated cell pool can be performed to detect the presence of the allele of interest from the parental cells and the allele from cells that have been targeted. This strategy will be effective

only if sensitive probes are available to detect the allele of interest and if a significant percentage of cells in the cell pool have been targeted.

3. Quantitative PCR analyses can be performed to determine the number of alleles in the cell pool that have been targeted vs those that have not been targeted using primers that are specific for each allele. To detect the targeted allele, it is essential to perform PCR across and beyond the region where the targeting DNA has integrated into the chromosomal allele.

4. For some alleles, no sensitive probes are available to use for Southern blotting, and suitable PCR primers cannot be prepared to amplify outside and through the crossover regions between the targeting DNA and the chromosomal DNA. Targeting at these alleles can be assessed by examining colonies produced after electroporation, as described in **Subheading 3.2.2.** However, it is best to at least determine the amount of targeting DNA that can be detected in the DNA of the cell pool about 1 wk after electroporation (*see* **Note 19**), before investing time to produce colonies and to analyze them. Primers can be designed to amplify short regions found only in the targeting DNA that could integrate into the chromosome by homologous recombination of the larger targeting DNA.

3.2.2. Assessment of Colonies

3.2.2.1. ISOLATION OF COLONIES BY LIMITING DILUTION

1. This method can be used for isolation of colonies after electroporating cells with a targeting DNA that contains no gene encoding a selectable marker. After cells have grown as pools in nonselective media (**Fig. 2D**), they are removed from the well of a six-well tissue culture cluster, as described in **Subheading 3.1.1., steps 3** through **6**. However, in step 5, cells should be well suspended in a 2-mL final volume (instead of 10 mL), using cell growth medium in a 15-mL disposable centrifuge tube.

2. According to the cell type of interest, the cells are then plated at 0.5–10 cells per well in 96-well dishes, as shown in **Fig. 2F** (*see* **Note 2**). If the cells of interest have never been plated at limiting dilution previously, the number of cells to plate per well is empirically determined. Begin by plating cells at 1, 5, and 10 cells per well in 100 μL cell culture medium.

3. Wells should be checked every day after plating to detect colonies forming from single cells. Wells that have no cells, or that have colonies growing from two or more cells, should be marked and excluded.

4. Expand colonies from single cells to 10^3–10^4 cells. Medium should not be changed soon after plating. An additional 50 μL medium should be added to the wells no later than 7 d after plating. Alternatively, some cell types grow best at limiting dilution using a supplement of filtered conditioned medium.

5. After expansion, harvest the cells for preparation of genomic DNA and for cryopreservation.

6. To identify targeted colonies, perform Southern blot or PCR analyses on genomic DNAs prepared from colonies chosen at random. If the frequency of homologous recombination is high, numerous targeted colonies can be detected. The percent-

age of colonies that are targeted can be calculated, and this percentage will reflect the absolute frequency of homologous recombination. Without growing cells in selection after electroporation, the author detected one in 10 colonies that had been targeted *(7)*. No colonies with nonhomologous recombination were detected.

7. If the frequency of homologous recombination is not high, and if the targeting DNA encodes a selectable marker that integrates into the chromosome along with the targeting DNA, or if the chromosomal allele is selectable, the isolated colonies can be grown for about 2 wk in the appropriate selective media. Genomic DNA can be prepared from colonies that survive selection, and these DNAs can be analyzed by Southern blotting or by PCR.

3.2.2.2. Isolation of Colonies by Co-Plating with Parental Cells

1. This method is used for experiments in which the targeting DNA encodes a selectable marker that integrates into the chromosome along with the targeting DNA, or if the chromosomal allele is selectable. Colonies can be formed from electroporated cells plated in high dilutions, along with nonelectroporated parental cells in 10 cm dishes. Use 10-, 100-, and 1000-fold dilutions of electroporated cells. The total number of cells plated should be about 7.2×10^6 cells (*see* **Note 13**). The surface area of the bottom of a 10-cm dish is approx 60 cm², and is six-fold greater than that of one well of a six-well tissue culture cluster. Prior to these experiments, perform control experiments to determine the selection procedures to use that will kill all parental cells within 3–6 d *(7)*.

2. Cells should be approx 70% confluent on the dish the day following plating.

3. Grow cells for at least 60 h in nonselective media. The medium may need to be changed 2–3× during this period.

4. The number of integrations that are nonhomologous vs homologous can be predicted by using double selection *(7,9)*.

5. The first selection is performed using selection for the gene product made by the marker gene. Colonies are counted after selection, and this count estimates the total number of colonies that have integrated the targeting DNA, either by homologous recombination or by nonhomologous recombination.

6. These colonies are then grown in the second selective media that positively selects for targeted colonies. After selection, the colonies are counted. The gene targeting frequency is determined by dividing the number of colonies counted after the second selection by the number of colonies counted after the first selection.

7. Colonies can be stained (*see* **Note 10**) and counted using a dissection microscope. For experiments that require cell culture after counting, as in double-selection, colonies are not stained after the first selection, and are counted using an inverted microscope. Colonies are counted in three 1-cm squares drawn at random in separate quadrants on the bottom of each dish. The counts are averaged and multiplied by the total surface area of the dish. To correct for any differences in colony density from the center to the edge of the plates, sequential fields spanning the full width of each plate are counted, using an eyepiece reticle and a guideline marked across the diameter of each plate. Based on the known area of the reticle field, the number of fields counted, and the total plate area, the total

number of colonies is calculated and compared to counts obtained by counting squares described above. The calculations should be identical. Furthermore, it is possible to count all colonies on the dish for the higher dilutions, 1000-fold, of electroporated cells.

8. The total number of targeted colonies produced from a specific number of electroporated cells is also calculated. After corrections for dilutions, the total number of colonies produced should be similar, and is reflective of the absolute frequency of homologous recombination.

3.2.2.3. ISOLATION OF COLONIES USING SELECTION OF CELL POOLS

1. After cells have grown as pools in nonselective media (**Fig. 2D**), they are grown in the appropriate selective media for about 2 wk for each selection (**Fig. 2E**).
2. Double selection (described above) can be used to predict the number of integrations that are homologous or nonhomologous. Colonies are counted after the first and second selections, and the gene targeting frequency is calculated as described above.

3.2.3. Assessment of DNA Delivery into the Nucleus

1. In order to optimize the gene targeting frequency, the DNA copy number delivered to the nucleus after using various electroporation conditions should be determined. This can be measured by performing quantitative Southern blot analyses or quantitative PCR analyses of DNA isolated from the nuclei of cells at different time-points after electroporation. Nuclei can be isolated by subcellular fractionation of the cells. Probes for Southern blotting and primers for PCR should be made from sequences found only in the targeting DNA, and not in the chromosomal DNA.
2. *In situ* DNA PCR can be used to determine the percentage of cells that have been transfected. PCR primers that are specific only to the targeting DNA should be used.
3. The DNA copy number in the nucleus after electroporation can be calculated by dividing the number of copies of targeting DNA isolated from a defined number of nuclei by the total number of cells that have been transfected (*see* **Note 20**).

4. Notes

1. Various genetic changes can occur as cells and cell lines are passed. For example, duplications can occur in the genomic region of interest. Therefore, it is essential to begin all gene targeting experiments with cells and cell lines that are similar in passage number, and use of cells of low passage number is preferred. If one is interested in studying cells of high passage number, then it is essential to start gene targeting experiments with cells of similar passage number.
2. Some cell types and cell lines require gelatin-coated tissue culture dishes. For growth of these cells, the dishes are coated with 0.1% (w/v) gelatin just prior to plating. The author prefers to use cell culture tested gelatin (Sigma, cat. no. G 1393).
3. These Nunc vials can be purchased from PGC Scientifics, Gaithersburg, MD. Conical-bottom, 1.0 mL, star foot cryotube vials with internal threads are PGC cat. no. 36-6576-03. Similar vials with external threads are PGC cat. no. 36-6576-15.

Star-foot cryotube vials can be easily opened and closed in a Nunc slotted rack (PGC Scientifics, cat. no. 36-6576-30). Conical bottom tubes are useful because mixtures of DNA and cells should not spread out over a large surface area just prior to electroporation.

4. The targeting DNA should be carefully designed. If possible, use longer lengths of homology. For example, a good targeting DNA used for correction of the *hprt* locus in male mouse embryonic stem cells, E14TG2a, contains 4.0 kb and 3.5 kb regions of homology to the genomic DNA *(7,9)*. The author is investigating the minimal lengths of homology required to produce high frequencies of homologous recombination. The regions of homology should have as few DNA base-pair mismatches as possible with respect to the chromosomal sequences.

5. The targeting DNA should be linearized by digestion with a restriction enzyme(s) just prior to use for gene targeting. Use restriction enzymes that produce sticky ends on the targeting DNA. In addition, the author prefers to use enzymes such as *Bam*H I and *Xho* I that produce recessed 3' termini. One end of the targeting DNA should contain only genomic DNA sequences that are homologous to the chromosomal DNA sequences.

6. For DNA purification, the author performs one phenol extraction followed by one chloroform extraction. The supernatant is precipitated and washed using the standard protocol for ethanol precipitation *(12)*. It is best not to use DNA that has been isolated from a gel after electrophoresis. Small amounts of agarose are thought to reduce the frequency of DNA integration. In addition, it is essential to obtain an accurate determination of DNA concentration in the stock. This concentration should be determined by OD_{260} using a spectrophotometer, and by gel electrophoresis using linearized DNA standards of known concentration. For a 15-kb targeting DNA, 5 nM DNA in a 25-μL final volume is about 1.2 μg. Therefore, for a DNA fragment of this size, 1.2 μL of a 1-μg/μL DNA stock would be used for one electroporation using the microelectroporation chamber. It is important that the final 25-μL vol consist of at least 23 μL cell growth medium. For transient expression and high frequency of nonhomologous recombination applications, the stock of supercoiled DNA must be more concentrated, approx 10 μg/μL. For a 7-kb reporter gene plasmid, 110 nM DNA in 25 μL is about 12 μg. Therefore, 1.2 μL of a 10-μg/μL DNA stock would be used to produce a final concentration of 110 mM in 25 μL. The DNA concentration for stocks at 10 μg/μL should be checked over time. Often the stock may become slightly more concentrated after many aliquots have been removed. It is helpful to vortex concentrated DNA stock solutions well just prior to removing each aliquot.

7. For cryopreservation, the author uses a commercially prepared dimethyl sulfoxide cell-culture-freezing medium sold by Life Technologies (cat. no. 11102-019). This medium can be used for a broad spectrum of mammalian cells, and often is superior to any freezing medium that can be made in the laboratory.

8. Materials numbered 3–7 and 13–20, listed under the gene targeting protocol, are also required for assessment of homologous recombination.

9. Particularly for analyses that require high sensitivity, the author prefers to use the following materials and reagents for Southern blotting: QuikHyb™ hybridization solution

(Stratagene, La Jolla, CA, cat. no. 201220), GeneScreen *Plus* hybridization transfer membrane (E.I. du Pont de Nemours, NEN Products, Boston, MA, cat. no. NEF-988), Random Primers DNA Labeling System (Life Technologies, cat. no. 18187-013).

10. The author prefers to use Diff-Quik Differential Stain (Scientific Products Division of Baxter Health Care, McGaw Park, IL, cat. no. B4132-1).

11. This section presents methods that can be used for many different cells and lines. Specific details for gene targeting in the mouse embryonic stem cell line, E14TG2a, have been described *(7)*.

12. Some cell types and cell lines should not be diluted to low concentrations when passing. For example, E14TG2a cells must be passed at a subcultivation ratio of 1:5 for optimal growth. Therefore, for some cell types and cell lines, optimal growth is dependent on the density of cells that grow on the tissue culture dish.

13. For cells such as E14TG2a, there are approx 10^7 cells on a 10-cm dish at 70% confluency; and each electroporation uses about 2×10^6 cells. If cells are much larger than E14TG2a, there are fewer cells on a 10-cm dish at 70% confluency. However, there should also be fewer cells used for each electroporation. If recovery of the cells from the 10 cm dish has been efficient, regardless of cell size, one-sixth of the concentrated cells should be used for each electroporation.

14. The final volume of cells mixed with DNA should be 25 µL per aliquot. Therefore, an allowance must be made for the addition of DNA that should be no greater than 2 µL. It is also important to note the volume of the cell pellet, in order to calculate the amount of media to use for resuspending the cells just prior to electroporation. Therefore, the maximum volume of 138 µL (6×23 µL) of cell growth medium should be reduced to compensate for the volume of the cell pellet.

15. Although the author has never tried using 37°C conditions throughout the gene targeting protocol, this may be an interesting variation to test.

16. For one well of a six-well tissue culture cluster with an inner diameter of 35 mm, the surface area at the bottom of the well is about 10 cm². Plating at the optimal cell density after electroporation was shown to be critical for increasing the frequency of homologous recombination *(7)*.

17. Before performing any gene targeting experiments, the amount of cell death that is produced after electroporation using various conditions should be determined by trypan blue exclusion experiments. The goal is to produce the least cell death and the highest frequency of homologous recombination.

18. When using conditions that produce much cell death, as in high frequency of nonhomologous recombination, plate the electroporated cells into smaller dishes, such as one well of a 12-well tissue culture cluster. This application is particularly useful for making stable cell lines that have been difficult to produce by other DNA transfer methods. For example, the author has been able to produce 5–10% of cells with stable integration of cDNAs of interest using these conditions.

19. The author could easily detect the targeting DNA in genomic DNA preparations made from cell pools 1 wk after electroporation *(7)*. Furthermore, the amount of specific targeting DNA sequences detected from cell pools grown in nonselective media was similar to that found in genomic DNA from cells of a targeted

colony that had been grown under selection and verified for homologous recombination by Southern blot analysis.

20. The author determined that approx 1–2 copies of DNA were delivered into each nucleus of E14TG2a mouse embryonic stem cells, using electroporation conditions that were optimized to produce efficient gene targeting *(7)*.

Acknowledgment

The author thanks David D. Roberts for reviewing this chapter and providing the artwork for **Figs. 1** and **2**.

References

1. Kunzelmann, K., Legendre, J.-Y., Knoell, D. L., Escobar, L. C., Xu, Z., and Gruenert, D. C. (1996) Gene targeting of CFTR DNA in CF epithelial cells. *Gene Therapy* **3,** 859–867.

2. Cole-Strauss, A., Yoon, K., Xiang, Y., Byrne, B. C., Rice, M. C., Gryn, J., Holloman, W. K., and Kmiec, E. B. (1996) Correction of the mutation responsible for sickle cell anemia by an RNA-DNA oligonucleotide. *Science* **273,** 1386–1389.

3. Fujita, A., Sakagami, K., Kanegae, Y., Saito, I., and Kobayashi, I. (1995) Gene targeting with a replication-defective adenovirus vector. *J. Virol.* **69,** 6180–6190.

4. Dieken, E. S., Epner, E. M., Fiering, S., Fournier, R. E. K., and Groudine, M. (1996) Efficient modification of human chromosomal alleles using recombination-proficient chicken/human microcell hybrids. *Nature Genet.* **12,** 174–182.

5. Yoon, K., Cole-Strauss, A., and Kmiec, E. B. (1996) Targeted gene correction of episomal DNA in mammalian cells mediated by a chimeric RNA-DNA oligonucleotide. *Proc. Natl. Acad. Sci. USA* **93,** 2071–2076.

6. Lasic, D. D. and Templeton, N. S. (1996) Liposomes in gene therapy. *Adv. Drug Del. Rev.* **20,** 221–266.

7. Templeton, N. S., Roberts, D. D., and Safer, B. (1997) Efficient gene targeting in mouse embryonic stem cells. *Gene Ther.* **4,** 700–709.

8. te Riele, H., Maandag, E. R., and Berns, A. (1992) Highly efficient gene targeting in embryonic stem cells through homologous recombination with isogenic DNA constructs. *Proc. Natl. Acad. Sci. USA* **89,** 5128–5132.

9. Reid, L. H., Shesely, E. G., Kim, H.-S., and Smithies, O. (1991) Cotransformation and gene targeting in mouse embryonic stem cells. *Mol. Cell. Biol.* **11,** 2769–2777.

10. Hooper, M. L. (1992) Introducing planned changes into the animal germline, in *Embryonal Stem Cells* (Evans, H. J., ed.), Harwood Academic, Switzerland.

11. Kogoma, T. (1996) Recombination by replication. *Cell* **85,** 625–627.

12. Sambrook, J., Fritsch, E. F., and Maniatis, T. (1989) Concentrating Nucleic Acids in *Molecular Cloning: a Laboratory Manual,* 2d ed. (Ford, N., Nolan, C., and Ferguson, M., eds.), Cold Spring Harbor Laboratory, Cold Spring Harbor, NY, pp. E.10–E.15.

5

Effective Gene Transfer Using
Viral Vectors Based on SV40

David S. Strayer

1. Introduction

To date, virus-mediated gene transfer has focused principally on murine leu-kemia virus and adenovirus as delivery vehicles *(1,2)*. It has become clear that these viral delivery systems are not adequate for the range of potential thera-peutic needs, and other vehicles are being developed for these purposes, including adeno-associated virus, herpesvirus, and others *(3,4)*. Each virus has advantages and disadvantages: The latter include inactivation by human complement, limited infectivity, low titers, short-lived expression, immunoge-nicity, contamination by replication-competent or helper virus, and so on.

The search continues for additional effective, safe gene transfer vectors. This chapter describes the experimental approaches to the application of another virus, simian virus-40 (SV40) to gene transfer. SV40 is a papovavirus, with a genome of 5.2 kb. It contains five genes encoding three structural proteins (VP1, VP2, VP3), large T (for transforming) antigen (Tag), and small t anti-gen. Tag is so named because it can immortalize cultured cells from many animal species. In contrast to this behavior in cultured cells, SV40 infection is not associated with tumor development in any animal except neonatal ham-sters. In its natural host, monkeys, it may cause a mild, transient infection. Other animals, including humans, show few, if any, clinical effects when given SV40 *(5)*.

(MHC-I) has been suggested as a receptor for SV40. The virus binds to cells, perhaps via MHC-I, and is endocytosed. Enclosed in an endosome, the virus is thereupon transported to the nucleus, where it is released and uncoats.

Because of its documented safety in humans who received live, wild-type SV40 as an unrecognized contaminant in early batches of the Salk polio vaccine

From: *Methods in Molecular Biology, vol. 133: Gene Targeting Protocols*
Edited by: E. Kmiec © Humana Press Inc., Totowa, NJ

Table 1
Advantages and Disadvantages of SV40 as a Gene Transfer Agent

Advantages	Disadvantages
May infect cells of diverse organ types and animal species of origin	Small genome size limits the size of potential DNA inserts to be transduced
May infect and express its genes in both resting and dividing cells. In particular, SV40 may infect and express its genes in resting peripheral blood mononuclear cells	Potential for reacquisition of Tag gene from packaging cell line, and hence reacquisition of replication competence, is of concern
May integrate into host DNA or be carried as episome	Titering SV40 can be cumbersome and is not always reproducible if *in situ* PCR is not available
Deleting Tag gene both removes replication competence and diminishes potential risk	
Deleting Tag gene substantially reduces immunogenicity of virus-infected cells	
Cloned virus genome is easily manipulated: replication-defective virus is easy to prepare	
Packaging cell lines are available, supplying needed gene products *in trans,* avoiding need for helper virus	
Integration of SV40 into host DNA is random, both with respect to viral and host genome sites of integration	
Integration of SV40 into host DNA has not been associated with cellular gene activation	
Virus can be made in stocks of 10^9 IU/mL, and may be concentrated to 10^{10} IU/mL	
Transduction efficiency may exceed 50%	
Safety of wild-type SV40 has been documented in humans	

(6), SV40 seems a reasonable possibility for a viral gene transfer vehicle. Based on prior experimental work, SV40 has a number of potential advantages (and disadvantages) in application as a gene transfer agent. Some of these are listed in **Table 1**, but several deserve emphasis.

Immunity to virus-infected cells is directed principally against Tag, which, though it is primarily a nuclear protein, inserts into the cell membrane, and serves as target for both antibody- and cell-mediated immune responses *(7)*. The constructs the author has devised delete Tag from the viral genome, thus greatly diminishing both predicted and observed immune responsiveness to virus-infected cells. Long-term expression of transduced genes is also possible in this setting, because, without evidence of immune elimination, infected cells may carry the viral genome integrated into host DNA, as well as in episomal form.

The authors have applied SV40-based viruses to deliver several genes, including reporter genes, as well as genes of therapeutic interest, to mice in vivo and to human cells in culture. Using luciferase reporter gene, an SV40-derived virus was delivered intratracheally *(8)*, intravenously, and to bone marrow cells *(9)*. Transgene expression and activity were documented for over 1 yr after virus administration in vivo. Furthermore, the author has transduced high levels of intracellular antibodies (single-chain Fv fragments), active ribozyme molecules (directed against endogenous cellular transcripts), and target cell membrane molecules for immunization purposes (D. S. Strayer, et al., in preparation).

Thus, SV40 has considerable potential as a gene delivery vehicle for a variety of applications. This chapter describes general approaches and selected specific methodologies that can be used to apply SV40-derived vectors to studies of gene transfer in vitro and in vivo.

1.1. Approaches

1.1.1. General Principles

The basic principles of using SV40-derived viral vectors for gene transfer in vivo have been described by the author *(8,9)*, and their applications to gene transfer in vitro have been published by others *(10,11)*. There are four basic steps involved:

1. Manipulation of the cloned SV40 genome for the intended purpose.
2. Excision of the modified genome from the carrier plasmid and transfection into a packaging cell line.
3. Production, isolation, titering of virus.
4. Use of the recombinant virus for the desired gene transfer application.

Approaches to each of these are described below.

1.1.2. Manipulation of Cloned Viral Genome

The author's approach to the construction of SV40-derivative viruses is illustrated in **Fig. 1**, and is described in this and the following subheadings. One of the advantages of SV40 that facilitates its adaptation to gene transfer studies is the ease with which the whole virus genome can be manipulated. The author received the SV40 genome as pBSV-1 (gift, J. S. Butel), in which plasmid the

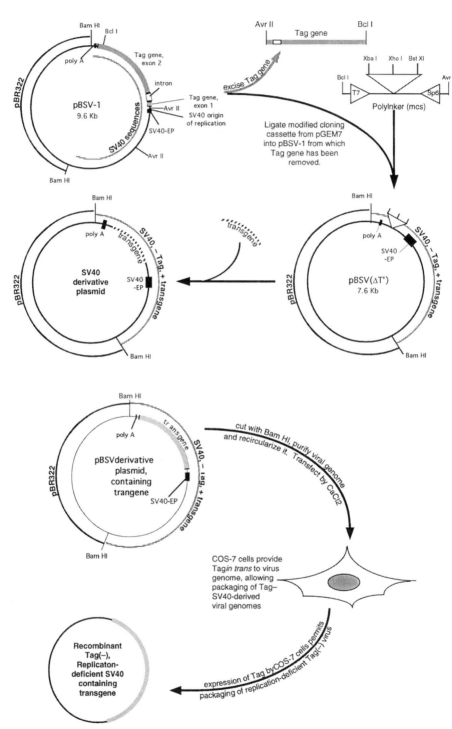

5.2 kb viral genome had been cloned as a *Bam*HI fragment into pBR322. To adapt this construct for use, the 2.4 kb *Tag* gene was excised and replaced with a polylinker derived from pGEM7® (Promega, Madison, WI). The SV40 early promoter (SV40-EP), immediately upstream of the *Tag* gene, and the polyadenylation signal, immediately downstream of the *Tag* gene, remained intact. The polylinker was flanked by bacteriophage promoters: Sp6 upstream (i.e., toward and with the same directionality as the SV40-EP) and T7 downstream. Any gene cloned into the polylinker in the correct orientation could be sequenced using the phage promoters, and would be expressed using the viral promoter. This plasmid, pBSV(ΔT'), was used effectively to produce replication-deficient virus that could express luciferase as a reporter gene, as described in the author's initial published gene transfer studies *(8,9)*.

1.1.3. Producing Virus

Packaging SV40-derivative virus requires a cell line that supplies *in trans* the necessary virus product that is lacking in the modified genomes described above. Tag is necessary for SV40 replication *(12)*. Because the *Tag* gene was deleted to make room for the multiple-cloning site, packaging cells must supply its encoded protein. COS-7 cells contain integrated SV40 DNA, which lacks a portion of the origin of replication, and so cannot produce virus *(13)*. Virus DNA is excised from the carrier plasmid, gel-purified, recircularized, and transfected into COS-7 cells. After 1–2 wk, an initial stock of virus is produced. It may be used either as a crude cell lysate or band purified *(see below)*. The SV40-derivative virus produced in this fashion is replication-defective *(8,9)*. No helper virus is used in this system.

Fig. 1. *(opposite page)* Construction of SV40-derivative viruses. SV40 genome, cloned as a *Bam*HI fragment into the unique *Bam*HI site of pBR322 (to produce pBSV-1), was re-engineered to produce a genome capable of incorporating foreign genes, yet incapable of replicating itself. To excise the *Tag* gene, pBSV-1 was digested with *Bcl*I, and partially digested with *Avr*II. This procedure left the SV40 early promoter, just upstream to the *Tag* gene, and the polyA site, just downstream from the *Tag* gene, intact. Into this opened plasmid was inserted a modified polylinker from pGEM7: modified to eliminate the *Bam*HI site and to incorporate *Bcl*I and *Avr*II restriction sites flanking the T7 and Sp6 bacteriophage promoters, respectively. Cloning this polylinker into the linearized Tag-deficient viral genome in pBR322 provided a potential target for gene transfer: pBSV(ΔT'). Potential transgenes cloned into this plasmid in orientation (5' → 3') Sp6 → T7 will be expressed under the control of the SV40 early promoter (SV40-EP). To produce virus from this construct, the viral genome is excised from the carrier plasmid using (in this case) *Bam*HI, gel-purified, and religated to itself. This recircularized viral genome is transfected into COS-7 cells, which supply the requisite Tag in *trans,* and allow packaging of a viral genome that is otherwise replication-defective.

1.1.4. Subsequent Plasmid Constructs

Although it worked well to express luciferase, pBSV(ΔT') had several limitations. pBR322 replicates to relatively low copy number in *Escherichia coli,* providing less plasmid for use in transfecting a packaging cell line. Because of existing restriction sites in both pBR322 and in SV40 genome, the inserted polylinker contained only three unique sites for use in cloning: *Bst*XI, *Xho*I, and *Xba*I. SV40-EP did not suit all uses, and other promoter constructs had to be devised. (SV40-EP was still necessary, however, because it overlapped the viral origin of replication.) More importantly, the need to use *Bam*HI to excise virus DNA from carrier plasmid for transfection limited inserted cDNAs to those lacking *Bam*HI sites.

Additional plasmid constructs were therefore produced, two of which are illustrated in **Fig. 2**. Both pSV5 and pT7A5 incorporate modifications that address these points. In both, the polylinker has been modified to include more unique restriction sites. Both of these include carrier plasmids (pGEM13 in the case of pSV5, and pT7 for pT7A5) that replicate in *Escherichia coli* more efficiently than pBR322. The virus genome is cloned into each, using unique restriction sites that were engineered into the constructs specifically for this purpose (*Not*I for pSV5 and *Pme*I for pT7A5). In addition, pT7A5 incorporates the cytomegalovirus intermediate early promoter. Other constructs have been generated, e.g., a pol III promoter and termination signal were added for expression or antisense and ribozymes, an intron was added to facilitate expression, specific flanking sequences were added to facilitate integration, and so on.

1.1.5. Titering Virus

Classically, SV40 has been titered in monkey cells using agar overlays containing neutral red *(14)*. Although the author has used this method successfully, it has a number of limitations. The author has found that it does not always provide reproducible titers. It also is cumbersome, and requires 2–3 wk for clear results. Only a cell line that supplies Tag can be used to titer replication-defective virus. Because the infectivity of a virus may vary from one target cell to another, titers derived from only the packaging cell line may not reflect the virus' infectivity for cells from different tissues and animals. Therefore, the author developed a rapid, reliable technique for titering replication-defective SV40, based on *in situ* polymerase chain reaction (PCR, *see below*). This technique can be applied to any DNA virus, and adapted to measuring infectivity in any target cell type *(15)*. In general, crude cell lysates, prepared as described below from SV40-infected cells, yield ≥10^9 infectious units (IU)/mL.

1.1.6. Applying SV40-Derivative Virus to Gene Transfer Studies

The author has used SV40-derived viruses for gene transfer both in vivo in mice and in cultured cells. Choice of route and dosage in vivo vary, depending on the individual application. SV40 infects almost every cell type examined. To infect cells grown in culture, the author has used SV40 at virus:cell ratios (multiplicity of infection [moi]) from 1 to 1000. Even at the highest moi, no more than minimal evidence of cytotoxicity has been detected with these replication-defective SV40 derivative viruses, as measured by levels of housekeeping transcripts, or by sustained cell viability.

2. Materials
2.1. Solutions for Purification of SV40

Solutions required:

1. Double detergent: 10% Triton X-100, 5% deoxycholate; store at RT.
2. 75% Sucrose: 75 g sucrose per 100 mL in 0.2 M Tris, pH 7.4: store at RT.
3. 20% Sucrose: 20 g sucrose per 100 mL in 0.02 M Tris, pH 7.4: store at 4°C.

All solutions are warmed carefully to dissolve sucrose. This step should be done carefully, avoiding overheating, because sucrose will carmelize at high temperatures. Filter-sterilize using a 0.45-µ filter.

Rotor: Beckman SW28 or equivalent. Sterilize the buckets by autoclaving. Tubes should be sterilized by soaking in 70% ethanol for at least 10 min.

2.2. In Situ PCR

Reagents, for 100 µL PCR cocktail mix: 10 µL 10X buffer with gelatin (Perkin-Elmer Cetus); 2.5 µL of each dNTP (250 µM each [final concentration]); primer pair 0.5 µM each (final concentration); 2 µL Taq polymerase, 0.1U/µL (final concentration); Dd H_2O to 100 µL.

The author chose a primer pair that would provide a PCR product derived from among the late virus genes, away from the transgene. Clearly, the choice of primer pair for this purpose is empirical. An oligonucleotide probe that has been biotinylated at the 5' end is also used *(see below)*. This can be commercially prepared, and obviously will also vary, depending on the virus and the sequence of the region amplified by PCR.

2.3. In Situ Hybridization

Hybridization solution (final concentrations): 50% formamide; 2X (SSC); 10X Denhardt's solution; 1 mg/mL Salmon sperm DNA; 0.1% sodium dodeoyl sulfate; 16 nM 5' biotinylated probe.

3. Methods
3.1. Production of Virus Stocks

1. Preparation of initial sample of recombinant SV40: COS-7 cells, subconfluent in a 60-mm tissue culture dish, are transfected using any desired protocol (the au-

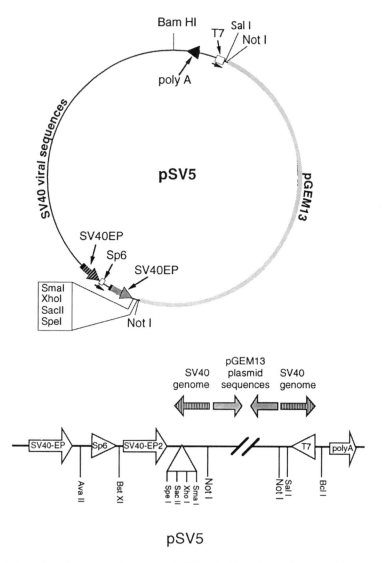

Fig. 2. *(continued on opposite page)* pSV5 and pT7A5 transfer plasmids for generating SV40-based expression vectors. This figure illustrates two of the several subsequent plasmids the author developed for SV40-mediated gene delivery. They were devised to be more flexible than pBSV(ΔT'), and to provide alternative possibilities for transgene expression. **(A)** The plasmid form of pSV5, with the cloning region illustrated underneath. **(B)** The plasmid form of pT7A5, again with the cloning region underneath.

thor generally uses standard CaCl$_2$ protocols *[16]*) with 10 μg gel-purified, recircularized, virus genome free of carrier plasmid. Cytopathic effect is observed within 1–2 d, and is extensive by 7 d.

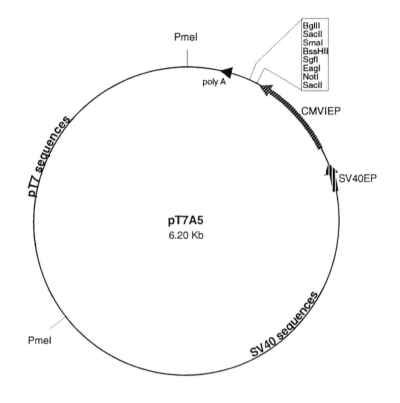

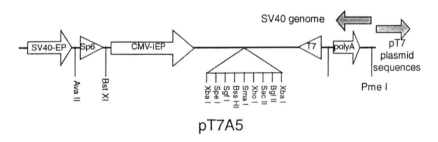

pT7A5

2. Harvest virus by removing medium: Because SV40 remains associated with the cell, most virus will be in the monolayer. Freeze-thaw the cell monolayer 3×. Add 1 mL Dalbecco's modified Eagle's medium (DMEM) 2% fetal calf serum (FCS) to the 60-mm dish, and scrape off the monolayer using a rubber policeman. Place the crude lysate in a conical tube, and sonicate it using a bath sonicator for 2 min. The crude lysate may be stored at –80°C. Most of the virus remains associated with cell cytoskeletal debris. Thus, the debris must not be removed. This initial sample is then used to generate a working virus stock.

3. Plate COS-7 Cells in 150-cm^2 Tissue Culture Flask, and allow them to achieve ≈80% confluence in DMEM-10% FCS. Remove medium and add 2 mL DMEM-2% FCS + 1 mL viral stock. Place flask on an orbital shaker for 2 h at room temperature (RT). Add 17 mL DMEM-2% FCS, and place at 37°C in an atmosphere of 5–7% CO_2 for about 2 wk. There should be noticeable foci within 1–2 d, and most cells will be infected, as judged by cytopathic effect, within 10–14 d, when the virus is ready to harvest.

4. Harvest the virus as in step 2 above, by removing the medium and freezing and thawing the monolayer 3×. Add 5 mL DMEM-2% FCS to each flask, and scrape the cells off with a rubber policeman. Place the crude lysate in a 15-mL conical tube, sonicate it in a bath sonicator for 2 min, and store at –80°C. **Do not discard cellular debris.** In cell lysates, SV40 is mostly associated with cytoskeletal aggregates and remnants. The virus may be used as crude lysate or after banding *(see below)*.

3.2. Band Purification of SV40 (Adapted from *ref. 14*)

1. From four 150-cm^2 flasks, 20 mL crude lysate should be obtained. Split this into two 10-mL aliquots, and add 1 mL of the double-detergent solution. This step dissociates the virus from cell cytoskeletal debris. Incubate on ice for 15 min. Spin at 16,000g for 20 min, at 4°C, to remove cellular debris. Remove supernatant, and bring aliquots to 13 mL.

2. Virus is concentrated from the supernatant on a discontinuous sucrose density gradient. Add 1.5 mL 75% sucrose to a sterile SW28 tube. Then carefully layer 2.5 mL 20% sucrose over it. Layer the 13 mL double-detergent supernatant over the sucrose solutions. Place tubes into buckets and spin 22,500 rpm for 3.5 h.

3. Pierce the bottom of the centrifuge tube with an 18-gage needle. Drip the gradient into sterile microcentrifuge tubes, 0.5 mL per fraction. Collect only the first eight fractions. The virus is usually in fractions 4, 5, or 6. Pool these, and dialyze sterilely (the author uses sterile dialysis cassettes for this purpose) against three changes of 1000 mL phosphate-buffered saline (PBS). You may detect the virus by ultraviolet spectrophotometery: the A_{260}:A_{280} ratio is usually 1.3–1.5.

3.3. Titering Replication-Defective SV40 Viruses

Titering replication-defective SV40 viruses is performed by *in situ* PCR. This technique, developed in conjunction with Omar Bagasra, Jefferson Medical College, measures only the ability of virus to infect (i.e., to release its DNA into) target cells *(15)*. The procedure must be standardized for each different target cell type, because each cell type is different, and, in particular, requires different times of proteinase K digestion. The approach described here is for TC7 cells. It is critical to determine the number of cells/well.

1. Plate TC7 cells (gift, J. S. Butel) in six-well cluster dishes, so that they will grow to about 80% confluence overnight. For TC7 cells, this means 1.5 × 10^5 cells/well. TC7 cells do not carry the virus genome, and therefore will not support replication of Tag-SV40-derivative viruses.

2. Make serial 10-fold dilutions of virus stock with DMEM-2% FCS. Be sure to include a negative control (no virus) and 100 μL straight viral stock. Remove medium from cultures. Plate 100 μL of each dilution + 400 μL DMEM-2% FCS. Be sure to completely cover the cell monolayer. Incubate for 2 h at RT, with shaking. Bring each well to 3 mL with DMEM-2% FCS, and incubate overnight at 37°C.

3. Cell removal and fixation: Prepare Teflon slides (Erie Scientific, Erie, PA) by precoating them with 3-aminopropyl-triethoxy-silane (AES). Remove cells from plate with 250 μL 10× trypsin (GIBCO), wash with 500 μL PBS, then place 750 μL cell suspension in 1.5-mL microcentrifuge tubes and spin 2 min in microcentrifuge, to remove supernatant. Resuspend cell pellet in 20 μL serum-free medium. Spread cell suspension onto the glass surface of AES-treated slides, and allow to dry. Heat-fix 1 min at 105°C, then soak in 4% paraformaldehyde for 3 h. Wash in 3X PBS for 10 min/wash, then twice in 1X PBS for 5 min in PBS. Store at 4°C until ready for *in situ* PCR.

4. Proteinase K Digestion: Place slides in PBS containing 6 μg/mL proteinase K (Boehringer Mannheim, Indianapolis, IN) for exactly 15 min at RT. This step is highly variable, and depends on the particular cell type used. The cells must be sufficiently treated to allow the PCR and *in situ* hybridization reagents to penetrate, but not treated so extensively that there is no cellular material left on the slide. In the author's experience, each and every cell line must be studied beforehand to optimize this step prior to attempting titering. Stop the reaction by heating the slides to 92°C for 1 min. Wash in 1X PBS, then in double-distilled water, and allow to air-dry.

3.4. In Situ *PCR*

1. Apply 13 μL PCR mixture to slide and place a cover slip over the reaction mixture, taking care to avoid air bubbles. Seal the cover slip with one light coat of clear nail polish, and allow it to dry, then apply another heavier coat of nail polish, and allow it to dry.

2. Cycle parameters: 94°C for 30 s, followed by 50°C for 1 min, then 72°C for 1 min, for a total of 40 cycles, followed by a soaking step at 4°C.

3. From PCR, place slide in 95% EtOH for 10 min, to remove cover slip. Be sure all nail polish has been removed from the slide. Heat 95°C 1 min, to fix the amplified DNA.

3.5. In Situ *Hybridization*

1. Hybridization: Soak slides in 2X salt-sodium citrate (SSC) for 5 min. Place 13 μL hybridization mix on the slide and coverslip. Heat 95°C for 5 min, then place in a humidified chamber 37°C overnight. Wash in 2X SSC for 5 min, then in 1X PBS for 5 min. Prepare a solution of strepavidin-peroxidase to 330 μg/mL final concentration in PBS. Place 13 μL on slide, coverslip, and keep at 37°C for 1 h. Wash in 1X PBS 2 min.

2. Development: Prepare reaction solution: 5 mL 50 m*M* sodium acetate, pH 5.0, + 25 μL 30% H_2O_2 + 250 μL aminoethylcarbamazole solution. Flood the slides

with this solution, and incubate at 37°C for 10 min. Check the color. When positive control is clearly red, mount in 50% glycerol–3.5% gelatin, and seal slide with clear nail polish.

3. Using a microscope, identify a slide with >1%, but <50%, positive (i.e., virus-infected) cells. Determine the fraction of total cells that are positive for virus infection. Using the dilution factor and the number of cells infected (both of which are known), the infectious titer of the virus stock can be determined using the following formula:

Titer [IU/mL] = [fraction of + cells] × [number of cells/well] ~ [dilution factor]

3.6. Transduction of Cultured Cells with SV40-Derived Viruses

Precise methods to be used for transducing cultured cells using SV40 vectors will vary, depending on the effect desired, the number and type of cells, and so on. The author has found that the approach described below is uniformly effective for his purposes, and routinely achieves high levels of virus infection and transgene infection.

1. Plate cells in a 60-mm tissue culture dish to about 80% confluence. Cells may be trypsinized and allowed to adhere in 3–5 mL DMEM-10% FCS just before infection.
2. Remove medium and add 0.4 mL DMEM-2% FCS + 0.1 mL viral stock at the appropriate dilution.
3. Place culture dish on an orbital shaker for 2 h at RT. **Do not remove virus-containing medium from the culture mixture.**
4. Add 2.5 mL DMEM-2% FCS, and place at 37°C overnight, or until desired assay time.

The author prefers to assay for transgene expression by immunocytochemistry, Northern analysis, Western blotting, and other techniques. The assay method chosen will depend on the nature of the transgene and its desired effect.

4. Notes

The development and use of SV40-based viruses as gene transduction vectors is in its infancy. Because of safety, high levels of infectivity, efficient transduction, longevity of expression in vivo, and ease of use, such vectors are attractive vehicles for gene transfer. Much work remains to be done, and several important parameters need to be optimized. The greatest limitation of the system at the moment is the size of the DNA insert that can be cloned into the virus without loss of efficiency in packaging. The author is currently investigating this question. Other pressing issues involve maintaining long term high levels of expression both in vitro and in vivo. Studies to date have used unselected cells, but selection ex vivo may provide additional assurance of high levels of sustained transgene expression.

In an atmosphere in which serious deficiencies in all of the commonly used gene transfer vectors are widely acknowledged, SV40-based vectors may be a useful addition to the gene therapy armamentarium.

Acknowledgments

The work described in this chapter has been done largely by Joe Milano, whose diligence and tenacity have been instrumental in its success. The contributions of other people in this laboratory, and of collaborators and colleagues, has proven invaluable in these efforts: Omar Bagasra, Ling-Xun Duan, Iwata Ozaki, Roger Pomerantz, and Mark Zern. The author gratefully acknowledges the help of Janet S. Butel, Baylor College of Medicine, for providing pBSV-1, wt SV40, and TC7 cells, and whose laboratory's accumulated expertise in growing and manipulating SV40 was generously shared. This work was supported by grant CA44800 from the U.S. Public Health Service. The use of SV40-derived viral vectors for gene transfer to animals and humans, or to cells to be administered to animals and humans, is the subject of pending U.S. and international patent applications.

References

1. Vile, R. G. and Russell, S. J. (1995) Retroviruses as vectors. *Br. Med. Bull.* **51,** 12–30.
2. Brody, S. L. and Crystal, R. G. (1994) Adenovirus-mediated in vivo gene transfer. *Ann. NY Acad. Sci.* **716,** 90–101.
3. Kotin, R. M. (1994) Prospects for the use of adeno-associated virus as a vector for human gene therapy. *Hum. Gene Ther.* **5,** 793–801.
4. Glorioso, J. C., Goins, W. F., Fink, D. J., and DeLuca, N. A. (1994) Herpes simplex virus vectors and gene transfer to the brain. *Dev. Biol. Stand.* **82,** 79–87.
5. Tooze, J., ed. (1981) *DNA Tumor Viruses: Molecular Biology of Tumor Viruses.* 2nd ed., Cold Spring Harbor Laboratory, Cold Spring Harbor, NY.
6. Shah, K. and Nathanson, N. (1976) Human exposure to SV40: review and comment. *J. Epidemiol.* **103,** 1–12.
7. Gooding, L. R. (1977) Specificities of killing by cytotoxic lymphocytes generated in vivo and in vitro to syngeneic SV40 transformed cells. *J. Immunol.* **118,** 920–927.
8. Strayer, D. S. (1996) SV40 as an effective gene transfer vector *in vivo. J. Biol. Chem.* **271,** 24,741–24,746.
9. Strayer, D. S. and Milano, J. (1996) SV40 mediates stable gene transfer *in vivo. Gene Ther.* **3,** 581–587.
10. Gething, M. J. and Sambrook, J. (1981) Cell-surface expression of influenza haemagglutinin from a cloned DNA copy of the RNA gene. *Nature* **293,** 620–625.
11. Asano, M., Iwakura, Y., and Kawade, Y. (1985) SV40 vector with early gene replacement efficient in transducing exogenous DNA into mammalian cells. *Nucleic Acids Res.* **13,** 8573–8586.

12. Eckhart, W. (1990) Polyomavirinae and their replication, in *Virology,* (Fields, B. N., et al., eds.), Raven, New York, pp. 1593–1607.

13. Gluzman, Y. (1981) SV40-transformed simian cells support the replication of early SV40 mutants. *Cell* **23,** 175–182.

14. Rosenberg, B. H., Deutsch, J. F., and Ungers, G. E. (1981) Growth and purification of SV40 virus for biochemical studies. *J. Virol. Methods* **3,** 167–176.

15. Strayer, D. S., Duan, L.-X., Owata, I., Milano, J., Bobraski, L. E., and Bagasra, O. (1997) Titering replication-defective virus for use in gene transfer. *Biotechniques* **22,** 447–450.

16. Sambrook, J., Fritsch, E. F., and Maniatis, T. (1989) *Molecular Cloning: A Laboratory Manual.* Cold Spring Harbor Laboratory, Cold Spring Harbor, NY.

6

Rapid Generation of Isogenic Mammalian Cell Lines Expressing Recombinant Transgenes by Use of Cre Recombinase

Bruce D. Bethke and Brian Sauer

1. Introduction

Mammalian cell lines expressing a recombinant gene of interest are conventionally generated by random genomic integration of exogenous DNA containing the recombinant gene and a selectable marker. In contrast, site-specific recombination targets the exogenous DNA to a preselected site in the mammalian genome *(1,2)*. Genomic targeting with Cre recombinase of phage P1 is relatively simple and results in reproducible gene expression from a single copy of the inserted DNA *(3)*. Thus, recombinase-mediated targeting can greatly speed the generation of stably transfected cell lines expressing a desired recombinant gene product. Because the cell lines obtained by Cre-mediated targeting are isogenic, one can eliminate the extensive functional screening required in conventional methods because of random integration and concomitant position and copy number effects on gene expression *(4)*. Precise single-copy gene delivery to a defined chromosomal position is particularly valuable to characterize mutant regulatory sequences driving a reporter gene or to evaluate mutant alleles and variant isoforms of a particular recombinant gene, as has been done, for example, with the angiotensin AT_1 receptor *(5)*.

Figure 1 shows the strategy for Cre-mediated targeting with a *lox-neo* fusion gene. The parental cell line contains the 34-bp *loxP* target fused to a defective neomycin phosphotransferase II gene (*neo*) lacking both a promoter and an AUG translational start signal. The *lox*-integration vector provides both a promoter and an AUG start fused in frame with the *lox* site. Because the *lox-neo* target and AUG-*lox* fusion are in the same reading frame, Cre-mediated recombination with the *lox*-integration vector regenerates a functional *neo* gene,

From: *Methods in Molecular Biology, vol. 133: Gene Targeting Protocols*
Edited by: E. Kmiec © Humana Press Inc., Totowa, NJ

A

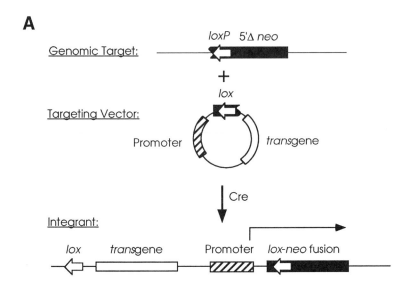

B

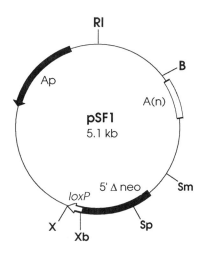

Fig. 1. (**A**) Cre-mediated *neo* gene activation by site-specific targeting. The genomic target is a neomycin phosphotransferase II gene (*neo*), in which the first five codons have been replaced with an in-frame *loxP* site, and which lacks both a promoter and an AUG initiation signal. The *lox*-integration vector carries a AUG-*lox* fusion sequence in the same reading frame as the *lox-neo* fusion. Cre-mediated integration restores *neo* gene function, thus allowing direct selection for recombinants by

thereby allowing direct selection of recombinants by resistance to G418. Note that, after integration, the resulting integrated DNA is flanked by directly repeated *lox* sites, and thus is itself a substrate for excisive recombination *(6,7)*. Hence, expression of Cre must be transient to prevent additional rounds of Cre activity that would excise the integrated targeting construct. This is simply achieved by co-transfection of the *lox-neo* cell line with both the *lox*-integration vector and a nonreplicating Cre-expression vector that is subsequently segregated and lost.

2. Materials

2.1. Cell Lines

Cell line 14-1-2 carries a single copy of the *lox-neo* target integrated into the genome, and was derived from Chinese hamster ovary (CHO) line DG46 *(8)* by complementation of a dihydrofolate reductase (DHFR) mutation *(3)*. The authors recommend maintaining 14-1-2 in nucleoside- and deoxynucleoside-free growth medium to ensure expression of the DHFR minigene positioned adjacent to the *lox-neo* target in this cell line. Following Cre-mediated targeting, selection and maintenance of G418-resistant transformants are performed in standard minimum essential medium (MEM).

1. CHO 14-1-2 cells. Cell line CHO 14-1-2 has been extensively used for Cre-mediated targeting *(3,5,10)*, and is suitable as a parental cell line for most purposes. Alternatively, the *lox-neo* target (from pSF1) can be placed into the genome of more specialized cell lines by standard gene transfer methods *(4)*, using a dominant marker, such as hygromycin-B-phosphotransferase *(14)*, puromycin acetyltransferase *(PAC) (15)*, or guanine phosphoribosyl transferase *(gpt) (16)*. For best results, the *lox-neo* target should be a single-copy integrant.

   The cDNA of the desired gene can be expressed under the control of either the strong constitutive cytomegalovirus (CMV) promoter or an inducible promoter by choosing the appropriate *lox*-integration vector (**Fig. 2**). Alternatively, genes having their own promoters and polyadenylation signals can be cloned into the *lox*-integration vector pBS226.

2. Medium A: MEM α-medium (contains L-glutamine, but no nucleosides or deoxynucleosides, Gibco, cat. no. 12561-023), supplemented with 10% dialyzed

---

resistance to G418. (**B**) *Lox-neo* target. Plasmid pSF1 contains the *lox-neo* target and both unique *Bam*HI and *Eco*RI sites for insertion of a selectable marker gene. Stable transformants carrying the *lox-neo* target can thus be made by standard gene-transfer methods. Cell line 14-1-2 carries a single copy of the *lox-neo* target, and was derived from a CHO DHFRΔ cell line by complementation with a DHFR minigene cloned into the *Bam*HI site of pSF1 *(3)*.

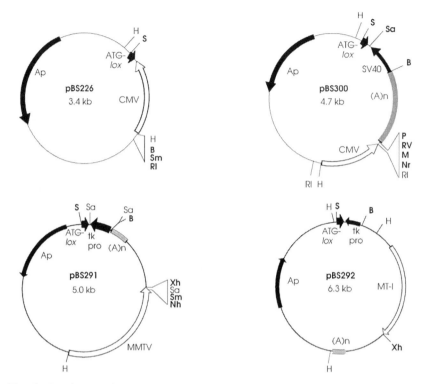

Fig. 2. *Lox*-integration vectors. The coding region of the gene to be expressed is cloned into pBS300 (*5*) for expression from the strong constitutive CMV promoter (*9*), or into either pBS291 or pBS292 for inducible cDNA expression from the MMTV (*18*) and MT-I (*19*) promoters, respectively. Genes having their own regulatory sequences can be introduced into pBS226 (*3*). Genetic elements: CMV, human cytomegalovirus major immediate early promoter; MMTV, mouse mammary tumor virus promoter; MT-I, mouse metallothionein I promoter; SV40 (A)n, simian virus-40 polyadenylation sequence; tk pro, thymidine kinase promoter of herpes simplex virus. Restriction sites: B, *Bam*HI; H, *Hind*III; M, *Mlu*I; Nh, *Nhe*I; Nr, *Nru*I; P, *Pst*I; RI, EcoRI; RV, *Eco*RV; S, *Sph*I; Sa, *Sal*I; Sm, *Sma*I; Xh, *Xho*I. Sites in boldface are unique.

    fetal bovine serum (FBS; Gibco, cat. no. 10440-048) and 50 µg/mL gentamicin sulfate (Gibco, cat. no. 15750-011).
3. Medium B: MEM, with L-glutamine (Gibco, cat. no. 11095-080), supplemented with 10% FBS (Gibco, cat. no. 10437-023) and 50 µg/mL gentamicin sulfate.
4. Dulbecco's phosphate-buffered saline (DPBS), calcium- and magnesium-free.
5. 0.1% Trypsin.
6. 100×20 mm Falcon Primaria® dishes (cat. no. 3803).
7. Humidified incubator ($37°C$, 5% CO_2).
8. G418 (Geneticin, Gibco, cat. no. 11811-031).

2.2. DNA Vectors

Vector pBS185 provides transient Cre expression from the human CMV major immediate early promoter *(1,9)*. The gene of interest to be expressed should be cloned into a *lox*-integration vector *(5)*.

1. Cre expression construct: pBS185 *(1)*.
2. *lox*-integration vectors (*see* **Fig. 2**).
3. Transfection efficiency reporter: CMV-lacZ (or related) vector.

2.3. Electroporation and Selection

A number of common methods of gene transfer (electroporation *[1,3,10]*, calcium-phosphate precipitation *[11]*, and lipofection *[10]*) have been used successfully for Cre-mediated targeting of *lox*-integration vectors. Here is presented an optimized electroporation protocol.

1. Gibco-BRL Cell Porator with chamber safe (*see* **Note 1**).
2. Electroporation cuvets (Gibco, cat. no. 11608-031).
3. Cytomix *(12)*: 120 mM KCl, 0.15 mM CaCl$_2$, 10 mM K$_2$HPO$_4$/KH$_2$PO$_4$, pH 7.6, 25 mM HEPES, pH 7.6, 2 mM EGTA, pH 7.6, 5 mM MgCl$_2$. Filter sterilize and store at room temperature. Just prior to use, add ATP to a concentration of 2 mM (from a 40-mM, pH 7.6, stock, filter-sterilized, and stored at –20°C), and glutathione to a concentration of 5 mM (from a 100-mM stock, prepared fresh).
4. Hemocytometer.
5. Benchtop centrifuge.
6. Inverted light microscope.

2.4. β-Galactosidase Transfection Control

Transfection efficiencies are monitored by inclusion of a CMV-lacZ control. The percentage of β-galactosidase (β-gal) positive cells is determined by X-gal staining *(13)*. The following solutions should be prepared fresh before each use.

1. Fixative: 2% formaldehyde, 0.2% glutaraldehyde, in PBS.
2. X-gal solution: 25 μg/mL X-gal (5-bromo-4-chloro-3-indoxyl-β-D-galactopyranoside), 5 mM potassium ferricyanide, 5 mM potassium ferrocyanide, 2 mM MgCl$_2$, in PBS.

2.5. Cloning of Transformants

G418-resistant colonies are subcloned and expanded to yield independent cell lines.

1. Whatman 3MM paper, cut into ~3 mm squares (autoclaved).
2. Fine-tipped forceps.
3. Four-well Falcon Primaria dishes (cat. no. 3847).

4. Ethanol.
5. Bunsen burner.

3. Methods

3.1. Electroporation and Selection

Optimal transfection efficiencies are obtained with cells at 40–60% confluence. DNA is electroporated into 1×10^7 cells (about six 100-mm dishes or three to four T-150 flasks) in a 1-mL cuvet.

1. Two days prior to electroporation, split near-confluent cells (grown in medium A) 1:10.
2. On day of electroporation, wash cells (40–60% confluent) twice with 10 mL DPBS (Ca^{++}-, Mg^{++}-free), and detach with 1 mL 0.1% trypsin (2–5 min 37°C) (*see* **Note 2**).
3. Add 3 mL growth medium to each plate to inactivate trypsin, then pool the cell suspensions into a 50-mL tube. Using a hemocytometer, determine the number of cells obtained.
4. Pellet the cells in a benchtop centrifuge (4 min at 1000g), resuspend with 40 mL DPBS, and repellet. Resuspend the cells with 20 mL DPBS and repellet. Completely aspirate the PBS, and resuspend the washed cells in cytomix to a density of 1.2×10^7/mL.
5. To an electroporation cuvet add 180 µL cytomix and 10–20 µg DNA in 20 µL TE or water.
6. Add 0.8 mL cell suspension to each electroporation cuvet, and mix by gently inverting three to four times.
7. Incubate cells with DNA for 10 min at room temperature, then electroporate with a single pulse of 350 V at 1600 µF capacitance. This yields a field strength of 875 V/cm.
8. Incubate cells at room temperature for 10 min to allow cell recovery (*see* **Note 6**). Aliquot the electroporated cells to four 10-cm dishes, each containing 10 mL Medium B. Rinse the cuvet twice with medium to recover any cells adhering to the electrodes, and add to dishes.
9. Incubate the dishes at 37°C. Two d after electroporation, split cells 1:4 into Medium B supplemented with 400 µg/mL G418. Re-feed with fresh G418 medium 3–4 d later.
10. Ten days after application of selection, resistant colonies are clearly visible.

3.2. β-Galactosidase Transfection Control

Transfection control plates are stained for β-gal 48 h after electroporation.

1. Wash each plate twice with 10 mL DPBS.
2. Apply 10 mL fixative, and incubate 5 min at 4°C.
3. Wash twice with 10 mL DPBS.
4. Add 10 mL X-gal solution, and incubate at 37°C for 2 h to overnight (a CO_2 environment is not required). Transfected cells will express β-gal, and hence stain

intensely blue. The percentage of β-gal-positive cells is easily determined using an inverted microscope. Approximately 15% of the electroporated cells express β-gal with this procedure.

3.3. Cloning of Transformants

Well isolated G418-resistant colonies should be chosen for cloning and expansion to avoid cross-contamination.

1. Aspirate the medium from the dish, and wash twice with 10 mL DPBS.
2. Identify colonies by circling them with a marking pen on the bottom of the dish.
3. Place sterile filter paper squares (one per circled colony) into 2 mL 0.1% trypsin in a small dish.
4. Aseptically, pick up filter paper squares with forceps and place on top of outlined colonies (dipping the forceps in alcohol and flaming between each pick up).
5. After 1 min, lift off filters with sterile forceps and place each filter in a separate well of a 24-well dish containing 1 mL medium B supplemented with 200 μg/mL G418.
6. Incubate the clones 3–4 d at 37°C, then trypsinize (150 μL) and transfer to 10 cm dishes containing 10 mL of the same medium. (*See* **Notes 7–11**).

4. Notes

1. Other electroporation devices can also be used. However, because of electrical design differences between these devices, voltage and capacitance settings may need to be modified to obtain maximal transfection efficiencies.
2. Trypsinization should be kept to a minimum. Extensive trypsinization reduces postelectroporation survival of the cells.
3. DNA for transfection should be prepared by cesium chloride centrifugation, or be of equivalent purity. Impure preparations containing bacterial proteins, and/or contaminated with resins or phenol, reduce the efficiency of transfection.
4. Electroporation should be performed with 10–20 μg DNA (20 μg gives the higher transfection efficiency). A ratio of *lox*-integration vector to Cre-expression vector of 3:1 gives optimal targeting efficiency. Using 5 μg pBS185 and 15 μg pBS226 (*lox*-integration vector), the authors obtained about 1200 G418-resistant colonies per $1 \times 10_{exp}7$ cfu/mL (*see* Fig. 3).
5. A standard HEPES electroporation buffer (for recipe, *see* ref. *17*) can be used for Cre-mediated targeting (*1,3,10*). However, cytomix increases cell viability approx fourfold, with a concomitant increase in the number of stable integrants.
6. The percentage of surviving cells after electroporation is determined by removing 4-μL pre- and postelectroporation aliquots from the cuvets to 5 mL Medium B. A 50-μL aliquot of these diluted cells is added to 10 mL Medium B in a 10-cm dish, and incubated at 37°C for 10 d. Colonies are stained with methylene blue solution (50% ethanol or methanol, 50% distilled water, 0.25% methylene blue [w/v]; filter through Whatman #1 before use) and counted to determine cell survival. Generally, successful electroporation results in 30–50% cell survival.

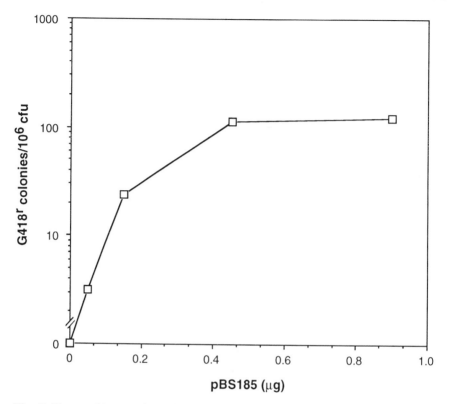

Fig. 3. Targeted integration of pBS226. CHO 14-1-2 cells were electroporated as described in **Subheading 3.**, with 15 μg of the pBS226 *lox*-integration vector and increasing amounts of Cre expression plasmid pBS185. G418-resistant colonies were scored by methylene blue staining at 10 d postelectroporation and are presented as the number of resistant colonies per 10^6 surviving cells. CFU, colony-forming unit.

7. Targeted insertion cell lines can be maintained in 200 μg/mL G418.
8. Southern analysis is required to confirm that targeted cell lines contain a single copy of the *lox*-integration vector. After digestion with restriction enzymes appropriate for the *lox*-integration vector used, Southern blots are hybridized with a vector-specific probe, such as the CMV promoter, to confirm that the predicted restriction fragments are present.
9. More than 96% transformants result from site-specific integration (**3**), although certain DNA sequences cloned into the *lox*-integration vectors can increase the incidence of additional illegitimate recombination events (**5**).
10. The efficiency of targeted insertion is on the order of 0.02–0.05%, thus 200–500 targeted recombinants are obtained per 10^6 surviving cells.
11. The frequency of targeted insertion is 5–15% that obtained by random integration of vectors such as pSV2neo.

References

1. Sauer, B. and Henderson, N. (1990) Targeted insertion of exogenous DNA into the eukaryotic genome by Cre recombinase. *New Biol* **2,** 441–449.
2. O'Gorman, S., Fox, D. T., and Wahl, G. M. (1991) Recombinase-mediated gene activation and site-specific integration in mammalian cells. *Science* **251,** 1351–1355.
3. Fukushige, S. and Sauer, B. (1992) Genomic targeting with a positive-selection *lox* integration vector allows highly reproducible gene expression in mammalian cells. *Proc. Natl. Acad. Sci. USA* **89,** 7905–7909.
4. Murphy, D. and Carter, D. A. (eds.) (1993) *Methods in Molecular Biology, vol. 18: Transgenesis Techniques: Principles and Protocols,* Humana Press, Totowa, NJ.
5. Sauer, B., Baubonis, W., Fukushige, S., and Santomenna, L. (1992) Construction of isogenic cell lines expressing human and rat angiotensin II AT$_1$ receptors by Cre-mediated site-specific recombination. *Methods: Companion Methods Enzymol.* **4,** 143–149.
6. Hoess, R. H. and Abremski, K. (1990) Cre-*lox* recombination system, in *Nucleic Acids and Molecular Biology,* vol. 4. (Eckstein, F. and Lilley, F. M. J., eds.), Springer-Verlag, Berlin-Heidelberg, pp. 90–109.
7. Sternberg, N. and Hamilton, D. (1981) Bacteriophage P1 site-specific recombination. I. Recombination between *loxP* sites. *J. Mol. Biol.* **150,** 467–486.
8. Urlaub, G., Kas, E., Carothers, A. M., and Chasin, L. A. (1983) Deletion of the diploid dihydrofolate reductase locus for cultured mammalian cells. *Cell* **33,** 405–412.
9. Fickenscher, H., Stamminger, T., Rüger, R., and Fleckenstein, B. (1989) Role of a repetitive palindromic sequence element in the human cytomegalovirus major immediate early enhancer. *J. Gen. Virol.* **70,** 107–123.
10. Baubonis, W. and Sauer, B. (1993) Genomic targeting with purified Cre recombinase. *Nucleic Acids Res.* **21,** 2025–2029.
11. Sauer, B. and Henderson, N. (1988) Site-specific DNA recombination in mammalian cells by the Cre recombinase of bacteriophage P1. *Proc. Natl. Acad. Sci. USA* **85,** 5166–5170.
12. van den Hoff, M. J. B., Moorman, A. F. M., and Lamers, W. H. (1992) Electroporation in 'intracellular' buffer increases cell survival. *Nucleic Acids Res.* **20,** 2902.
13. Sanes, J. R., Rubenstein, J. L. R., and Nicolas, J.-F. (1986) Use of a recombinant retrovirus to study post-implantation cell lineage in mouse embryos. *EMBO J.* **5,** 3133–3142.
14. Gitz, L. and Davies, J. (1983) Plasmid-encoded hygromycin B resistance: the sequence of the hygromycin B phosphotransferase gene and its expression in *Escherichia coli* and *Saccharomyces cerevisiae. Gene* **25,** 179–188.
15. Vara, J. A., Portela, A., Ortin, J., and Jimenez, A. (1986) Expression in mammalian cells of a gene from *Streptomyces alboniger* conferring puromycin resistance. *Nucleic Acids Res.* **14,** 4617–4624.
16. Mulligan, R. C. and Berg, P. (1981) Selection for animal cells that express the *Escherichia coli* gene coding for xanthine-guanine phospho-ribosyltransferase. *Proc. Natl. Acad. Sci. USA* **78,** 2072–2076.

17. Chu, G., Hayakawa, H., and Berg, P. (1987) Electroporation for the efficient transfection of mammalian cells with DNA. *Nucleic Acids Res.* **15,** 1311–1327.

18. Lee, F., Mulligan, R., Berg, P., and Ringold, G. (1981) Glucocorticoids regulate expression of dihydrofolate reductase cDNA in mouse mammary tumour virus chimaeric plasmids. *Nature* **294,** 228–232.

19. Pavlakis, G. N. and Hamer, D. H. (1983) Regulation of a metallothionein-growth hormone hybrid gene in bovine papilloma virus. *Proc. Natl. Acad. Sci. USA* **80,** 397–401.

7

Site-Directed Alteration of Genomic DNA by Small-Fragment Homologous Replacement

Kaarin K. Goncz and Dieter C. Gruenert

1. Introduction

The site-directed alteration of genomic sequences by homologous replacement *(1,2)*, psoralen mutation *(3)*, or site-directed repair-mediated correction *(4)* is a technology that can be used to achieve a number of different ends, including: the introduction of specific mutations into vectors, development of transgenic animals, and gene therapy. Homologous replacement is versatile, in that sequences can be directly targeted and altered, inserted, or deleted. As such, it shows great potential for gene therapy to treat inherited genetic disorders for which the sequence information is known. Treatment involves direct conversion of mutant sequences to a wild-type genotype, thereby restoring the normal phenotype. Small-fragment homologous replacement (SFHR) is a technique that has shown promise in this application *(5)*. SFHR has been used to correct the most common mutation associated with cystic fibrosis (CF), a 3-bp deletion in the CF transmembrane conductance regulator *(CFTR)* gene, resulting in the loss of a phenylalanine at amino acid position 508 (ΔF508) *(6–8)*.

Transformed human epithelial cells from CF individuals homozygous for the ΔF508 mutation were used to test the efficacy of SFHR *(9,10)*. Correction of mutant genomic sequences by SFHR was accomplished by the introduction of small fragments (~500 nt) of single-stranded (ss) DNA into cells. The desired change in the target sequence was flanked on either side with sequence homologous to the endogenous sequence. After entering the cell, the fragment paired its homolog and replaced the endogenous sequence with the exogenously introduced fragment sequence, through an undefined process. This replacement resulted in the desired alteration of the CFTR sequence, as determined by

From: *Methods in Molecular Biology, vol. 133: Gene Targeting Protocols*
Edited by: E. Kmiec © Humana Press Inc., Totowa, NJ

polymerase chain reaction (PCR) amplification analysis of genomic DNA and mRNA-derived cDNA, as well as by functional analysis of the protein.

The SFHR technique can be used to alter any genomic or recombinant DNA, as long as the sequence has been defined. However, the success of such site-directed mutagenesis will depend on the system to be altered, as well as other factors including the length of sequence homology contained in the fragment *(11,12)*, the degree of nonhomology *(11)*, the proliferative transcriptional state of the gene to be altered, and how the fragment is delivered into cells. Each system will require different conditions to achieve the desired sequence replacement. The protocol outlined here was used to replace mutant sequences in transformed CF ΔF508 epithelial cells with wild-type sequence. The rationale behind many of the steps is explained in the notes, and can be used as a reference to develop individual protocols.

2. Materials

2.1. Tissue Culture

1. Simian virus-40 (SV40): transformed CF tracheobronchial, ΣCFTE29o- *(9)* cell line, homozygous for the ΔF508 mutation (ΔF508/ΔF508), as well as SV40 transformed normal cell lines, 56FHTE8o- *(13)*, and 16HBE14o- *(14)*.
2. Eagle's minimal essential medium (MEM) supplemented with 10% fetal bovine serum (FBS), 1X penicillin/streptomycin, and 2 mM L-glutamine.
3. Dulbecco's modified Eagle's/Ham's F12 medium (DMEH-16/F-12) with 10% FBS, 1X penicillin/streptomycin, and 2 mM L-glutamine.
4. HEPES buffered saline, pH 7.4–7.6 (HBS). 19.04 g HEPES, 28.52 g NaCl, 0.8 g KCl, 6.8 g Glucose, 15 g Na$_2$HPO$_4$·7H$_2$O, 1 mL 0.5% phenol red, ddH$_2$O to 4 L *(15)*.
5. (PET): 5 mL 10% polyvinylpyrrolidone (BioFluids, Rockville, MD), 5 mL 0.2% EGTA in HBS, 4 mL 0.25% trypsin with 0.02% EDTA (Versene) (UCSF cell culture facility, San Francisco, CA), 36 mL HBS *(15,16)*.
6. General tissue culture supplies, pipets, flasks, Pasture pipets and so on.

2.2. Preparation of Small Fragment

1. DNA sequence for the *CFTR* gene *(17,18)*.
2. Genomic DNA containing wild-type CFTR sequence.
3. DNA oligonucleotides CF5 and CF1A (*see* **Table 1** and **Fig. 1**).
4. Polymerase chain reaction (PCR) solution: 10X PCR buffer (10 mM Tris-HCl, pH 8.4, 500 mM KCl, 20 mM Mg^{2+}, 0.01% gelatin), 2.5 mM dNTP, oligonucleotide primers (5 µM), Ampli-Taq polymerase, 5 U/µL (Perkin-Elmer, Branchburg, NJ).
5. Tris-borate buffer (TBE): 0.9 M Tris-borate, 2 mM EDTA.
6. Agarose (Bio-Rad, Hercules, CA).
7. Orange G loading buffer (Sigma, St. Louis, MO) and 123-bp DNA ladder (Gibco-BRL, Gaithersburg, MD).

Table 1
Oligonucleotide Primers

Primer	Sequence (5'-3')	Sense/antisense	Allele-specific
CF1A	GCAGAGTACCTGAAACAGGAAGTA	Sense	No
CF1B	CCTCTCTGTGAACCTCTATCA	Sense	No
CF5	CATTCACAGTAGCTTACCCA	Antisense	No
CF6	CCACATATCACTATATGCATGC	Antisense	No
CF7C	ATAGGAAACACCAAAGATGA	Antisense	Yes
CF8C	ATAGGAAACACCAATGATAT	Antisense	Yes
CF17	GAGGGATTTGGGGAATTATTTG	Sense	No
CF22	CTTGCTAAAGAAATTCTTGCTC	Antisense	No
oligo N	CACCAAAGATGATATTTTC	Antisense	Yes
oligo ΔF	AACACCAATGATATTTTCTT	Antisense	Yes

8. Gel electrophoresis equipment.
9. TA cloning kit (Invitrogen, San Diego, CA).
10. MAX Efficiency DH5α competent cells (Gibco-BRL).
11. Lauric Broth (LB) Medium: 10 g tryptone, 5 g yeast extract, 10 g NaCl, ddH$_2$O to 1 L.
12. LB ampicillin plates: LB Medium, 14 g agar, 1 mL ampicillin (50 mg/mL).
13. 3 *M* Na-acetate, pH 5.2.
14. Ethanol: 100% and 70%.
15. Pyrogen-free H$_2$O.

2.3. DNA/DOTAP Liposome Complex

1. DNA fragment.
2. (DOTAP) cationic lipid transfection-reagent (Boehringer Mannheim, Indianapolis, IN).
3. RecA protein (Pharmacia, Piscataway, NJ), 4.8 m*M* ATPγS, 2 m*M* Mg-acetate, reaction buffer (100 m*M* Tris-acetate, pH 7.5, at 37°C; 10 m*M* dithiothreitol; 500 m*M* Na-acetate).
4. Serum-free (SF) medium: MEM, 2 m*M* L-glutamine.

2.4. Transfection

1. DNA/DOTAP liposome complex.
2. SF medium.
3. HBS.
4. MEM or DMEH-16/F-12 complete medium.

2.5. DNA and RNA Isolation

1. Cell pellet.
2. Phosphate-buffered saline (PBS).

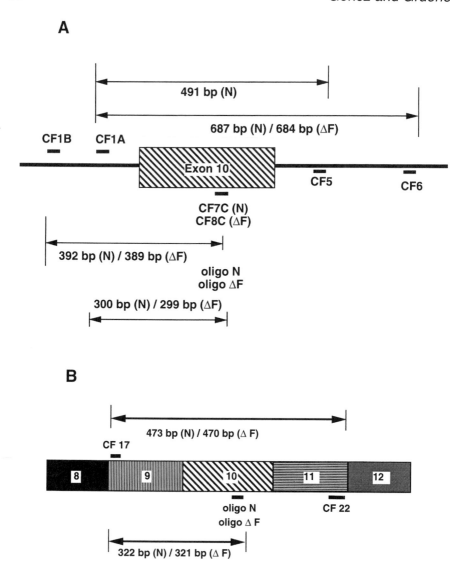

Fig. 1. Relative location of oligonucleotide primers used for PCR analysis of genomic DNA and mRNA-derived cDNA from SFHR experiments. The small fragment used for transfection (491 bp) is manufactured using primers CF1A and CF5. For RT-PCR, primers in exon 9 (CF17) and allele-specific (normal, oligo N or ΔF508, oligo ΔF) primers in exon 10 are used. These primers span intron–exon boundaries, and assure that only CFTR mRNA-derived cDNA is amplified. Amplification with primers CF17/oligo N yields a 322-bp normal DNA fragment, only if transcription of homologously recombined DNA has occurred. A 321-bp fragment would be generated, if the ΔF508 mutation were present.

3. RNA lysate buffer: 0.14 M NaCl, 1.5 mM MgCl$_2$, 10 mM Tris-HCl, pH 7.6.
4. 20% NP-40, 20% sodium dodecyl sulfate (SDS), 0.5 M EDTA, 10 mg/mL pro-teinase K, Tris-saturated phenol, chloroform:isoamyl alcohol (24:1), 5 M NaCl, 0.25 M MgCl, 100% ethanol, 75% ethanol.
5. DNA lysate buffer: 10 mM Tris-HCl, 400 mM NaCl, 2 mM EDTA, pH 7.6.
6. 10% SDS, 10 mg/mL RNase A, 6 M NaCl.

2.6. PCR and Reverse Transcriptase PCR

1. Isolated genomic DNA or RNA.
2. Oligonucleotide primers: CF1B, CF6, CF7C, CF8C, CF17, CF22 (*see* **Table 1** and **Fig. 1**).
3. PCR and reverse transcriptase (RT)-PCR solutions: 10X PCR buffer (10 mM Tris-HCl, pH 8.4), 500 mM KCl, 20 mM Mg^{2+}, 0.01% gelatin), 2.5 mM dNTPs, oligonucleotide primers (5 µM), Ampli-Taq polymerase, 5 U/µL (Perkin Elmer).
4. Reverse transcription solutions: 5X First Strand Buffer and Superscript II RNase H Reverse Transcriptase (Gibco-BRL), 2.5 mM dNTPs, 0.1 M dithiothreitol (DTT), 50 µM Random Hexamers (Pharmacia), diethyl pyrocarbonate (DEPC) H$_2$O.
5. TBE: 0.9 M Tris-borate, 2 mM EDTA.
6. Agarose (Bio-Rad).
7. Orange G loading buffer (Sigma) and 123 bp DNA ladder (Gibco-BRL).
8. Gel electrophoresis equipment.

2.7. Southern Hybridization

1. Isolated genomic DNA or RNA.
2. Oligonucleotide primers: CF1B and CF6 (see **Table 1** and **Fig. 1**).
3. PCR solutions: 10X PCR buffer (10 mM Tris-Cl, pH 8.4, 500 mM KCl, 20 mM Mg^{2+}, 0.01% gelatin), 2.5 mM dNTPs, oligonucleotide primers (5 µM), Ampli-Taq polymerase, 5 U/µL (Perkin-Elmer).
4. Oligonucleotide N and ΔF (*see* **Table 1** and **Fig. 1**).
5. Adenosine 5'-triphosphate [γ-^{32}P], 4000 Ci/mmol (ICN Pharmaceuticals, Costa Mesa, CA).
6. T4-polynucleotide kinase, 10 U/µL (Gibco-BRL), 1 M Tris-HCl, pH 7.5, 200 mM MgCl$_2$, 100 mM Cleland's reagent, NucTrap® Probe Purification Columns (Stratagene, La Jolla, CA).
7. Agarose (Bio-Rad), TBE: 0.9 M Tris-borate, 2 mM EDTA.
8. Nylon hybridization membrane, GeneScreen*Plus*® Hybridization Transfer Mem-brane (Biotechnology Systems, NEN® Research Products, Boston MA).
9. 6X, 2X, and 0.1X SSC (20X SSC is 175.3 g NaCl and 88.2 g sodium citrate in 1 L, pH 7.0), 1% SDS, Ficoll (Type 400, Pharmacia), bovine serum albumin (Fraction V, Sigma), polyvinylpyrrolidone, salmon sperm.
10. X-ray film.
11. GS 300 Scanning Densitometer (Hoefer Scientific Instruments, San Fran-cisco, CA).

3. Methods

3.1. Tissue Culture

1. All cell lines are grown under humidified conditions in a 5% CO_2 atmosphere at 37°C.

3.2. Preparation of Small Fragment

1. A 491-bp fragment of wild-type CFTR is generated by PCR from the region of the gene spanning exon 10 (192 bp) and the 3' and 5' flanking introns, using the CF1A and CF5 oligonucleotides (**Table 1** and **Fig. 1**), with genomic DNA from wild-type epithelial cells as a template.
2. For a 10-µL reaction: 1 µL DNA (100 µg/mL), 1 µL 10X PCR Buffer, 1 µL dNTPs, 1 µL of each oligonucleotide, 1 µL of a 1:10 dilution of Taq, 4 µL ddH₂O. The PCR amplification conditions are as follows for a Perkin-Elmer 9600 machine: initial denaturation, 94°C, 2 min.; amplification, 94°C, 20 s (denaturation)/58°C, 20 s (annealing)/72°C, 1 min (extension) for 30 cycles; final extension, 72°C, 5 min.
3. Fragment size is confirmed by electrophoresis of 10 µL of the PCR reaction on a 1% agarose gel.
4. The fragment is cloned into the TA cloning vector (Invitrogen), according to manufacturer's instructions.
5. MAX efficiency DH5α-competent bacterial cells are transformed with the resulting vector, and plated onto LB agar plates *(19)*.
6. Blue colonies are selected and screened by restriction enzyme digest and sequence analysis *(17)*.
7. The vector containing the correct sequence (pCRII-491) is grown up and harvested by standard Maxi prep protocol *(19)*, and can then be used as a template for subsequent PCR reactions to make fragment.
8. Preparative quantities of fragment are produced with 96 separate 100 µL PCR amplifications.
9. For a 100-µL reaction: 1 µL pCRII-491 (1 ng/µL), 10 µL 10X buffer, 10 µL dNTPs, 4 µL of each oligonucleotide primer, 0.3 µL Taq, 70.7 µL ddH₂O. The PCR amplification conditions are as follows for a Perkin-Elmer 9600 machine: initial denaturation, 94°C, 2 min; amplification, 94°C, 20 s (denaturation)/58°C, 20 s (annealing)/72°C, 1 min (extension) for 25 cycles, final extension 72°C 5 min.
10. Approximately 1–3 µg of fragment will be produced per 100 µL reaction.
11. Individual PCR amplifications are pooled and the DNA fragment precipitated by the addition of one-tenth vol 3 *M* Na-acetate and 2 × the volume of 100% ethanol.
12. The mixture is placed at –20°C for 1 h or overnight (ON). The DNA is then pelleted by centrifugation in an Eppendorf microcentrifuge tube at high speed (16,000*g*) for 10 min.
13. The resulting pellet is washed once with 70% ethanol and then air-dried for 10 min.
14. The DNA pellet is suspended in pyrogen free water at a concentration of 1 µg/µL.

3.3. Fragment Delivery Complex Construction

1. A stock amount of DNA fragment (>50 µL) is denatured by boiling for 10 min, then immediately placed in an ice-water bath. Denatured DNA (5 µL) is added to 95 µL SF medium. A 35-µL aliquot of DOTAP is suspended in 65 µL SF medium. The lipid mixture is then added dropwise to the DNA mixture, and left at room temperature for 15–30 min. The complex-forming reaction is carried out in polystyrene tubes.

2. RecA coating *(3,5,20–22)* of the DNA fragment before forming the complex with DOTAP involves the following: 5 µg denatured DNA is added to 63 µL reaction buffer containing 200 µg recA protein, 4.8 m*M* ATPγS, 2 m*M* Mg-acetate, and 1.7 µL 10X reaction buffer for a final volume of 67 µL, and incubated for 10 min at 37°C. To stop the RecA coating reaction, the Mg-acetate concentration is increased to 20 m*M* by adding 7 µL 200 m*M* Mg-acetate. Under these conditions, the ssDNA fragments are coated with RecA protein at a molar ratio of 3 bases per 1 Rec A molecule. After coating, the fragments are immediately placed on ice at 4°C until they are complexed with DOTAP, as described above.

3.4. Transfection

1. Cells (1×10^5–1×10^6) are plated into a T25 flask the day before transfection.
2. The cells are given fresh medium several hours before transfection.
3. Immediately before transfection, the medium is removed and the cells are washed 1× with HBS.
4. SF media (1.5 mL) is added to the flask.
5. The DNA–DOTAP complex is added to the media in the flask.
6. Cells are then incubated for 4 h. After this time period, the transfection solution is removed and the cells are washed 1–2× with HBS before feeding with 3.5 mL complete MEM or DMEH-16/F-12.

3.5. DNA and RNA Isolation

1. Genomic DNA and RNA is isolated 2–4 d after transfection, depending on how long it takes the cells to become confluent.
2. Growth medium is removed and the cells washed once with HBS. Cells are detached by incubation with 1.5 mL of PET at 37°C for 10 min. The trypsin is neutralized by the addition to the flask of 1.5 mL complete medium.
3. Cells in suspension are pelleted by centrifugation at low speed for 5 min in a 15-mL conical tube. If the transfected cells are to be subcultured, the cell suspension is divided in half prior to centrifugation, and one pellet is resuspended in 3.5 mL complete medium and replated into a T25 flask.
4. For both DNA and RNA isolation, the cell pellet is washed 1× in cold PBS and resuspended in 300 µL RNA lysate buffer in an eppendorf tube. Cell membranes are lysed by the addition of 15 µL 20% NP-40 solution, followed by incubation on ice for 5 min. The suspension is then centrifuged for 5 min at 5,000*g* at 4°C. The supernatant is transferred to a fresh microcentrifuge tube for RNA isolation; the pellet is reserved for DNA isolation *(14)*.

5. To the RNA supernatant, the following are added: 20 μL 20% SDS, 6 μL 0.5 *M* EDTA and 5 μL proteinase K. The mixture is incubated for 10 min at 50°C, and then extracted twice with 100 μL phenol/150 μL chloroform:isoamyl alcohol by centrifugation at 14,000*g* at room temperature (RT) for 5 min. The aqueous phase is transferred to a fresh tube containing 10 μL 5M NaCl, 10 μL 0.25 *M* MgCl$_2$, and 2.5 vol of 100% ethanol, and incubated at –20°C for 2 h (or ON). The RNA is precipitated by centrifugation at 14,000*g* for 10 min at 4°C. The RNA pellet is washed 1× with 75% ice-cold ethanol and is resuspended in 50–100 μL DEPC water. Measure the concentration by spectrophotometer. Adjust the concentration to 1 μg/μL, and run 300 ng on a 1% agarose gel to assess purity.

6. The DNA pellet is resuspended in 300 μL of DNA lysate buffer. Add 30 μL 10% SDS and 1–2 μL RNase A solution. Vortex, and incubate at 37°C for 2 h (or ON). Add 10 μL proteinase K, vortex, and incubate at 55°C for 2 h or 37°C ON. Add 130 μL saturated NaCl (6 *M*), shake as vigorously as possible for 20 s to break down protein debris, and let sit 0.5 h. Centrifuge at 16,000*g* for 10 min, transfer supernatant by pouring into a fresh tube. Add 2 vol 100% ethanol, and invert several times to precipitate DNA. Centrifuge at 16,000*g* for 5 min, wash with 70% ethanol, air-dry, and dissolve the pellet in 50–100 μL ddH$_2$O. Measure the concentration by spectrophotometer. Adjust the concentration to 100 ng/μL and run 100 ng on a 1% agarose gel to assess purity.

3.6. PCR and RT-PCR

1. DNA PCR: Successful replacement of endogenous ΔF508 DNA sequences with wild-type sequences is first ascertained by PCR with allele-specific oligonucleotide primers. Genomic DNA from transfected cells is amplified with two sets of oligonucleotide primers: CF1B and CF7C or CF1A and oligo N, and CF1B and CF8C or CF1A and oligoΔF. Amplification with CF1B and CF7C or CF1A and oligo N, respectively, will result in a 392-bp or 300-bp wild-type product, only if wild-type DNA is present; amplification with CF1B and CF8C or CF1A and oligo ΔF, respectively, will yield a 389-bp or 299-bp product, only if ΔF508 DNA is present (*see* **Fig. 1A** and **Fig. 2**). PCR amplification (10 μL) is performed on sample DNA, along with three controls; DNA from normal cells, ΔF508/ΔF508 DNA and H$_2$O. The amplification conditions are as follows: 1 μL DNA (100 μL/mg), 1 μL 10X buffer, 1 μL dNTPs, 1 μL of each oligonucleotide primer, 1 μL of a 1:10 dilution of Taq, 4 μL ddH$_2$O. Initial denaturization, 94°C; 2 min; amplification, 94°C, 20 s (denaturation)/59°C, 20 s (annealing)/72°C, 1 min (extension) for 30 cycles; final extension, 72°C for 5 min.

2. PCR amplification products (10 μL) are separated by electrophoresis on a 1% agarose gel. A 123-bp ladder is used as a marker.

3. RNA RT-PCR: The presence of mRNA transcribed with endogenous wild-type sequence is assessed by PCR amplification from mRNA-derived cDNA. First-strand cDNA is made from RNA, following manufacturer's directions for Superscript II RNase H Reverse Transcriptase.

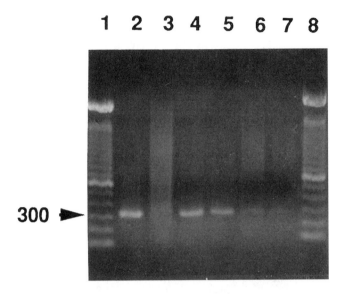

Fig. 2. DNA allele-specific PCR. PCR analysis of ΣCFTE29o- cells. Genomic DNA from transfected cells was amplified with CF1A/oligo N primers. The PCR product in each lane is from the following: lane 2, nontransfected normal (16HBE14o-) control cells; lane 3, non-transfected ΣCFTE29o- cells, lanes 4 and 5, cells transfected by electroporation with RecA-coated DNA fragments; lanes 6, cells transfected by gramicidin S-lipid complexes with RecA-coated DNA; lane 7, cells transfected by gramicidin S-lipid complexes with uncoated DNA; lanes 1 and 8, 100 bp marker DNA.

4. PCR amplification is performed on cDNA using two sets of allele-specific oligonucleotide primers. Amplification with CF17 and oligo N will result in a 322-bp product, only if wild-type RNA is present; amplification with CF17 and oligo ΔF will result in a 321-bp product only if ΔF508 RNA is present (*see* **Fig. 1B** and **Fig. 3**). A 100 μL PCR reaction is performed on sample RNA-derived cDNA, along with three controls: cDNA from normal cells, ΔF508/ΔF508 cDNA and H_2O, as follows: 2 μL cDNA, 10 μL 10X buffer, 10 μL dNTPs, 4 μL of each oligonucleotide primer, 0.5 μL Taq, 29.5 μL ddH$_2$O. Initial denaturation, 94°C, 2 min; amplification 94°C, 20 s (denaturation)/59°C, 20 s (annealing)/72°C, 1 min (extension) for 30 cycles; final extension, 72°C, 5 min.
5. PCR amplification products (10 μL) are separated by electrophoresis on a 1% agarose gel. A 123-bp ladder is used as a marker.

3.7. Southern Hybridization

1. PCR amplification is performed on isolated genomic DNA using nonallele-specific oligonucleotide primers, CF1B and CF6, according to the protocol given in step 1 above. These oligonucleotide primers will amplify DNA with both wild-type and ΔF508 sequences.

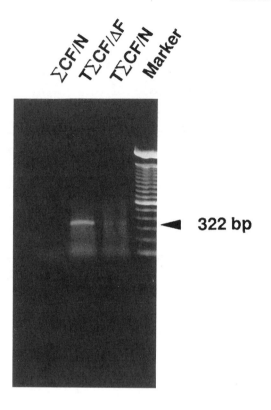

Fig. 3. Analysis of DNA fragments amplified from first-strand CFTR cDNA of transfected ΣCFTE29o- (TΣCF) cells. The cells were electroporated with the Rec A coated 491-bp fragment, and cytoplasmic RNA was isolated 7 d after transfection. The CFTR mRNA was reverse transcribed into first-strand CFTR cDNA. The cDNA was then amplified with primer CF17 (exon 9) and either allele specific primers for normal (oligo N) (322-bp fragment) or mutant (oligo ΔF) (321 bp fragment) sequences. As expected, a 321-bp fragment was observed in transfected ΣCFTE29o- cells when the cDNA was amplified with CF17/ΔF (lane TΣCF/ΔF). In addition, transfected cells amplified with CF17/N gave a 322-bp band (lane TΣCF/N). No band was observed when the cDNA from nontransfected cells was amplified with the CF17/N primers (lane ΣCF/N).

2. PCR products are run separately on parallel 1.4% agarose gels, and transferred to GeneScreen*Plus* membranes for Southern hybridization, as previously described *(9,23)*.
3. Oligonucleotide probes, oligo N and oligo DF, are radioactively labeled by mixing 50 pmol of each oligonucleotide primer with 50 μCi [γ-^{32}P], 1 μL Tris-HCl, pH 7.5, 1 μL MgCl$_2$, 1 μL DDT, 1 μL T4 polynucleotide kinase ddH$_2$O to 20 μL. The reaction is incubated for 30 min at 37°C, and heat inactivated for 10 min at 65°C. The unincorporated radioactive nucleotides are removed by column purification.

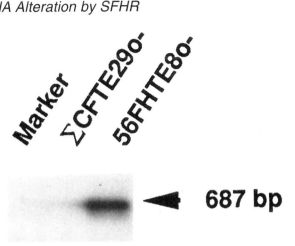

Fig. 4. An example of allele-specific Southern hybridization analysis of a nonallele-specific PCR amplification with primers CF1A/CF6 of DNA from ΣCFTE29o- and 56FHTE8o- cells. The PCR product of the amplifications was probed with ^{32}P-labeled oligo N.

4. The membranes are hybridized ON at 37°C, separately, with each labeled oligo-nucleotide in a solution containing 6X SSC, 1% SDS, 1 g Ficol/L, 1 g/L bovine serum albumin, 1 g polyvinylpyrrolidone, and 100 µg/mL sonicated salmon sperm DNA.
5. The following day, the membranes are then washed twice at 45°C in 2X SSC/0.1% SDS for 30 min, and once at room temperature in 0.1% SSC for 30 min.
6. The membranes are then exposed to X-ray film, and positively hybridized bands can be visualized autoradiographically (**Fig. 4**).
7. Analysis of autoradiographs can be carried out with a GS 300 Scanning Densito-meter (Hoefer) to determine the efficiency of homologous replacement.
8. The relative efficiency of hybridization of the oligo N and oligo ΔF probes is determined by comparing the intensity of transmission after hybridization to PCR fragments derived from heterozygote (ΔF/N) lymphocyte controls. For normal-ization, band intensities of all samples are multiplied by a factor that gives equal signals from oligo N and oligo ΔF hybridization of the ΔF/N control.

The relative frequency of the wild-type CFTR in the population of CF1B/CF6 fragments is then determined as $(D_N-D_B)/(D_N-D_B)+D_{\Delta F}$, where D_N = the densitometric value for the oligo N, D_B = the densitometric value for the back-ground hybridization by the oligo N probe, and $D_{\Delta F}$ = the normalized densito-metric value for the oligo ΔF hybridization.

4. Notes

1. The small DNA fragment for our *CFTR* targeting was designed to be ~500 bp, to incorporate an intact exon 10, in which the ΔF508 mutation was located.

Flanking intron sequences were also included, i.e., the ends of the fragment code for intron sequences and the middle of the fragment codes for the exon. Such a fragment has a greater chance of accommodating any unexpected or nonhomologous exchanges that may occur at the ends of the fragment. As the ends of the fragment code for intron sequences, base alterations are less likely to be detrimental to the coding regions.

2. In other experiments not discussed here, an *Xho*I restriction site was incorporated into the 491-bp fragment by PCR with a silent mutation (G > C at base 34 in exon 10). The introduction of a unique restriction enzyme cleavage site can be useful for further verification that homologous replacement has occurred.

3. The exogenous fragment can be isolated a number of ways including: gel purification, Qiagen column (Chatsworth, CA) purification, or purification by Gene Clean (La Jolla, CA). However, it is possible that some problems may arise by using these approaches. In particular, others have found a lower transfection efficiency using DNA isolated by Qiagen, and restriction digestion of DNA purified by Gene Clean has been inconsistent.

4. A net charge ratio of one negative to three positive charges has been used successfully to transfect human airway epithelial cells with the DNA:DOTAP complexes. The efficiency of transfection will depend on the charge ratio and the cell type to be transfected.

5. Other components can be used to complex with the DNA prior to transfection. These include other cationic lipids (e.g., Lipofectamine, Gibco-BRL), lipid–protein complexes *(24)*, Starburst Dendrimer™ *(25)*, poly-L-lysine *(26,27)* or calcium phosphate precipitation. Physical methods, such as electroporation *(28,29)* or microinjection may also be used in ex vivo experiments.

6. The DNA fragment was first denatured prior to transfection, to reduce the number of random incorporation events. Theoretically, if the fragment is single-stranded, it will preferentially pair with homologous sequences, thus greatly inhibiting the ability to integrate randomly. Double-stranded DNA is able to more readily integrate into the genomic DNA at random sites. Such random integration can result in insertional mutagenesis and the obstruction of gene expression or cell death.

7. The amount of fragment used for SFHR transfections was based on the rate of homologous recombination in other systems. Currently, this rate is considered to be ~ 10^{-6} *(1,2,30)*. To compensate for this frequency, the authors postulated that each cell should be exposed to 2×10^{-6} dsDNA fragments, if SFHR was to occur in the nucleus. This translates to ~5 µg of fragment, if approx 10^7 cells are transfected, assuming a 100% transfection efficiency.

8. Three sets of oligonucleotides were designed for the experiments. The first set (CF5 and CF1A) were used to make the DNA fragment via PCR amplification. A second set (CF1B and CF7C or CF1B and 8C) are allele-specific oligonucleotides that distinguish between the presence of wild-type or ΔF508 sequences in isolated genomic DNA samples. The third set of oligonucleotides are nonallele-specific (CF1B and CF6) and outside the region of homology. They will amplify

both wild-type and ΔF508 CFTR sequences, and encompass the homologous region of the DNA. These oligonucleotide primers will ensure that any randomly integrated or free-floating fragment will not amplify; only replacement of endogenous sequence by the exogenous fragment will be detected. In addition, allele-specific PCR can be performed as nested PCR of the non-allele specific PCR product. PCR products resulting from the nonallele-specific amplification can be probed with allele-specific probes to assay for homologous replacement.

9. Because much of the analysis of SFHR is performed using PCR, it is important to control for artifacts associated with PCR to avoid false positive results. First, appropriate control samples must always be run, along with any experimental samples, i.e., a positive control, a negative control, and water. In addition, RNA can be treated with DNase to eliminate nonspecific amplification. Finally, reconstitution experiments should be performed to determine if the presence of free-floating fragment will result in a false-positive, as a consequence of crossover between the exogenous fragment and the genomic DNA *(31,32)* under the PCR amplification conditions used.

10. The isolation of a clonal population of cells that have undergone SFHR is ultimately desirable. This can be accomplished in a system that is under investigation in which the alteration of the genomic sequence leads to a selectable phenotypic change in the cell, e.g., cell survival. At present, no such selection is possible in the CF system. Cells that have undergone successful SFHR are indistinguishable from those that have not. Therefore, a limiting dilution must be performed to separate a clone.

11. The authors' experiments indicate that, within a population of proliferating cells transfected by the above protocol, ~1–10% have undergone SFHR *(5)*. This frequency represents the number of cells within the population of transfected cells that have undergone at least one replacement event. However, at the DNA level, the frequency of replacement must have been significantly lower, because each locus was exposed to ~10^6 fragments (opportunities) for replacement.

12. Stability of SFHR over time. The correction of the sequence should be a permanent correction. However, it is possible that DNA repair machinery will correct the exogenously introduced DNA after replacement. In addition, if the transcribed strand is transiently replaced by the exogenous DNA, a temporary correction would be detected. The mismatch would be transiently transcribed and expressed as functional protein. However, the sequence would eventually revert to the original endogenous form.

References

1. Boggs, S. S. (1990) Targeted gene modification for gene therapy of stem cells. *Int. J. Cell. Cloning* **8,** 80–96.
2. Capecchi, M. R. (1989) Altering the genome by homologous recombination. *Science* **224,** 1288–1292.
3. Cheng, S., Van Houten, B., Gamper, H. B., Sancar, A., and Hearst, J. (1988) Use of psoralen-modified oligonucleotides to trap three-stranded rec A-DNA com-

plexes and repair of these cross-linked complexes by ABC exonuclease. *J. Biol. Chem.* **263**, 15,110–15,117.

4. Yoon, K., Cole-Strauss, A., and Kmiec, E. B. (1996) Targeted gene correction of episomal DNA in mammalian cells mediated by a chimeric RNA-DNA oligonucleotide. *Proc. Natl. Acad. Sci. USA* **93**, 2071–2076.

5. Kunzelmann, K., Legendre, J.-Y., Knoell, D., Escobar, L. C., Xu, Z., and Gruenert, D. C. (1996) Gene targeting of CFTR DNA in CF epithelial cells. *Gene Ther.* **3**, 859–867.

6. Cystic Fibrosis Genetic Analysis Consortium (1990) World-wide survey of ΔF508 mutation. *Am. J. Hum. Genet.* **47**, 354–359.

7. Kerem, B., Rommens, J. M., Buchanan, J. A., Markiewicz, D., Cox, T. K., Chakravarti, A., Buchwald, M., and Tsui, L. C. (1989) Identification of the cystic fibrosis gene: genetic analysis. *Science* **245**, 1073–1080.

8. Tsui, L.-C. (1992) Mutations and sequence variations detected in the cystic fibrosis transmembrane conductance regualtor (CFTR) gene: report from the Cystic Fibrosis Genetic Analysis Consortium. *Hum. Mut.* **1**, 197–203.

9. Kunzelmann, K., Schwiebert, E., Kuo, W.-L., Stanton, B. A., and Gruenert, D. C. (1993) Immortalized cystic fibrosis tracheal epithelial cell line homozygous for the ΔF508 CFTR mutation. *Am. J. Respir. Cell. Mol. Biol.* **8**, 522–529.

10. Kunzelmann, K., Lei, D. C., Eng, K., Escobar, L. C., Koslowsky, T., and Gruenert, D. C. (1995) Epithelial cell specific properties and genetic complementation in a ΔF508 cystic fibrosis nasal polyp cell line. *In Vitro Cell Dev. Biol.* **31**, 617–624.

11. Morrison, C. and Wagner, E. (1996) Extrachromosomal recombination occurs efficiently in cells defective in various DNA repair systems. *Nucleic Acids Res.* **24**, 2053–2058.

12. Fujitani, Y., Yamamoto, K., and Kobayashi, I. (1995) Dependence of frequency of homologous recombination on the homology length. *Genetics* **140**, 797–809.

13. Gruenert, D. C., Basbaum, C. B., Welsh, M. J., Li, M., Finkbeiner, W. E., and Nadel, J. A. (1988) Characterization of human tracheal epithelial cells transformed by an origin-defective simian virus 40. *Proc. Natl. Acad. Sci. USA* **85**, 5951–5955.

14. Cozens, A. L., Yezzi, M. J., Kunzelmann, K., Ohrui, T., Chin, L., Eng, K., et al. (1994) CFTR Expression and chloride secretion in polarized immortal human bronchial epithelial cells. *Am. J. Respir. Cell. Mol. Biol.* **10**, 38–47.

15. Lechner, J. F. and LaVeck, M. A. (1985) A serum-free method for culturing normal human bronchial epithelial cells at clonal density. *J. Tissue Culture Methods* **9**, 43–48.

16. Gruenert, D. C., Basbaum, C. B., and Widdicombe, J. H. (1990) Long-term culture of normal and cystic fibrosis epithelial cells grown under serum-free conditions. *In Vitro Cell Dev. Biol.* **26**, 411–418.

17. Xu, Z. and Gruenert, D. C. (1996) Human CFTR sequences in regions flanking exon 10: simple repeat sequence polymorphism in intron 9. *Biochem. Biophys. Res. Commun.* **219**, 140–145.

18. Zielenski, J., Rozmahel, R., Bozon, D., Kerem, B., Grzelczak, Z., Riordan, J. R., Rommens, J., and Tsui, L. C. (1991) Genomic DNA sequence of the cystic

fibrosis transmembrane conductance regulator (CFTR) gene. *Genomics* **10,** 214–228.

19. Sambrook, J., Fritsch, E. F., and Maniatis, T. (1989) *Molecular Cloning: A Laboratory Manual.* Cold Spring Harbor Laboratory Press, Cold Spring Harbor, NY.
20. Ferrin, L. J. and Camerini-Otero, R. D. (1991) Selective cleavage of human DNA: recA assisted restriction endonuclease (RARE) cleavage. *Science* **254,** 1494–1497.
21. Sena, E. P. and Zarling, D. A. (1993) Targeting in linear DNA duplexes with two complementary probe strands for hybrid stability. *Nature Genet.* **3,** 365–371.
22. Hunger-Bertling, K., Harrer, P. and Bertling, W. (1990) Short DNA fragments induce site specific recombination in mammalian cells. *Mol. Cell Biochem.* **92,** 107–116.
23. Cozens, A. L., Yezzi, M. J., Chin, L., Finkbeiner, W. E., Wagner, J. A., and Gruenert, D. C. (1992) Characterization of immortal cystic fibrosis tracheobronchial gland epithelial cells. *Proc. Natl. Acad. Sci. USA* **89,** 5171–5175.
24. Legendre, J.-Y. and Szoka, F. C. (1993) Cyclic amphipathic peptide-DNA complexes mediate high efficiency transfection of adherent mammalian cells. *Proc. Natl. Acad. Sci. USA* **90,** 893–897.
25. Haensler, J. and Szoka, F. C. (1993) Polyamidoamine cascade polymers and their use for efficient transfection of cells in culture. *Bioconjugate Chem.* **4,** 85–93.
26. Ferkol, T., Perales, J. C., Eckman, E., Kaetzel, C. S., Hanson, R. W., and Davis, P. B. (1995) Gene transfer into the airway epithelium of animals by targeting the polymeric immunoglobulin receptor. *J. Clin. Invest.* **95,** 493–502.
27. Ferkol, T., Kaetzel, C. S., and Davis, P. B. (1993) Gene transfer into respiratory epithelial cells by targeting the polymeric immunoglobulin receptor. *J. Clin. Invest.* **92,** 2394–2400.
28. Iannuzzi, M. C., Weber, J. L., Yankaskas, J., Boucher, R., and Collins, F. S. (1988) Introduction of biologically active foreign genes into human respiratory epithelial cells using electroporation. *Am. Rev. Respir. Dis.* **138,** 965–968.
29. Zimmermann, U. (1982) Electric field-mediated fusion and related electrical phenomena. *Biochim. Biophys. Acta.* **694,** 227–277.
30. Capecchi, M. R. (1989) New mouse genetics: altering the genome by gene targeting. *Trends Genet.* **5,** 70–76.
31. Meyerhans, A., Vartanian, J.-P. and Wain-Hobson, S. (1990) DNA recombination during PCR. *Nucleic Acids Res.* **18,** 1687–1691.
32. Kim, H.-S., Popovich, B. W., Shehee, W. R., Shesely, E. G., and Smithies, O. (1991) Problems encountered in detecting a targeted gene by the polymerase chain reaction. *Gene* **103,** 227–233.

8

Mutation Correction by Homologous Recombination with an Adenovirus Vector

Ayumi Fujita-Kusano, Yasuhiro Naito, Izumu Saito, and Ichizo Kobayashi

1. Introduction

Gene targeting, the designed alteration of genomic information by homologous recombination, has provided a powerful means of genetic analysis of mammalian systems *(1)*. Its wider application, especially to human gene therapy, is, however, hampered by its low level of efficiency. Only a very small fraction of the treated cells will acquire the designed change. The overall inefficiency may result from the rarity of precise homologous recombination and from the low frequency of appropriate gene transfer.

In the method described here, a replication-defective adenovirus (Ad) vector is used for delivery of donor DNA, in order to bypass these problems. Homologous recombination is selected between a donor *neo* gene inserted in the adenovirus vector and a target mutant *neo* gene on a nuclear papillomavirus plasmid *(2)*. These recombinant Ad can allow gene transfer to 100% of the treated cells without impairing their viability. Homologous recombinants are obtained at a level of frequency much higher than that obtained by electroporation or a calcium-phosphate procedure. The structure of the recombinants is analyzed in detail after recovery in an *Escherichia coli* strain *(3,4)*.

Figure 1A illustrates target and donor plasmids. The target mammalian plasmid (pIK423) consists of bovine papillomavirus type 1 (BPV-1), an *E. coli* plasmid, the hygromycin phosphotransferase gene *(hph)*, and a neomycin phosphotransferase gene *(neo)* with a deletion at its C terminus. BPV-1 is a mammalian-bacterial shuttle vector, and replicates in cultured mouse cells as an extrachromosomal plasmid. In this protocol, BPV-1 is regarded as a model

From: *Methods in Molecular Biology, vol. 133: Gene Targeting Protocols*
Edited by: E. Kmiec © Humana Press Inc., Totowa, NJ

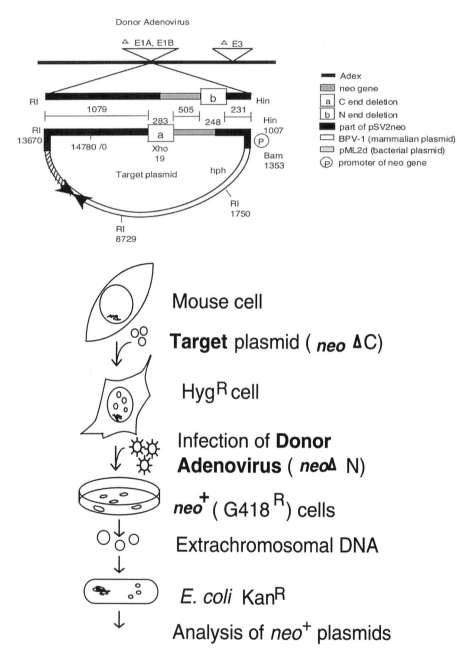

Fig. 1. Experimental system. (**A**) The donor virus and the target plasmid. The donor is a *neo* gene without a mammalian promoter, either with a deletion (deletion b) [AdexΔneo(Δp), shown here], or without a deletion [Adex*neo*+(Δp), not shown here], inserted into an adenovirus vector [Adex]. The target plasmid pIK423 carries a *neo*

chromosome, because it exists as a chromatin-like structure in nuclei (*5*). A replication-defective adenovirus vector, Adex, was used for gene transfer (*6*). It cannot replicate its genome in mouse cells, and does not kill these host cells. An intact *neo* gene without a mammalian promoter, or a *neo* gene with another nonoverlapping deletion, was inserted into this vector to generate the donors, Adex*neo*$^+$Δ(p) and AdexΔ*neo*(Δp).

Figure 1B illustrates establishment of the target cell line, infection with the donor Ad and identification of target gene restoration by homologous recombination. First, to establish the target cell line, the target plasmid (pIK423) is transferred to the C127 cell line, taking advantage of the phenotype of hygromycin resistance conferred by the *hph* gene. Second, the donor Ad is delivered to this cell line. Homologous recombination between the two *neo* genes should restore a functional *neo* gene (*neo*$^+$) and should make the cell resistant to drug G418. Third, these *neo*$^+$ plasmid molecules are recovered in a recA strain of *E. coli* by selecting for kanamycin resistance, which the *neo*$^+$ gene confers. The structure of the recovered plasmids is analyzed by restriction mapping and sequencing. There are other attempts of gene targeting with Ad vectors (*7,8*).

2. Materials
2.1. Establishment of Target Plasmid in Cells

1. Mouse cell line C127.
2. Target plasmid pIK423 (**Fig. 1A**): It was made from pIK30, which contains the coding region of the *neo* gene from pSV2neo, pML2, a deletion derivative of pBR322, and the full-length genome of BPV-1. pHYG, carrying the *hph* gene with the herpes simplex virus thymidine kinase promoter was digested with *Nsp*7524V and *Bst*PI, end-filled with Klenow fragment, ligated with a *Bam*HI linker (5'-CGGATCCG-3'), and then inserted into the *Bam*HI site of pIK30 (pIK325). pIK423 was made from pIK325 by deleting the 283-bp fragment between two *Nae*I sites of the *neo* region.
3. Target plasmid pIK454: It contains a *neo* gene with a 248-bp deletion between two *Nar*I sites, the *cml* gene (*Hae*II–*Hae*II fragment) from pACYC184, and a

---

gene with another deletion mutation (deletion a) on a shuttle vector consisting of a mammalian plasmid (BPV-1) and a bacterial plasmid (pML2). Homologous regions between the donor and the target are drawn as parallel lines, and the lengths of the sequences are noted. The direction of the arrows indicates the direction of the major transcription. Triangles indicate the region deleted from wild-type Ad5. Bam, *Bam*HI; RI, *Eco*RI; Hin, *Hin*dIII; X, *Xho*I; hph, the *hph* gene. Numbers below the restriction enzymes indicate the cleavage sites. 14780/0 is the coordinate of the start/end of the target plasmid. (**B**) Diagram of the experimental procedure. *See* the text.

*Hin*dIII–*Bam*HI fragment of λ dv (pKC31). pIK434 contains a *neo* gene with a 248-bp deletion between two *Nar*I sites, the *hph* gene with the herpes simplex virus thymidine kinase promoter, and pML2.

4. 2X HEPES buffer: 16.4 g NaCl, 11.9 g HEPES acid, 0.21 g Na_2HPO_4, dissolved in 800 mL H_2O. Titrate to pH 7.05 with 5 N NaOH. Add H_2O to 1 L. Filter-sterilize through a 0.45–μm nitrocellulose filter.
5. 2.5 M $CaCl_2$.
6. 20% glycerol.
7. Phosphate-buffered saline (PBS).
8. Hygromycin-B.
9. *E. coli* DH10B: an *E. coli* recA strain.

2.2. Construction of Donor

1. Plasmids, pIK23 and pIK29. The donors of *neo* gene fragments.
2. Restriction enzymes: *Apa*I, *Hin*dIII, *Swa*I, and *Eco*T22I.
3. GeneClean II kit (Bio 101).
4. Oligonucleotide linker: *Eco*RV linker.
5. Cassette cosmid pAdex1w (provided by Y. Saito [*see* **ref. 6**]).
6. T4 DNA ligase.
7. Gigapack XL in vitro packaging kit (Stratagene, La Jolla, CA).
8. *E. coli* DH5α.
9. LB-Amp plate: 10 g tryptone, 5 g yeast extract, 10 g NaCl, 15 g Bacto-agar, dissolved in 1 L H_2O, and autoclaved. Cool the solution to about 50°C, add ampicillin (50 μg/mL final), mix by swirling, and pour plates.
10. Parent adenovirus Ad5-dlX (provided by I. Saito on request [*see* **ref. 6**]).
11. Absolute ethanol.
12. 10 mM Tris-HCl, pH 7.5, 1 mM EDTA (TE).
13. LB media: 10 g tryptone, 5 g yeast extract, 10 g NaCl, dissolved in 1 L H_2O, and autoclaved.
14. Sephadex G-50 spin column.
15. HeLa cell.
16. 10 mM Tris-HCl, pH 8.0.
17. CsCl.
18. 8 M guanidine hydrochloride.
19. Ethidium bromide solution: 1 μg/mL.
20. Proteinase K solution: 10 mg/mL.
21. Roux bottle.
22. Bioruptor 200: a sealed-type sonicator (CosmoBio, Tokyo).
23. Beckman SW28 tube.
24. Beckman SW50.1 tube.
25. Beckman VTi65 tube.
26. Beckman SW28 rotor.
27. Beckman SW50.1 rotor.
28. Beckman VTi65 rotor.

29. Human kidney cell line 293, which constitutively expresses the E1A and E1B proteins of Ad type 5.
30. Dulbecco's modified Eagle medium supplemented with 5% fetal calf serum (DMEM-5% FCS).
31. DMEM-10% FCS.
32. 50 mM Tris-HCl, pH 7.5, 100 mM NaCl, 10 mM EDTA (TNE).
33. 10% sodium dodecyl sulfate.
34. Phenol-chloroform.
35. Chloroform.
36. TE containing 20 µg/mL pancreatic RNase.
37. CellPhect transfection kit (Pharmacia, Piscataway, NJ).
38. 6-cm φ-diam culture dish.
39. 10 cm φ-diam culture dish.
40. 96-well collagen-coated tissue culture plate.
41. 24-well collagen-coated tissue culture plate.
42. 225 cm^2 flask.
43. 5-mL freezing tube.
44. Dry ice.
45. PBS: 137 mM NaCl, 2.7 mM KCl, 4.3 mM Na$_2$HPO$_4$·1.4 mM KH$_2$PO$_4$, pH ~7.3.
46. Eight-channel pipet.
47. 2.2 M CsCl-10 mM HEPES.
48. 4 M CsCl-10 mM HEPES.
49. PBS-10% glycerol.

2.3. Infection Efficiency of Adenovirus

1. 0.25% glutaraldehyde solution.
2. 5-bromo-4-chloro-3-indolyl-, β-D-galactopyranoside (X-Gal).

2.4. Gene Targeting to Plasmid DNA

G418. Prepare in a highly buffered solution (e.g., 100 mM HEPES, pH 7.3).

2.5. Product Classification, Sequence Determination, and Analysis

1. Gene pulser system (Bio-Rad, Hercules, CA).
2. LB-Kan plate: 10 g tryptone, 5 g yeast extract, 10 g NaCl, 15 g Bacto-agar, dissolved in 1 L H$_2$O, and autoclaved. Cool the solution to about 50°C, add kanamycin (30 µg/mL final), mix by swirling, and pour plates.
3. pUC19 cloning vector.
4. M13 universal primer (5'-CGACGTTGTAAAACGACGGCCAGT).
5. M13 reverse primer (5'-CAGGAAACAGCTATGAC).
6. Gene Works (Intelli Genetics, Mountain View, CA) computer software package.

3. Methods
3.1. Establishment of Target Plasmid in Cells

1. Seed exponentially growing C127 cells at 4×10^5 cells/6-cm dish) the day before transfection.

2. On the day of transfection, dissolve 5–500 µg target plasmid (pIK423 or pIK454) DNA into 80 µL 2X HEPES buffer. Wash the cells with 2 mL DMEM-5% FCS 15 min before transfection, and incubate. Add 8 µL 2.5 M CaCl$_2$, mix quickly by vortex for 20 s, and incubate at room temperature for 5 min. Add the DNA solution to 6-cm dish, and incubate.

3. After 4 h of incubation, remove medium, and add 20% glycerol. Incubate at room temperature for exactly by 1 h. Add 5 mL PBS. Wash the cells with 5 mL PBS, add 4 mL DMEM-5% FCS.

4. 72 h after transfection, start selection by changing medium to selection medium (hygromycin-B, 400 µg/mL final).

5. Isolate a number of hygromycin-resistant (Hyg^r) colonies 3 wk after transfection. Isolate extrachromosomal plasmid DNA and recover it in an *E. coli recA* strain (DH10B) by electroporation. Isolate plasmid DNA by miniprep, assess the size of the restriction fragments by gel electrophoresis, and analyze by Southern hybridization, with pIK423 as a probe, after cleavage with a single-site enzyme *(Eco*RV*)* and a no-site enzyme *(Sac*I*)*.

3.2. Construction of the Donor

Details are described in **ref. 6.**

1. To obtain the fragment of pSV2neo (pIK29) or its derivative lacking 248 bp, including the N-terminus, of *neo* gene (pIK23), digest pIK23 or pIK29 with *Apa*I and *Hin*dIII. Purify the *neo* gene fragment using GeneCleanII. Prepare blunt ends by ligation with an *Eco*RV linker.

2. Digest the cassette cosmid pAdex1w with *Swa*I. Ligate *Swa*I-linearized pAdex1w and the blunt-ended *neo* gene fragment with T4 DNA ligase. Digest the DNA sample with *Swa*I to remove self-ligated pAdex1w.

3. Package the DNA sample in vitro using Gigapack XL. Mix the packaged reaction with *E. coli* DH5α, and plate onto LB-Amp plate. Pick a number of individual colonies, and isolate their cosmid DNA. Analyze the size of the restriction fragments by gel electrophoresis, and select the clones containing the desired insert.

4. Purify virions of the parent adenovirus Ad5-dlX through a buoyant CsCl gradient. Disintegrate virions by addition of an equal volume of 8 M guanidine hydrochloride. Isolate the released DNA-terminal protein complex (TCP) through a buoyant density gradient of 2.8 M CsCl/4 M guanidine hydrochloride, by centrifugation in a VTi65 rotor (Beckman) for 16 h at 55,000 rpm. Identify DNA-TPC-containing fractions by the ethidium bromide spot test, pool, and dialyze. Digest the DNA-TPC with *Eco*T22I, and purify by gel filtration through a Sephadex G-50 spin column.

5. Mix 1 µg digested DNA-TPC with 8 µg cassette cosmid bearing the *neo* fragment, and transfect the human embryonic kidney 293 cells with the mixed DNA in a 6-cm dish by the calcium phosphate method using a CellPhect transfection kit (Pharmacia).

6. After 1 d incubation, spread the cells in three 96-well plates at a 10-fold serial dilution mixed with untransfected 293 cells. After cultivation for 10–15 d, isolate virus clones, and propagate further to assess restriction analysis.

7. To purify the recombinant Ads, infect 293 cells (3×10^7 cells/225-cm^2 flask) with Ad at a multiplicity of infection (MOI) of 20, and culture. After 3-d incubation, harvest the infected cells, sonicate at 200 W for 3 min (30 s $\times$ 6) with a sealed type sonicator, Bioruptor 200, and centrifuge (10,000 rpm, 10 min, 4°C). Ultracentrifuge the supernatant in a step gradient of CsCl (2.2 M and 4.0 M CsCl in 10 mM HEPES [N-2-hydroxyethylpiperazine-N'-2-ethanesulfonic acid], 25,000 rpm, 2 h, 4°C, SW28 rotor). Collect the virus band, and centrifuge again in a step gradient (2.2 M and 4.0 M CsCl in 10 mM HEPES, 35,000 rpm, 3 h, 4°C, SW41 rotor). Dialyze the virus band overnight against PBS-10% glycerol.

8. Determine titers of virus stocks by an end point cytopathic-effect assay. Dispense 50 µL DMEM-5% FCS medium into each well of a 96-well tissue culture plate, and then prepare eight rows of a threefold serial dilution of the virus, starting from a 10^{-4} dilution. Add 3×10^5 cells to each well, incubate the plate, and add 50 µL DMEM-5% FCS medium to each well every 3 d. Twelve d later, determine the end point of the cytopathic effect by microscopy, and calculate the median tissue culture infection's dose (TCID$_{50}$).

3.3. Infection Efficiency of Adenovirus

1. Seed the target cell line carrying the target plasmid (C127 [pIK423–2-3]) at 4×10^5/6-cm dish.
2. Add the Ad (AdexCA*lacZ*, titer 1.3×10^8/mL) at an MOI of 4, 40, or 400 (d 0), and incubate.
3. After 3 d of incubation, wash the cells twice with PBS, fix with 0.25% glutaraldehyde solution, wash twice with PBS, stain with X-Gal, and incubate for more than 3 h. Photograph under a microscope, and count the stained and unstained cells.

3.4. Gene Targeting to Plasmid DNA

1. Seed the cells of C127 carrying pIK423 at 4×10^5/6-cm dish the day prior to infection.
2. On the day of infection, remove media from dish by aspiration. Add the donor Ad Adex*neo*ΔN or Adex*neo*$^+$ at an MOI of 4–400 (day 0). Shake the dish gently 3× every 20 min. Add 1 mL DMEM-5% FCS medium. Wash the cells with DMEM-5% FCS medium.
3. Start G418 selection on d 3 at 500 µg/mL (final).
4. After 19–24 d of incubation, count G418^r colonies and trypsinize.
5. Isolate extrachromosomal DNA by Hirt method 1 mo after the infection.

3.5. Product Classification, Sequence Determination, and Analysis

1. Transform the extrachromosomal DNA prepared by the Hirt method to *E. coli* DH10B by electroporation, using a Bio-Rad gene pulser at 2.5 kV, 25 µF, and 200 Ω), plate onto LB-Kan plate. Count kanamycin-resistant (Kan^r) colonies.
2. Analyze plasmid molecules in each of these transformants with restriction enzymes.
3. Analyze those products carrying nonhomologous joints by Southern hybridization with Ad5 DNA digested, with *Bgl*II as a probe.

4. Subclone fragments containing nonhomologous joints in pUC19, and determine DNA sequences with T7 DNA polymerase, by using the M13 universal primer or the M13 reverse primer in a Pharmacia sequencer. Analyze the sequence data with Gene Works, a computer software package. Analyze the DNA homology and palindromes by DNA Alignment and DNA Motif, respectively ("Minimum stem" is set to 6 bp).

4. Notes

1. For the authors, most of the transformants (33 of 45) from one Hyg^r clone (C127 [pIK423–2]) were indistinguishable from pIK423 when cut with a single site enzyme (*Bam*HI). Six subclones were isolated from this Hyg^r clone, and their extrachromosomal DNA was analyzed by Southern hybridization. One subclone (C127 [pIK423–2–3]) with extrachromosomal DNA indistinguishable from pIK423 was chosen as the target cell line. The copy number of the target plasmid was estimated to be 93 dimer equivalents per cell in the above-described Southern hybridization experiments. Most of them were in dimeric form.

2. The cassette cosmid for constructing recombinant Ad of the E1-substitution type, pAdex1w, is an 11-kb charomid vector bearing an Ad5 genome spanning (mu) 0–99.3 map units, with deletions of E1 (mu 1.3–9.3) and E3 (mu 79.6–84.8). The unique *Swa*I site was created by linker insertion at the E1 deletion.

3. Gigapack XL prefers to package DNA exceeding the vector size of 42 kb, and to select the cosmid containing the insert.

4. Ad5-dlX has an E3 deletion (mu 79.6–84.8), and is used as parent virus for recombinant adenovirus construction. The *Eco*T22I-digested DNA-TPC was stable at –80°C.

5. 293 is a human embryonic kidney cell line transformed by Ad5 E1A and E1B genes, and supports propagation of E1-deleted recombinant Ad. The desired recombinant adenovirus is generated by overlapping recombination.

6. Obtained donor adenovirus vector, Adex*neo*Δ*neo*(Δp) (**Fig. 1A**), and its *neo*$^+$ version, Adex*neo*$^+$(Δp), are Ad5, with deletions of the El and E3 regions. An *Apa*I-*Hin*dIII fragment of pSV2neo or its derivative, lacking 248 bp, including the N terminus, of the *neo* gene, was inserted into the El-deleted position. AdexCA*lacZ* carrying the *E. coli lacZ* gene, was constructed similarly.

7. One TCID$_{50}$/mL corresponds to approx 1 PFU/mL.

8. At an MOI of 40, essentially all (96%; 127 of 132 and 129 of 136) of the treated cells were stained. The authors also assessed cell survival after infection with the donor virus AdexΔ*neo*(Δp) by trypan blue staining. Essentially all infected cells excluded the dye, even at an MOI of 400.

9. Continue the selection until extrachromosomal DNA is prepared.

10. We infected the target cells (C127 [pIK423–2–3]) with the donor Ad vectors, AdexΔ*neo*(Δp) and Adex*neo*$^+$(Δp), at various MOIs. The G418^r colonies were obtained at high frequencies (~8.3×10^{-4}/infected cell). Their production required the presence of both the target and the donor DNA. Their number increased as the MOI increased from 4 to 400.

11. The number of *neo*$^+$ transformants does not increase linearly with the increase in MOI of the virus particles. This result is expected if, once all cells are infected,

the number of the viral DNA molecules is not the only limiting factor in the recombination reaction.

12. G418^r clones could be produced by integration of the donor DNA near chromosomal promoters, especially when the donor is with the promoterless, but otherwise intact *neo* gene. The authors examined this possibility by Southern hybridization of the total DNA of the mixture of the mouse G418^r colonies, with the full-length genome of Ad5 DNA as a probe. No hybridizing material (<0.1 copy per diploid genome was detected.

References

1. Capecchi, M. R. (1989) Altering the genome by homologous recombination. *Science* **244,** 1288–1292.
2. Fujita, A., Sakagami, K., Kanegae, Y., Saito, I., and Kobayashi, I. (1995) Gene targeting with a replication-defective adenovirus vector. *J. Virol.* **69,** 6180–6190.
3. Kitamura, Y., Yoshikura, H., and Kobayashi, I. (1990) Homologous recombination in a mammalian plasmid. *Mol. Gen. Genet.* **222,** 185–191.
4. Sakagami, K., Tokinaga, Y., Yoshikura, H., and Kobayashi, I. (1994) Homology-associated non-homologous recombination in mammalian cells. *Proc. Natl. Acad. Sci. USA* **91,** 8527–8531.
5. Rösl, F., Waldeck, W., Zentgraf, H., and Sauer, G. (1986) Properties of intracellular bovine papillomavirus chromatin. *J. Virol.* **58,** 500–507.
6. Miyake, S., Makimura, M., Kanegae, Y., Harada, S., Sato, Y., Takamori, K., Tokuda, C., and Saito, I. (1996) Efficient generation of recombinant adenoviruses using adenovirus DNA-terminal protein complex and a cosmid bearing the full-length virus genome. *Proc. Natl. Acad. Sci. USA* **93,** 1320–1324.
7. Wang, Q. and Taylor, M. W. (1993) Correction of a deletion mutant by gene targeting with an adenovirus vector. *Mol. Cell. Biol.* **13,** 918–927.
8. Mitani, K., Wakamiya, M., Hasty, P., Graham, F. L., Bradley, A., and Caskey C. T. (1995) Gene targeting in mouse embryonic stem cells with an adenoviral vector. *Somatic Cells Mol. Genet.* **21,** 221–231.

9

Site-Specific Targeting of DNA Plasmids to Chromosome 19 Using AAV *Cis* and *Trans* Sequences

Samuel M. Young, Jr., Weidong Xiao, and Richard Jude Samulski

1. Introduction

Adeno-associated virus (AAV) is of the genus *Dependovirus* and a member of the family Parvoviridae *(1)*. AAV is unique, in that it requires co-infection of a second helper virus (i.e., adenovirus [Ad] or herpesvirus) to undergo productive infection. In the absence of a helper virus, AAV will integrate preferentially into the host chromosome (ch). Targeting of AAV to ch19.13.3 qter locus has been documented at a frequency of 70% or greater *(2)*. Because of AAV's unique ability to integrate site-specifically, extensive research has been devoted to understanding how AAV integrates, with the hope of creating targeting vectors for gene therapy.

1.1. AAV Genes Required for Integration

AAV carries two elements, *cis* and *trans* sequences, which are required for targeted integration. The *trans* functions encode the AAV Rep proteins; the *cis* elements include the 145 inverted terminal repeats (ITRs) *(1,2)*. Of the two open reading frames (ORFs) that make up the AAV genetic map *(1)*, the left ORF encodes four nonstructural proteins, referred to as Rep78, 68, 52, and 40. The gene products from the Rep ORF are important for site-specific integration at the ch19 locus *(3)*. Samulski et al. first showed that all *rep+* viruses were capable of integrating into the ch19 locus, but *rep–* viruses appeared to integrate randomly. It was also demonstrated that the larger Rep proteins were responsible for targeted integration, which could be supplied in *trans (4,5)*. Though site-specific integration can be carried out by either of the large Rep proteins, the AAV ITR appears to be the only *cis* element required for

From: *Methods in Molecular Biology, vol. 133: Gene Targeting Protocols*
Edited by: E. Kmiec © Humana Press Inc., Totowa, NJ

integration *(6–8)*. The AAV ITR is thought to promote targeted integration in the presence of Rep, and random integration in the absence of Rep, demonstrating their essential role in viral integration. Integration in the absence of Rep is random, as mentioned above, and occurs via a cellular recombination pathway generating viral cellular junctions identical to wild type (deleted ITRs at the chromosomal junction) without specificity for ch19. Recently, research using recombinant vectors has corroborated this observation, and no targeting viral vectors to date have been developed *(9,10)*.

1.2. Chromosome 19 Target Locus

When the ch19 preintegration site (the ch 19.13.3qter) was cloned and sequenced, it was found to contain a Rep-binding Element (RBE) and a Rep-nicking site terminal resolution site *(trs) (11–13)*. These elements are identical to the sequences found in the AAV terminal repeats, which are required for viral replication, packaging, and integration. The present of these elements on ch19 provides a plausible explanation of why Rep targets AAV genomes to this locus. Rep tethering AAV to the ch19 locus via Rep-binding sites provides a simple mechanism for site-specific integration. Weitzman et al. *(14)* using in vitro-translated Rep68, biotin-labeled AAV terminal repeats, and a ^{32}P-labeled fragment from the ch19 site containing the RBE (Rep-binding element), demonstrated that Rep68 was able to mediate complex formation between the AAV ITR and the ch19 site. Although this provided a working explanation for AAV targeted integration, it is now known that Rep also binds sequences that are degenerate relative to its nominal binding element within the ITR *(15,16)*, and Rep binds other sequences within the human genome with higher affinity than the ch19-binding sequence *(17)*. For this reason, the simple model of ch19, carrying essential *cis* sequences (RBE and *trs*) required for targeted integration, remains doubtful. Recent data by Young et al. (manuscript submitted) have shown that there may be other elements unique to ch19 that facilitate the targeting integration. These elements, when compared to the other potential RBE within the human genome, ensure that the ch19 site is a preferred target. In addition to these studies, Linden et al. *(18)* have utilized an Epstein-Bars Virus CEBU Shuttle Vector (EBNA)-based vector system to demonstrate critical *cis* elements required for site-specific integration. In this system, targeted integration was dependent on a *trs* site present on ch19, as well as the RBE sequence. All of these observations clearly suggest that questions remain unanswered concerning Rep targeting and ch19 *cis* elements.

1.3. Integration Model

The exact mechanism for AAV integration is not known. When one analyzes the structure of integrated provirus, specific features can be identified.

Most proviruses contain 2–4 tandem copies that are arranged in head-to-tail fashion *(2)*. This implies that AAV may potentially replicate during integration using a rolling-circle mechanism. This is intriguing because it is opposite to viral replication seen in a lytic infection (hairpin model generating head to head or tail-to-tail concatamers) *(1)*. However, no experimental evidence for a replication intermediate that would allow rolling-circle replication has been observed in Rep-dependent replication. A number of AAV—ch19 junctions have been sequenced that display incomplete ITR sequences joined to cellular DNA, usually with microhomology at the junction. Identical features (incomplete ITRs with microhomology) have been found for AAV vectors that integrated randomly *(19,20)*.

From these observations, AAV integration (whether targeted or random) appears to utilize a cellular recombination pathway. In addition, the only intact AAV proviruses isolated to date, and characterized in detail, have involved single copy proviruses attached to chromosome DNA. For this reason, it is not clear whether these examples represent the majority of AAV integrants (head-to-tail provirus) that have been characterized by restriction digest only. Several models have been generated to explain the above data.

Many agree that the larger Rep proteins are important for targeted integration, and these proteins must contain all biochemical activities for targeting to occur *(18)*. Mutants of Rep that are unable to bind DNA, or are negative for ITR nicking activity, are also unable to confer site-specific integration *(21)*. In addition, it appears that replication occurs during integration, but how and when this happens is debatable. The authors' model (**Fig. 1**) is built on the premise that AAV will circularize prior to integration. This circularized substrate is essential for providing the template needed for rolling-circle replication, which in turn would generate the head-to-tail concatamers commonly seen with wild-type AAV and vector integration. In this model, when AAV infects a cell in the absence of helper virus, cleavage of the 3' ITRs takes place generating the intermediate shown in **Fig. 1B**.

Although Rep would be the ideal candidate to carry out this reaction, this would require *de novo* Rep expression or the presence of Rep protein that enters the cell with the virus. Both of these possibilities are viable, but neither have been demonstrated. However, it is also likely that a cellular protein(s) may facilitate this step, because resolution of AAV ITRs have been observed in vivo in the absence of Ad infection *(8)*. The likelihood of a cellular protein carrying out this step is supported by gel shift experiments using cellular extracts that demonstrate specific binding to the AAV ITRs *(22)*. The free 3' end of the virus then ligates to the 5'-terminal repeat, forming a single stranded circular molecule containing one unique terminal-repeat sequence (**Fig. 1C**). This unique ITR (DABB'CC'A'D') is a substrate that has been characterized

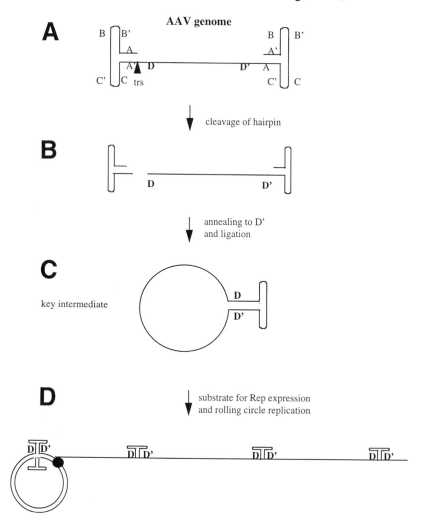

Fig. 1. Model for Rep-mediated integration. (**A**) AAV genome, which contains two inverted terminal repeats (ITR), and is single-stranded. (**B**) Cleavage of the ITR, which contains the D element. The cleaved ITR then becomes disassociated from the viral genome. (**C**) The free D element of the virus will anneal to the D' element and the cellular machinery will then fill in and ligate the nicked D element to the A' element. This will create a ITR that contains two D elements and a large single-strand region, which is capable of generating head to tail concatamers via a rolling-circle mechanism. This molecule will also serve as the substrate for Rep transcription. (**D**) Replication of the integration substrate by a rolling circle mechanism via the cellular replication machinery. This mechanism will generate head to tail concatamers of the virus. (**E**) The ch19 preintegration site. (**F**) Unwinding and nicking of the ch19 preintegration site by the newly synthesized Rep. (**G**) Rep-mediated complex forma-

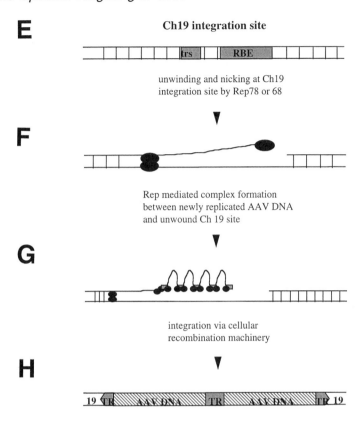

Ch19 integration site

unwinding and nicking at Ch19
integration site by Rep78 or 68

Rep mediated complex formation
between newly replicated AAV DNA
and unwound Ch 19 site

integration via cellular
recombination machinery

tion between the newly replicated AAV DNA and the unwound ch19 integration site. Rep78 or 68 will tether the two substrates together via Rep–Rep interaction. Rep would be able to bind the ITRs of the newly replicated viral DNA. This would create a compact substrate for integration. (**H**) Final integrated AAV DNA, which contains head-to-tail concatamers. This final step will take place via the cellular recombination machinery. It is likely that the opposite strand of DNA is nicked, so that the chromosome can accommodate the integrating viral DNA. The integrating viral DNA would then be used as the template to fill in this newly created gap.

both in vitro and in vivo and is referred to as a double-D ITR *(8)* because of flanking copies of the AAV-D sequence element (**Fig. 1C**). In this model, the double-D ITR is present on a single-strand AAV DNA molecule. This substrate then serves as a template for rolling-circle replication and Rep expression (**Fig. 1D**). Rolling-circle replication from this molecule probably takes place via cellular replication machinery, because Rep-mediated replication supports a tail-to-tail and head-to-head formation of replication intermediates *(1,23)*. In the case of wild-type virus, newly synthesized Rep from this intermediate would facilitate targeting to ch19 (**Fig. 1E**) via the RBEs. AAV-targeted integration utilizing Rep would initiate by nicking the preintegration site on ch19, followed by complex formation between the newly replicated AAV DNA and nicked ch19 site (**Fig. 1F,G**). Whether replication and recombination are separate or coupled remains to be determined, but it is clear that host machinery is essential for integration to take place. In this model, a break on the opposite strand of ch19 cellular DNA is necessary to insert the AAV DNA. This would create a DNA molecule with a gap, and the AAV DNA would be used as the template to repair this gap (**Fig. 1H**). Experiments are under way to test this AAV targeted integration model.

1.4. Protocol for AAV Targeting Integration

Although little is known about the mechanism of AAV integration and how targeting takes place, the authors have developed a targeting assay in which >70% of the integrants are located on ch19 *(4)*. This chapter will describe this assay in detail (**Fig. 2**). Essentially, Rep78 or 68 is supplied in *trans* through a rep construct driven by the HIV promoter. This plasmid substrate is co-transfected into Hela cells, along with the double-D-ITR *neo* vector described *(8)*. The double-D *(8)* plasmid behaves much like the standard AAV genome. In the presence of Rep and Ad, this circular molecule is converted to a linear substrate with covalently closed hairpins that replicate by the AAV model, generating monomers, dimers, and higher multimers that are indistinguishable from wild-type AAV replication intermediates. In the absence of Ad, these substrates are resolved to linear molecules with covalently closed hairpin ITRs, which in the presence of G-418 selection, form stable colonies by integration into the host chromosome. The integrants are then analyzed using a PCR technique optimized to replicate through the secondary structure of the AAV ITR. In conjunction with PCR analysis, Southern blot using vector- and ch19-specific probe are used to confirm targeted integration.

In addition, the authors have developed a Rep filter-binding assay (**Fig. 3**) that can be used to enrich for the integrated provirus. The Rep filter-binding

---

Fig. 2. Targeted integration protocol. Targeting integration assay substrates. (**A**) The pDD-2-*neo* plasmid. This plasmid has been shown to behave like the recombinant genome in terms of integration, replication, and rescue. The plasmid must be modified to contain the gene of interest. The *neo* gene serves as a means of selection for the integration event. (**B**) The pHIV-Rep78 plasmid. This plasmid contains the Rep78 protein. Rep78 has been shown to be sufficient for targeted integration. Rep78 is under the control of the HIV promoter. (**C**) One must then co-transfect both of these plasmids into HeLa cells. Most human cell types should be permissive for integration, but in this protocol, HeLa cells are used. The protocol can be modified to use cells of choice.

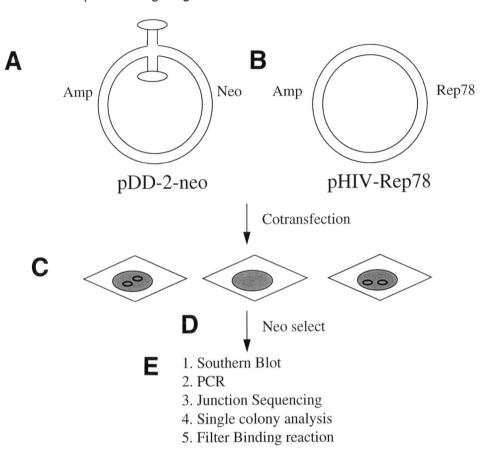

A Amp pDD-2-neo Neo

B Amp pHIV-Rep78 Rep78

Cotransfection

C

D Neo select

E
1. Southern Blot
2. PCR
3. Junction Sequencing
4. Single colony analysis
5. Filter Binding reaction

Co-transfection is carried out using Lipofectamine (Gibco-BRL), according to the manufacturer's instruction. (**D**) Place transfected cells under neo selection, using G418 at 200 μg/mL in DMEM plus 10% FBS. Selection usually takes approx 2 wk to get colonies. When colonies are approx 20–100 cells, they are ready to clone out. Expand the clones. (**E**) When one has expanded the isolated clones, one has many options to choose from to analyze for targeted integration: (1) Southern blot analysis can be carried out using a ch19 integration site-specific probe (pRE2) and a probe to the pDD-2-neo vector. One should see a shift in the size of the integration site, compared to the uninfected cells. Southern blot analysis protocol is found in *Current Protocols (24)*. PCR analysis and junction sequencing can also be carried out on single clones or pooled clones. The authors recommend that junction sequencing be performed with single clones. The junction-sequencing protocol is found within **Subheading 2.4.** PCR analysis for integration can be carried out with either pooled or single clones. (5) Filter-binding reactions can be carried out to enrich for integration events. This creates a decrease in background, and can yield cleaner results.

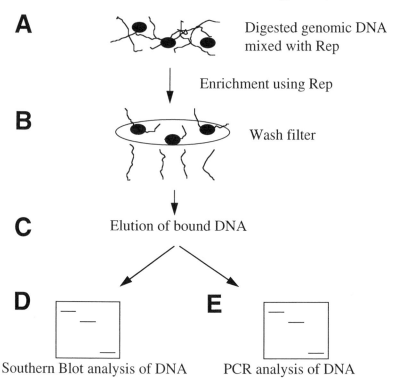

A   Digested genomic DNA
         mixed with Rep

Enrichment using Rep

B   Wash filter

C   Elution of bound DNA

D   **E**

Southern Blot analysis of DNA   PCR analysis of DNA

Fig. 3. Filter-binding reaction. (**A**) Genomic DNA isolated from single cell colonies are pooled; colonies that were neo-selected are cut with appropriate restriction enzymes, and are mixed with 20 pmol of purified Rep68. The reactions are allowed to incubate at RT for 30 min. (**B**). Reactions are passed over a prewetted Millipore HAWP 25-mm 0.45-μm pore size filter under gentle suction. The filters are then washed with 10 mL nonelution buffer, as described in **Subheading 4.2.** (**C**) Washed filters are then placed in an elution buffer, as described in **Subheading 4.2.**, and heated at 65°C for 30 min. Reactions are then ethanol-precipitated. (**D**) Southern blot analysis of reaction, as described in **Subheading 4.2.** (**E**) PCR analysis of bound material, as described in **Subheading 4.2.**

assay is dependent on highly purified Rep68 protein, which minimizes the amount of background DNA retained because of specific binding to the AAV ITR and ch19 RBE. However, because Rep68 is extremely degenerate in its binding, approx 25% of the genome will be retained, in addition to the ch19 integration event. Through multiple filter binding assays, one can enrich for the integration event, while decreasing the complexity of the background genomic DNA. This step facilitates the PCR analysis, while decreasing background commonly observed in genomic Southern blot analysis.

2. Materials

2.1. Targeted Integration

1. pDD-neo plasmid DNA (provided by the authors on request).
2. pRE2 plasmid DNA (provided by the authors on request).
3. pHIV-Rep78 or pHIV-Rep68, Rep expression plasmids (provided by the authors on request).
4. Lipofectamine (Gibco-BRL, Grand Island, NY).
5. Phosphate-buffered saline (PBS).
6. G418.
7. Dulbecco's modified Eagle's medium (DMEM) containing 10% fetal bovine serum (FBS).
8. Tissue culture hood.
9. Sterile 24-well tissue culture plates, 6-well tissue culture plates, and 10-cm tissue culture dishes.
10. HeLa cells grown to 60–80% confluency (*see* **Note 1**).
11. Trypsin-EDTA.
12. Sterile cloning rings.
13. Sterile pipets.
14. Phenol:chloroform:isoamyl alcohol 25:24:1 .
15. Chloroform:isoamyl alcohol 24:1.
16. HotStart PCR reagents (*see* **Note 2**).
17. dNTPs.
18. 7-deaza-dGTP.
19. PCR machine (Perkin-Elmer, Norwalk, CT) (**Note 3**).

2.2. Purification of Rep68H6 Protocol

1. Stump68 cells (provided by the authors on request) (*see* **Note 14**).
2. Rainin (Woburn, MA) high-pressure liquid chromatography machine or equivalent.
3. Bio-Rad (Hercules, CA) EP-1 Econo Pump or equivalent.
4. Bio-Rad Model 2110 Fraction Collector, or equivalent.
5. Hoefer, Pittsburgh, PA, gradient makers, or equivalent.
6. Luria-Bertani media.
7. Ampicillin and kanamycin.
8. Isopropylthiogalactose (IPTG).
9. Spectrophotometer.
10. Sorvall GS-3 or equivalent (Newtown, CT).
11. NaPO$_4$ monobasic.
12. 1 *M* Tris-HCl, pH 8.0.
13. Pepstatin A.
14. Leupeptin.
15. NiNTA agarose resin (Qiagen, Chatsworth, CA) (*see* **Note 15**).
16. MonoQ column (Pharmacia, Princeton, NJ).
17. Branson Sonifier, or equivalent.

18. Lysozyme (VWR Scientific, West Chester, PA) 1 mg/mL.
19. β–mercaptoethanol.
20. Imidazole.
21. Glycerol.
22. Tween-20.
23. Phenylmethylsulfonyl fluoride.
24. pH meter.
25. Silver Stain Plus Kit (Bio-Rad).

2.3. Filter-Binding Assay Protocol

1. Purified Rep68H6.
2. Millipore (Baltimore, MD) HAWP filters. 0.45-μm pore size. 25 mm.
3. Purified genomic DNA from cell lines.
4. Appropriate restriction enzymes.
5. Vacuum.
6. 25-mm Glass microanalysis vacuum filter holder and support.
7. 1 *M* Tris-HCl, pH 8.0.
8. 3 *M* KCl.
9. Glycerol.
10. BME.
11. 1 *M* HEPES-NaOH, pH 7.8.

3. Methods

3.1. Assessment of Targeted Integration

1. Co-transfect both pDD-2-neo (*see* **Note 4**) and pHIV78 or pHIV68 into Hela cells that are between 60 and 80% confluent, using Lipofectamine (Gibco-BRL) according to manufacturer's instructions (*see* **Note 5**).
2. Select cells containing integrated rAAV, using 400 μg/mL G-418 in DMEM plus 10% FBS.
3. Change the media every 3–5 d depending on the cell growth rate.
4. When the cells have grown to the size of 20–100 cells/colony, they are ready to clone out (*see* **Note 6**)
5. To pick the single cell colonies using a cloning ring, remove the media from the plate.
6. Wash the cells gently with PBS.
7. Place cloning rings with sterilized grease around the cell colonies.
8. Apply 50 μL 1X trypsin EDTA to each sealed cloning ring.
9. Incubate for 1 min at room temperature.
10. Transfer the trypsinized cells to a 24-well dish and incubate in 500 μL DMEM containing 10% FBS and 200 μg/mL G418.

3.2. Southern Blot Analysis

1. Isolate genomic DNA from pooled clones or single cell clones.
2. Isolate genomic DNA from uninfected cells to serve as control.
3. Cut the DNA with appropriate restriction enzymes (**Note 7**).

4. Carry out Southern blot analysis (*see* **Note 8**).
5. Probe uninfected DNA and *neo* selected colonies using the pRE2 plasmid (*see* **Note 9**).
6. Strip blots and probe with pDD-2-neo to confirm integration.

3.3. PCR Amplification of Junctions

1. When there are enough cells, prepare genomic DNA (*see* **Note 10**).
2. To minimize background, hot-start PCR method is employed (*see* **Note 11**).
3. Add component of PCR reaction in three steps.
4. Add the lower reagent mix (1.25 µL GeneAMP 10X PCR buffer II, 5 µL 25 m*M* MgCl$_2$ solution, 1 µL 10 m*M* dNTP, 1 µL primers to the AAV terminal repeats and 0.25 µL ddH$_2$O (*see* **Note 12**).
5. Add one AmpliWax™ PCR Gem 50 (Perkin-Elmer) to the tube, and heat to 80°C for 10 min.
6. Allow sample to cool to RT.
7. After the formation of a wax layer at RT, the upper reagent mix, (5 µL Gene Amp 10X PCR buffer II, 0.25 µL (1.25 U) AmpliTaq DNA polymerase, and 22.25 µL ddH$_2$O) was added to the tube.
8. Add 10 µL template DNA (about 100 ng) to the tube.
9. Perform PCR by linking the following four programs together: (1) two cycles at 97°C for 15 s, 58°C for 45 s, 72°C for 2 min; (2) 30–50 cycles: 94°C for 45 s, 58°C for 45 seconds, 72°C for 2 min; (3) 1 cycle 94°C for 45 s, 58°C for 45 s, 72°C for 7 min; (4) 4°C forever.
10. Clone into a TA vector and sequence the appropriate products (*see* **Note 13**).

3.4. Preparation of Stump68 Cell Extract

1. Use 5 mL LB to start an overnight culture of Stump68 cells. Grow in the presence of 25 µg/µL kanamycin and 100 µg/µL ampicillin (*see* **Note 16**).
2. Use overnight culture to grow 1 L of Stump68 cells in LB media at 37°C in the presence of 25 µg/µL of kanamycin and 100 µg/µL of ampicillin.
3. Grow the cells to an OD$_{600}$ of 0.8.
4. Induce the cells for 1 h with 0.1 m*M* IPTG.
5. Pellet the cells at 6000 rpm in a Sorvall GS-3, or equivalent, for 20 min at 4°C.
6. Resuspend the cell pellet in 50 m*M* NaPO$_4$ monobasic pH 8.1, 1 *M* NaCl, and pellet again.
7. Resuspend the cell pellet in 20 mL 50 m*M* NaPO$_4$ monobasic, pH 8.1, 1 *M* NaCl, 0.1% Tween-20, 10 m*M* β-mercaptoethanol (BME), 50 m*M* Imidazole, pH 7.0, 0.5 µg/mL leupeptin, 0.7 µg/mL pepstatin A, 0.1 m*M* phenylmethylsulfonyl fluoride (PMSF). pH the buffer to a final pH of 8.1 at 4°C.
8. Freeze thaw the cells on a dry-ice ethanol bath, and repeat again.
9. Incubate the cells on ice in the presence of 1 mg/mL lysozyme for 30 min.
10. Sonicate the cells for 30 s on ice at an output of 6 and duty cycle of 50 on a Branson Sonifer 250 (VWR Scientific). Cells should be viscous.
11. Spin the cells at 25,000 rpm in a Beckman (Fullerton, CA) SW41 at 4°C for 30 min, collect supernatant.

12. Add glycerol to a final concentration of 20% to the soluble cell lysate.
13. Divide the soluble lysate into 5-mL aliquots (*see* **Note 16**).

3.5. Purification of Rep68H6

1. Equilibrate a 2-mL (bed vol 2 mL; diameter 1.0 cm) Ni-NTA agarose (Qiagen) column in 50 mM NaPO$_4$, 1 M NaCl, 0.1% Tween-20, 10 mM BME, 50 mM Imidazole, pH 7.0, 20% glycerol (equilibration buffer) at a flow rate of 0.5 mL/min (*see* **Note 18**).
2. Apply a 5-mL aliquot of the soluble Stump68 extract to a Ni-NTA (Qiagen) column (bed vol 2 mL; diameter 1.0 cm) at flow rate of 0.20 mL/min.
3. Wash with 5 column volumes of 50 mM NaPO$_4$, 1 M NaCl, 0.1% Tween-20, 10 mM BME, 100 mM Imidazole, pH 7.0, 20% glycerol, 0.5 µg/mL leupeptin, 0.7 µg/mL pepstatin A, 0.1 mM PMSF, pH 6.0 at 4°C (wash buffer), at flow rate of 0.5 mL/min.
4. Elute the protein at a flow rate of 0.5 mL/min in an ascending linear gradient of 0.1 to 1 M Imidazole in the wash buffer, except that the final buffer pH is adjusted to 8.1 at 4°C.
5. Identify the fractions that contain the Rep68H6 using a sodium dodacyl sulfate-polyacrylamide gel electrophorises (SDS-PAGE) gel and a silver stain. (Bio-Rad Silver Stain Plus) (*see* **Note 19**).
6. Pool the fractions that contain the Rep68H6 and dialyze into 25 mM Tris-HCl, pH 8.0, 100 mM NaCl, 0.1% Tween-20, 0.1 mM EDTA, 10 mM BME, 15% glycerol, final pH of 8.1 at 4°C (MonoQ equilibration buffer).
7. Equilibrate a 1-mL MonoQ column (Pharmacia) in 5 column volumes MonoQ equilibration buffer.
8. Apply the equilibrated pooled fractions to a 1-mL MonoQ column (Pharmacia) at a flow rate of 0.5 mL/min.
9. Wash the column with 5 column volumes of MonoQ equilibration buffer at flow rate of 1.0 mL/min.
10. Elute the protein in a linear ascending 0.1–1.0 M NaCl gradient in MonoQ equilibration buffer.
11. Identify the peak fractions of Rep68H6 by running a SDS-PAGE gel and performing a silver stain (*see* **Note 20**).
12. The Rep68H6 peak is pooled and dialyzed into 25 mM Tris-HCl pH 8.0, 200 mM NaCl, 1 mM DTT, 0.1% Tween-20, and 20% glycerol and is stored at –80°C.
13. The protein should be >95% pure and possesses all wild type activities (*see* **Note 21**).

3.6. Filter-Binding Reaction

1. To an Eppendorf tube add 10 µg genomic DNA that has been digested with appropriate enzymes (*see* **Note 22**).
2. To the same Eppendorf tube add KCl, HEPES-NaOH, pH 7.8, glycerol, 20 pmol Rep68H6, BME and ddH$_2$O. The final reaction volume should be 300 µL. The final concentration of KCl should be 200 mM HEPES-NaOH, pH 7.8 10 mM, glycerol 10%, and 10 mM BME.

3. Mix the reaction mixture by gently tapping the sides.
4. Incubate reaction at RT for 30 min.
5. Prewet a Millipore 25-mm HAWP 0.45-µm pore size filter in the vacuum holder with 1 mL wash buffer (25 mM Tris-HCl, pH 8.0, 200 mM KCl, 10% glycerol).
6. Using gentle suction, pass the 300-µL reaction mixture over the filter.
7. Wash the filter with 10 mL wash buffer under gentle suction.
8. Remove filter and place in enough elution buffer (50 mM Tris-HCl pH 7.5, 10 mM EDTA, 0.5% SDS, 0.5 M NaOAC) to sufficiently cover the filter.
9. Heat the filter and buffer at 65°C for 30 min.
10. Remove the elution buffer and place in a fresh Eppendorf tube.
11. Precipitate the eluted DNA with 2.5 vol ethanol.
12. Perform PCR as described previously, or carry out Southern blot analysis.

4. Notes

1. HeLa cells are grown in 10 cm plates. Though transfection of HeLa cells is described in this protocol, other cell types can be used in this assay. Almost all human cell types are permissive for AAV integration. However, transfection efficiency may decrease in comparison to HeLa cells.
2. HotStart PCR reagents can be purchased from Perkin-Elmer (Norwalk, CT).
3. This is the Perkin Elmer GeneAmp 9600, which has a heated lid. If one does not have a machine that had a heated lid, then one will have to use mineral oil in PCR reactions.
4. pDD-2-*neo* can be modified to contain the gene of interest. However, studies have not been carried to determine the effects of increasing the size of pDD-2-neo on integration frequency. However, increasing double D vector size does not impair its ability to replicate *(8)*.
5. Lipofectamine (Gibco-BRL) is used in the assays described, but other transfection methods may be used, though transfection efficiency may decrease with different kits or methods.
6. Colonies may be pooled to check for integration, but if one is interested in obtaining junction information, then the authors recommend using clones made from single-cell colonies.
7. Because, AAV integrates as a concatamer, analysis is made easier by using an enzyme that is a no cutter for the pDD-2-*neo* plasmid. One should see a band that is bigger than the vector size and integrated in a head to tail fashion.
8. Southern Blot protocol can be found in *Current Protocols (24)*.
9. The pRE2 plasmid contains a cloned fragment from the ch19.13.3 qter. The fragment is 2.6 kb and contains the Rep-binding site and nicking site. To decrease background of Southern blots, the authors we recommend using a *Eco*RI-*Bam*HI digestion or *Pvu*II-*Bam*HI digestion of the plasmid, to decrease the amount of background signal. Regarding site-specific integration, one should see an increase in the preintegration site size in the co-transfected cells.
10. Prepare genomic DNA according to *Current Protocols (24)*.
11. The terminal repeats containing several palindromic repeats are able to form secondary structures, which makes PCR with Taq polymerase difficult. To ensure

that the terminal repeats are amplified properly, the hot start technique is employed to minimize background associated with genomic DNA.

12. Primers should be specific to the pDD-2-neo plasmid and ch19 preintegration region. The dNTP mix contains 7-deaza-dGTP because this has been shown to be efficient in reducing the secondary structure of the terminal repeats. The 10 mM dNTP mix containing 7-deaza-dGTP was made by mixing 10 mM dATP, 10 mM dCTP, 10 mM dTTP, 7.5 mM 7-deaza-dGTP, and 2.5 mM dGTP.

13. TA cloning kits can be purchased from Invitrogen.

14. Stump68 cells contain the pStump68 plasmid, which contains eight extra amino acids, RSHHHHHH, and a single amino acid change at position 536 at the carboxy end of Rep68H6. pStump68 is ampicillin resistant. pRep4 (Qiagen) produces the lacI repressor protein, and is kanamycin resistant.

15. Ni-NTA agarose resin can be purchased from Qiagen. Though there are other nickel resins from other companies, the authors recommend the Qiagen resin, because it permits stringent washing conditions.

16. Always use a fresh stab of cells that are uninduced. Never induce cells, remove IPTG, and then use these cells to start a new culture.

17. The soluble cell lysate can be frozen at –80°C and stored indefinitely or used immediately.

18. The buffer had a final pH of 8.1 at 4°C.

19. The authors have usually found a contaminating protein that stains negatively with the Silver Stain Plus Kit. The protein migrates at approx 25 kDa and overlaps with the Rep68H6 peak. The protein is approx 90% pure at this point. It is active for all biochemical activities.

20. The Rep68H6 peak is sharp and elutes before the negative staining protein.

21. The purified Rep68H6 protein has a half life of approximately 2 wk for nicking activity but DNA binding seems to remain stable. The DNA binding, trs endonuclease, and DNA helicase assay protocols can be found in ref. *25*.

22. Use enzymes that are no cutters for the pDD-2-neo plasmid.

Acknowledgments

The authors would like to thank Doug McCarty for careful reading and comments regarding this manuscript.

References

1. Berns, K. I. (1996) Parvoviridae: The viruses and their replication, in *Fields Virology,* vol. 2 (Fields, B. N., ed.), Raven, Philadelphia, pp. 2173–2197.

2. Muzyczka, N. (1992) Use of adeno-associated virus as a general transduction vector for mammalian cells. *Curr. Top. Microbiol. Immunol.* **158,** 97–129.

3. Samulski, R. J. (1993) Adeno-associated virus: integration at a specific chromosomal locus. *Curr. Opin. Genet. Dev.* **3,** 74–80.

4. Xiao, W. (1996) Characterization of cis and trans elements essential for the targeted integration and recombinant adeno-associated virus plasmid vectors, in

Curriculum in Genetics and Molecular Biology, University of North Carolina-Chapel Hill, Chapel Hill, NC, pp. 179.

5. Surosky, R. T., Urabe, M., Godwin, S. G., McQuiston, S. A., Kurtzman, G. J., Ozawa, K., and Natsoulis, G. (1997) Adeno-associated virus Rep proteins target DNA sequences to a unique locus in the human genome. *J. Virol.* **71**, 7951–7959.

6. Samulski, R. J., Chang, L.-S., and Shenk, T. (1989) Helper-free stocks of recombinant adeno-associated viruses: normal integration does not require viral gene expression. *J. Virol.* **63**, 3822–3828.

7. McLaughlin, S. K., Collis, P., Hermonat, P. L., and Muzyczka, N. (1988) Adeno-associated virus general transduction vectors: analysis of proviral structures. *J. Virol.* **62**, 1963–1973.

8. Xiao, X., Xiao, W., Li, J., and Samulski, R. J. (1997) A novel 165-base-pair terminal repeat sequence is the sole cis requirement for the adeno-associated virus life cycle. *J. Virol.* **71**, 941–948.

9. Kearns, W. G., Afione, S. A., Fulmer, S. B., Pang, M. G., Erikson, D., Egan, M., et al. (1996) Recombinant adeno-associated virus (AAV-CFTR) vectors do not integrate in a site-specific fashion in an immortalized epithelial cell line. *Gene Ther.* **3**, 748–755.

10. Walsh, C. E., Liu, J. M., Xiao, X., Young, N. S., Nienhuis, A. W., and Samulski, R. J. (1992) Regulated high level expression of a human gamma-globin gene introduced into erythroid cells by an adeno-associated virus vector. *Prac. Natl. Acad. Sci. USA* **89**, 7257–7261.

11. Kotin, R. M., Siniscalco, M., Samulski, R. J., Zhu, X. D., Hunter, L., Laughlin, C. A., et al. (1990) Site-specific integration by adeno-associated virus. *Proc. Natl. Acad. Sci. USA* **87**, 2211–2215.

12. Kotin, R. M., Linden, R. M., and Berns, K. I. (1992) Characterization of a preferred site on human chromosome 19q for integration of adeno-associated virus DNA by non-homologous recombination. *EMBO J.* **11**, 5071–5078.

13. Samulski, R. J., Zhu, X., Xiao, X., Brook, J. D., Housman, D. E., Epstein, N., and Hunter, L. A. (1991) Targeted integration of adeno-associated virus (AAV) into human chromosome 19 [published erratum appears in *EMBO J* 1992 Mar;11(3):1228]. *EMBO J.* **10**, 3941–3950.

14. Weitzman, M. D., Kyostio, S. R., Kotin, R. M., and Owens, R. A. (1994) Adeno-associated virus (AAV) Rep proteins mediate complex formation between AAV DNA and its integration site in human DNA. *Proc. Natl. Acad. Sci. USA* **91**, 5808–5812.

15. McCarty, D. M., Pereira, D. J., Zolotukhin, I., Zhou, X., Ryan, J. H., and Muzyczka, N. (1994) Identification of linear DNA sequences that specifically bind the adeno-associated virus Rep protein. *J. Virol.* **68**, 4988–4997.

16. Chiorini, J. A., Yang, L., Safer, B., and Kotin, R. M. (1995) Determination of adeno-associated virus Rep68 and Rep78 binding site by random sequence oligonucleotide selection. *J. Virol.* **69**, 7334–7338.

17. Wonderling, R. and Owens, R. (1997) Binding sites for adeno-associated virus Rep proteins within the human genome. *J. Virol.* **71**, 2528–2534.

18. Linden, R. M., Winocour, E., and Berns, K. I. (1996) The recombination signals for adeno-associated virus site-specific integration. *P.N.A.S.* 93, 7966–7972.
19. Rutledge, R. A. and Russell, D. W. (1997) Adeno-associated virus vector integration junctions. *J. Virol.* **71,** 8429–8436.
20. Yang, C. C., Xiao, X., Zhu, X., Ansardi, D. C., Epstein, N. D., Frey, M. R., Matera, A. G., and Samulski, R. J. (1997) Cellular recombination pathways and viral terminal repeat hairpin structures are sufficient for adeno-associate virus integration in vivo and in vitro. *J Virol.* **71,** 9231–9247.
21. Linden, R. M., Ward, P., Giraud, C., Winocour, E., and Berns, K. (1996) Site-specific integration by adeno-associated virus. *Proc. Natl. Acad. Sci. USA* **93,** 11,288–11,294.
22. Qing, K., Wang, X., Kube, D., Ponnazhagan, S., Bajpai, A., and Srivistava, A. (1997) Role of tyrosine phosphorylation of a cellular protein in adeno-associated cirus 2-mediated transgene expression. *Proc. Natl. Acad. Sci. USA* **94,** 10,879–10,884.
23. Ni, T. H., Zhou, X., McCarty, D. M., Zolotukhin, I., and Muzyczka, N. (1994) In vitro replication of adeno-associated virus DNA. *J. Virol.* **68,** 1128–1138.
24. Ausubel, F. M., Brent, R., Kingston, R. E., Moore, D. D., Seidman, J. G., Smith, J. A., and Struhl, K. (1998) *Current Protocols in Molecular Biology.* John Wiley, New York, NY.
25. Im, D.-S. and Muzyczka, N. (1990) The AAV origin binding protein Rep68 is an ATP-dependent site-specific endonuclease with DNA helicase activity. *Cell* **61,** 447–457.

10

Adeno-Associated Virus Based Gene Therapy in Skeletal Muscle

Richard J. Bartlett and Jesica M. McCue

1. Introduction

Gene therapy, with the promise of symptomatic relief and curative potential, is being considered for a treatment of a wide variety of genetic and acquired diseases, with over 100 protocols approved by the National Institutes of Health since 1989. Skeletal muscle is an especially attractive target for gene therapy, because of its accessibility and capability to uptake, maintain, and express recombinant protein from plasmid DNA *(1–7)*. Transduction of muscle has been considered for systemic delivery of recombinant proteins for treatment of anemia, inherited coagulopathies, endocrinologic disorders, and metabolic storage diseases, as well as localized delivery to treat dystrophinopathies and cardiovascular disorders *(6–15)*. Numerous studies have already demonstrated expression in muscle of such transgenes as various reporter enzymes and relevant therapeutic proteins *(1,3–5,16–18)*.

For gene therapy to be successful, a candidate gene must be identified, cloned, and subsequently delivered to a high percentage of target cells. Efficient transduction must also result in an appropriate level of expression for a satisfactory duration; characterization of the individual disease state governs the specific requirements for level and duration of transgene expression. Further, an inherent need to avoid problems, such as toxicity of the delivery vehicle or elicitation of host immune responses resulting in inflammation and elimination of transduced cells, also exists. Despite tremendous progress in this field, development continues of delivery systems allowing for safe, persistent expression of proteins with therapeutic value.

A variety of delivery systems, including both viral- *(19–21)* and nonviral-based vectors *(1)*, has been investigated, each with great potential, yet with

From: *Methods in Molecular Biology, vol. 133: Gene Targeting Protocols*
Edited by: E. Kmiec © Humana Press Inc., Totowa, NJ

defined limitations as well. Nonviral-based systems have included plasmid DNA alone (naked *[14–16]*), or associated with carrier molecules (proteins *[22–24]* or liposomes *[25–27]*). These strategies minimize safety concerns, are associated with low immunogenicity, are easy to produce, and are capable of delivering large gene-expression cassettes; however, most nonviral delivery systems are associated with low transduction efficiencies, and only transient transgene expression in vivo *(28)*. Viral agents that have been manipulated for gene therapy have included retrovirus (RV), herpesvirus (HSV), lentivirus (LV), adenovirus (Ad), and adenoassociated virus (AAV). RV has perhaps been best characterized and has the potential of providing efficient, long term expression of transgenes in dividing cells *(29–31)*. However, RV is incapable of infecting nondividing cells such as muscle and neurons, and is associated with concerns of insertional mutagenesis, because it integrates randomly into the host genome *(32)*. HSV and LV have the potential of efficiently transducing a wide variety of eukaryotic cells, but are less well understood, and are potentially pathogenic *(33)*. Use of Ad in gene therapy strategies has received great attention, because of its high transduction efficiency in both dividing and nondividing cells in vivo *(20,21)*. Current-generation Ad vectors elicit strong host immune responses to viral proteins and recombinant proteins alike, usually resulting in a short duration of transgene expression *(34–35)*.

2. AAV Biology

AAV has become the gene delivery system of choice in many gene therapy protocols *(36–40)*. AAV has a broad range of infectivity, including both dividing and nondividing cells, and appears to be nonpathogenic *(36,41–45)*. Greater than 80% of adults are seropositive for antibodies to AAV *(46)*, yet no disease has been attributed to infection *(47–48)*. Wild-type AAV demonstrates a proclivity for site-specific integration in healthy host cells *(49)*, a particularly attractive feature for applications in gene therapy. The AAV genome is small, easy to manipulate, and substitution of all viral-encoded genes with a transgene of choice has been possible *(36,50)*. The cloning of such recombinant AAV (rAAV), and development of in vitro packaging systems *(51–56)*, have opened the doors for the development of an efficient DNA carrier system, free from concerns of recombination with wild-type virus, toxicity, and immunologic host response *(57–59)*.

AAV is a member of the family Parvoviridae *(60,61)*, and is assigned to the genus *Dependovirus*, so named because of its first identification as a contaminant in purified Ad stocks *(62–63)*. In most instances, AAV does not productively infect cells (i.e., replicate and produce infectious virus particles), unless there is co-infection with an unrelated helper virus such as Ad or HSV. AAV

AAV Genomic Structure

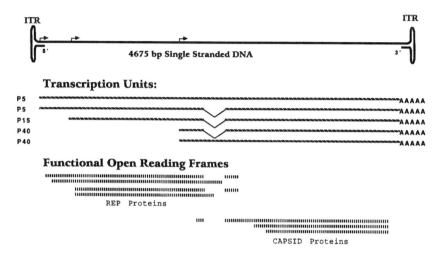

Fig. 1. AAV genomic structure. The single strand DNA genome is depicted with inverted terminal repeats (ITR) at either end. The three small arrows indicate approximate positions for the three functional promoters, p5, p19, and p40, and the middle portion depicts the transcripts from each promoter, with and without splicing of the viral intron. At the bottom, the functional open reading frames are shown as vertical hashed lines, and are grouped according to the Rep and capsid proteins.

was long considered to be a defective virus, even designated "Almost-A-Virus" at times, but recent studies have demonstrated that, rather than being defective, AAV preferentially establishes a latent infection in healthy host cells (integration occurs) *(64,65)*, and only undergoes productive replication when the host cell is stressed *(66–69)*. AAV has a broad host range; many serotypes have been isolated from a variety of invertebrate and vertebrate species; five serotypes in humans alone have been identified. All rAAV vectors currently in use are based on AAV type 2, but characterization of other serotypes is underway *(70)*. Recent identification of the AAV2 receptor as a membrane-associated heparin sulfate proteoglycan has provided insight for the broad host range of this virus *(71)*.

AAV is a single-strand, nonenveloped DNA virus with a genome of 4.7 kb *(72)*. Both plus and minus strands are packaged into virus particles and are equally infectious (*see* **Fig. 1**). The genome consists of two open reading frames (ORFs) flanked by inverted terminal repeats (ITR) *(59,72)*. The one ORF encodes three structural proteins involved in encapsidation of virus particles (cap). Differential splicing and an unusual initiation codon allow for production of the three cap proteins from p40, a single promoter at map unit 40

(73–75). The other ORF encodes four nonstructural proteins with overlapping amino acid sequences *(76)*. Frame-shift mutations in any region of this ORF inhibit AAV replication *(77,78)*; hence, these proteins have been designated, based on their perceived mol. wt, as Rep78, 68, 52, and 40 *(77,79,80)*. Rep78 and 68 are expressed from alternatively spliced transcripts from the promoter at map unit 5 (p5); Rep52 and 40 are derived from alternatively spliced transcripts from the promoter at map unit 19 (p19). Rep proteins function in regulation of viral gene expression, site-specific integration into and rescue from the host genome, and replication and encapsidation of viral genomes. Flanking the AAV coding region are two 145-nt ITR sequences, which are the minimal *cis*-acting elements necessary for integration, replication, and encapsidation of AAV *(59,80–85)*. The terminal 125 nucleotide (nt), when folded on itself, forms a palindromic hairpin structure, which serves as the primer for replication *(47,86–88)*. The remaining 20 bp represent the D sequence, binding of which by D sequence binding protein (D-BP) appears to mediate transduction efficiency *(89–91)*. The terminal resolution site (TRS) within the ITR, which is cleaved by Rep in a site-specific, strand specific manner during replication, is also an essential component of the AAV genome *(92)*.

The life cycle of AAV has been characterized *(48,93)*. Upon virus entry, presumably through receptor-mediated endocytosis by binding-membrane-associated proteoglycan *(71)*, particles are uncoated and the genome delivered to the nucleus. The fate of the viral genome is dependent on the host cell environment. Under nonpermissive conditions, low levels of Rep protein are expressed, which serves to suppress any further viral transcription from p5 and p19 *(94–96)*, and integration of the AAV genome into the q arm of human chromosome 19 ensues *(65,97–102)*. Thus, a latent infection has been established. Under permissive conditions, the AAV genome can subsequently be rescued from the integrated state to undergo productive infection. Productive infection is characterized by enhanced viral transcription, replication, and production of progeny virus *(47)*. Although host cell death is also associated with productive infection, this fate has been attributed to factors determining the permissive state of the cell, rather than AAV replication.

Those factors that elicit a permissive state of the cell include Ad or HSV infection *(42,103)*, as well as treatment of cells with a variety of genotoxic stimuli, such as heat shock, hydroxyurea, UV light, or carcinogenesis *(66–68,104)*. Thus, a working model has been established in which helper viral proteins have no direct role in AAV replication. Rather, proteins required for complete helper function, which, in the case of Ad co-infection, involve E1A, E1B, E4, E2A, and VA gene products *(34,59)*, maximize synthesis of the AAV gene products and various host cell factors necessary for AAV replication. The AAV gene products necessary for viral replication clearly involve the Rep proteins

(105). AAV harboring mutations in the Rep-binding site (RBS) of the p5 promoter, which blocked suppression (i.e., enhancing) of p5 transcripts normally occurring in latent infection, are capable of productive infection in nonpermissive 293 cells, further implicating Rep78 and/or 68 in AAV replication *(106)*.

Rep 78/68, although necessary, are not sufficient for AAV replication. Recent observations that HeLa cells are only able to support productive infection of AAV when grown at high density has enabled identification of cellular enzymes involved in AAV replication *(107)*. Through the use of chemical inhibitors, monoclonal antibodies, and fractionation of uninfected HeLa extracts targeting the cellular enzymes necessary for simian virus-40 replication, the following proteins were implicated in AAV replication: single-strand DNA-binding protein, replication protein A (RFA), the 3' primer-binding complex, replication factor C (RFC), and proliferating cell nuclear antigen (PCNA) *(107)*. Furthermore, in vitro replication of AAV has been accomplished utilizing Rep78, RPA, RFC, PCNA, and a phosphocellulose chromatography fraction (IIA) that contained DNA polymerase activity. Neither polymerase Δ or ε, nor a combination of both, was capable of substituting the DNA polymerase activity in fraction IIA, suggesting that a novel cellular protein or modification not yet identified is the remaining cellular component(s) necessary for AAV replication.

3. AAV Targeting

The ability of AAV to integrate into the genome of infected cells is a unique feature among mammalian viruses for two reasons: Integration occurs within a specific locus on chromosome 19 in humans *(49)*, designated AAVS1; and integration is independent of mitosis *(97–100,108)*. In the absence of productive infection, AAV penetrates the nucleus and is uncoated. The low levels of Rep78/68 produced are believed to inhibit viral transcription, repress viral DNA synthesis, and mediate integration into the host genome *(94–96)*. Integration into the AAVS1 occurs with a high frequency in wild-type AAV-infected cells *(49)*. In fact, a 510-nt fragment of AAVS1 has been identified that is sufficient to direct site-specific integration *(97,109)*. This sequence contains both a RBS *(110,111)* and TRS *(112)*, in the appropriate orientation and spacing in relation to the RBS and TRS present in the AAV ITR. Mutations involving 2–3 nt in the RBS or TRS of this fragment have been shown to block site-specific integration *(97)*. Furthermore, a 33-nt oligonucleotide containing these two signal sequences has been sufficient to direct the integration process. The current model for integration involves localized replication within AAVS1, in which single-strand displacement, and the ability of the elongating strand to switch templates, are key features *(97,112)*. Identification of RBS has been noted at multiple sites in the human genome *(113)*, but the proper conjunction of RBS and TRS, which appears to be required for Rep-mediated integration, has only been found once in the human genome, at the AAVS1 *(97)*. Although Rep protein is requirement for integration into AAV1 *(114)*, it has been suggested that all 145 nt of the ITR may not be necessary for targeted integration *(97)*. The uncoupling of targeted integration and rescue may be possible, and in fact desirable, for gene therapy vector development, in which efficient rescue and replication of recombinant provirus may be deleterious. However, all Rep encoding genes have been eliminated in current AAV vectors developed for gene therapy; integration of rAAV will probably be random and occur through a totally different mechanism mediated by host-cell proteins.

4. rAAV Transduction

With an understanding of the molecular biology of AAV and the ability to package foreign DNA flanked by ITRs into infectious virions *(36,47)*, rAAV became an attractive vehicle for gene therapy. Efficient transduction by AAV of a variety of cell lines, as well as tissues in vivo, has been demonstrated, including muscle *(57,116–120)*, brain *(121,122)*, heart *(123)*, retina *(124)*, lung *(125,126)*, and liver *(127,128)*. Current applications of rAAV-based therapies include antisense inhibition *(129,130)* and homologous recombination *(131)*, in addition to traditional gene therapies for delivery of therapeutic proteins *(123,132–134)*. Optimization of rAAV for use in gene therapy in the areas of integration, immunogenicity of individual and repeated administration, and substantial constraints on transgene size continues.

Stable transgene expression is a key feature for effective gene therapy of many diseases. Long term expression from rAAV has been demonstrated in vivo in such tissues as muscle *(57,116,118,120)* and neurons *(121,122)*, despite the elimination of Rep-encoding genes from these vectors. One possible mechanism for transgene stability is integration, but it has been difficult to resolve this issue definitively in nondividing cells. Rep-deficient AAV has been demonstrated to be successfully integrated into dividing cells, albeit nonspecifically *(135,138)*. However, because of limited material for analysis when studying nondividing cells, putative episomal replication or undefined concatamers of episomal form could not be ruled out as sources for stable gene expression *(58,118,126)*. Neither detection of rAAV by Southern analysis associated with high mol wt DNA nor PCR detection of rAAV head-tail concatamers (which can only occur through postulated mechanisms of integration, not replication *[135]*) has been evidence enough to confirm integration in nondividing tissue *(58,118,126)*. Wu et al. *(139)* recently described an Alu-PCR strategy, previously used to examine flanking sequences of integrated hepatitis B virus *(140)*, which may resolve this issue. Briefly, Alu sequences are interspersed repeat DNA in humans, which appear approximately every 4 kb in the human genome

(30). Thus, integrated transgenes can be amplified using a series of Alu- and transgene-specific primers. Integration was apparent following Southern analysis of Alu-PCR products from human NT neurons and alveolar macrophages transduced in vitro. The Alu-equivalent sequence B1, which is present in the rodent genome, was also used to identify rAAV integration into the rat hippocampus. Even when mixed cell populations were analyzed, relatively few PCR products were detected, indicating that AAV integration was not entirely random (it is unlikely that, with random integration, equal spacing from Alu sequences would occur). However, this may be the result of selective amplification of preferred integrated transgenes in the Alu-PCR procedure. The possibility of Rep-mediated integration still exists. Possible sources of Rep protein could be low-level wild type-AAV contamination, or several investigators have suggested an association, even encapsidation, of Rep with AAV particles *(141,142)*. Whether Rep was present and/or involved in integration into the genome of nondividing cells remains unclear; however, in no instance was the sequenced vector–cellular junction specific for AAVS1 *(139)*. Because the vector–cellular junction sequence was targeted in this assay, it can be concluded that the transgene associated with high-mol-wt DNA was not episomal in these cells. Furthermore, the combination of nested PCR and sequencing employed in these studies allows for analysis of the integration site and elucidation of sequence rearrangement. Although not yet demonstrated, quantification (i.e., copy number per cell) may also be possible if the transgene represents an endogenous gene, allowing intensities of each to be compared.

5. rAAV Transduction: Limiting Factors

The single-strand nature of the viral genome necessitates second-strand synthesis, which appears to be a rate-limiting step in transduction of cells by AAV *(143–146)*. A cellular tyrosine phosphoprotein has been identified that interacts specifically with the D-sequence of the 3' end of the AAV genome *(89–91)*. This protein, designated D-sequence binding protein (D-BP) has been postulated to prevent viral second-strand synthesis in nonpermissive HeLa cells. Qing et al. *(90)* have recently characterized the phosphorylation state of D-BP in various cell lines, as well as in murine tissues, and found that high transduction efficiency correlated with the phosphorylation state of D-BP; cells with higher levels of dephosphorylated D-BP are associated with higher transduction efficiencies. Expression of the adenoviral E4[orf6] protein, which is known to induce AAV gene expression *(143)*, also correlated with dephosphorylation of D-BP. Notably, of all murine tissues examined, the ratio of dephosphorylated to phosphorylated D-BP was highest in skeletal and brain tissue, which demonstrate high AAV-transduction capacity in vivo *(90)*. Spleen and thymus contained high levels of phosphorylated D-BP, providing evidence for a possible postentry block to AAV transduction in cells of these tissues *(143,144)*.

Specific immune responses to transduced cells in vivo have limited the progress of gene therapy for treatment of chronic diseases *(148,149)*. Somatic gene transfer is so effective at eliciting cellular immune responses *(150)* that it has been exploited for the development of vaccines for cancer and infectious disease *(29,151–156)*. Most gene therapy strategies are designed to promote prolonged gene expression, however, and immune responses to corrected cells is a substantial problem *(35,157–159)*. Expression of β-galactosidase following adenoviral infection in vivo has been demonstrated to elicit strong cellular and humoral immune responses that result in inflammation and loss of target cells *(35,160–162)*. However, rAAV delivered to skeletal muscle has not elicited such immune responses, but rather has yielded a surprisingly high stability of gene transfer *(57,116–118)*. Although there are differences in viral proteins expressed in these two systems (rAAV has no viral-encoded genes) *(163,164)*, recent work suggests fundamental differences in immunogenicity of transgene-encoded proteins following Ad vs AAV infection, as well *(165)*. In short, AAV-infected muscle evades destructive immune responses because of inefficient Antigen Presenting Cell (APC) transduction, specifically dendritic cells (Joos, 1998). Although dendritic cells are readily infected by AAV, a postentry block is evident by perinuclear localization of AAV in infected cells. Efficiency of second-strand synthesis, mediated by D-BP, may contribute to this effect *(90)*.

AAV does not appear to evade the immune system following repeated administration. Transgene expression has not been detected following intramuscular injection of rAAV vectors harboring the same or different transgenes into mice *(115,116,166)*. Utilizing class I MHC-, class II MHC-, or CD40L-deficient mice, it has been determined that the hosts humoral immune response to the vector prevented effective second administration *(166)*. However, readministration of rAAV may be possible with transient immunosuppression by anti-CD4 antibody treatment at the time of the initial injection, to attenuate AAV capsid-antibody and neutralizing-antibody titers *(166)*. Because repeated administration of the same AAV vector or subsequent delivery of different AAV vectors may be required for treatment of certain diseases, continued development of effective immunomodulatory paradigms is warranted.

Packaging constraints on genome size is a substantial limitation of the utility of rAAV for gene therapy. Virions harboring genomes greater than 120% the size of the wild-type AAV genome are not packaged efficiently *(36)*, thus transgenes (including regulatory region and coding sequence) must be less than 4.8 kb. The selection of a small and efficient promoter may be crucial for successful rAAV transduction with proteins whose cDNA size alone approaches the packaging limit. The AAV ITR itself may have transcriptional activity

(167), but more attention has been given to utilizing the p5 promoter in rAAV *(50,168)*. Baudard et al. *(168)* have demonstrated that a 234-nt region (nt 1–234 of wild-type AAAV) has promoter activity similar in strength to the entire p5 promoter and the retrovirus, Harvey murine sarcoma virus, long terminal repeat in NIH 3T3 cells. This promoter activity was seen in the absence of rep, from both episomal and integrated forms for the transgene. The 5' end of the wild type-AAV genome contains several regulatory elements that may confer transcriptional activity: binding sites for MTLF *(169)* YY1 *(170)*, SP1 and an Inr-like sequence *(171)* and a cryptic TATA box *(169)*. Further investigation will be required to determine the function of this promoter in various cell types.

The development of bicistronic rAAV vectors is a novel strategy for expressing multiple gene products from a single promoter *(168,172)*. Internal ribosome entry sites (IRES) from encephalomyocarditis (EMCV) and hepatitis C virus (HCV) have been investigated. Coordinate expression of hMDR-1 and hGC in stably selected NIH-3T3 cells, using the EMCV-IRES, has heightened the possibility of expanding a population of GC-expressing cells by MDR-1 drug selection for the treatment of Gaucher's disease *(168)*. The HCV-IRES has also been used to allow co-expression of a therapeutic gene and a selectable marker gene, in a manner comparable to vectors with the EMCV-IRES *(172)*. Urable **(172)** successfully obtained luciferase-expressing, blasticidin (bcr)-resistant 293 cells following either transfection or transduction. A substantial benefit of this bicistronic vector is that because HCV-IRES-bcr is only 650 bp, a therapeutic gene up to 3.6 kb can be co-expressed *(172)*.

The proficient expression capabilities of rAAV have been well demonstrated, but the fact remains that the production of rAAV particles is a relatively inefficient, tedious process *(51–56)*. Additionally, the packaging constraints on transgene size render rAAV useless for treatment of diseases that require highly regulated expression of large cDNAs. Thus, the pursuit of the ideal delivery system for gene therapy continues. Because the ITR sequence is the essential portion of the AAV genome required for replication, encapsidation, and integration into the host genome, novel strategies have emerged, combining ITR-flanked transgenes with alternative nonviral- and viral-delivery vehicles.

6. AAV ITR: Special Properties

The relevance of flanking a transgene with AAV-ITRs has been described in numerous reports *(50,168,172–178)*. In the presence of identical backbone plasmids, expression cassettes, and transfection methods, plasmids containing ITRs have consistently resulted in increased levels of transient and stable gene expression, compared to those lacking AAV sequences. Up to 10-fold increases in transient expression with plasmids harboring ITR sequences (pAAV) in various cell types have been reported *(50,172–175,178)*. Of greater interest is the apparent stability of pAAV in transfected cells. Transgene expression from cells transfected with pAAV has been detected for up to 4 mo; typical transfection procedures resulted in diminished expression within 1 wk *(168)*. In all reported cases, the level of expression from pAAV did decrease with time *(173–175)*, especially with removal of selection pressure *(168)*. Furthermore, enhancing/stabilizing effects of ITRs on plasmid DNA may be cell-specific, because Doll *(174)* reported high transient expression with pAAV in CNS-derived cells, which dropped dramatically within days. Whether transfection efficiency of pAAV correlates with transduction efficiency of rAAV in various cell types remains to be determined. Possible mechanisms for ITR-mediated prolonged gene expression from pAAV have not yet been identified, but may include stabilizing episomal DNA, enhancing expression from heterologous promoters, or promoting integration into the host genome. Further investigation is crucial to address these issues, as well as to demonstrate prolonged gene expression from pAAV in vivo. Evidence of pAAV plasmid 7 wk after administration via tail-vein injection of mice has been reported for several tissues by PCR analysis *(168)*, but relative efficiency and expression data have been limited.

Novel hybrid vectors have also been developed recently with the common feature that ITR-flanked transgenes are packaged into alternative virus particles, namely adenovirus (Ad/AAV) *(177)*, herpesvirus (HSV/AAV) *(179,180)*, and baculovirus (BV/AAV) *(181)*. Limited data is available on the utility of hybrid virions for gene therapy, but each has been efficiently produced at high titer, which may allow for transduction of a high number of cells. The greatest advantages of these systems include the increase in packaging limits of these viruses and the ability to transiently co-express Rep protein, upon infection with hybrid virions, to promote site-specific integration seen with wild-type AV, as reported recently in BV/AAV-infected–293 cells *(181)*.

7. AAV-Based Therapeutics

Wild-type AAV has the ability to infect a broad range of eukaryotic cell types *(36)*, but efficient and stable transduction with rAAV may be restricted to such tissues as muscle *(57,116,118,)* and brain *(121)*; transgene expression in other tissues is often poor *(182–184)*. Skeletal muscle is an attractive target for gene therapy, because muscle cells are readily accessible, have a large capacity for protein synthesis (including secreted products), and have the unique ability for uptake, expression, and maintenance of plasmid DNA *(1–7,18)*. There is significant interest in targeting muscle for the treatment of serum protein deficiencies *(8–13)* and local muscle disorders *(14,15)*. Moderate successes have been achieved with transplantation of modified myoblasts *(8,184,185)*, direct injection of plasmid DNA *(28)*, liposome-complexed DNA *(57)*, and various viral delivery systems *(9,186,187)*. However, gene expression with these strategies is often limited to a small percentage of cells, or occurs only transiently, precluding long-term correction *(3,4,12,15)*. Adenoviral vectors hold great promise for efficiently infecting nondividing cells, but transduction of mature muscle is much less efficient than that of neonatal muscle *(161,189,190)*, limiting their utility.

AAV-based recombinant vectors have now been tested in several experimental models of muscle targeted gene therapy *(57,116–121,191)*, and the reality of their transduction abilities has surpassed expectations. Efficient transduction of skeletal muscle by rAAV has been reported in vitro, as well as in mice *(57,116–119,191)*, rats *(146)*, dogs *(120)*, and rhesus monkeys *(118)*. Heart *(192)* and vascular smooth muscle cells *(193–195)* have also been successfully targeted. The reported efficiency of transient transduction has ranged from 10 to 70%; delivery techniques and variations in transducing-unit titers of rAAV preparations probably account for this variability. Stable gene expression has also been obtained following intramuscular injection with rAAV. β-galactosidase in mice has been detected in transduced skeletal muscle for up to 1.5 yr *(116)*; in transduced pig hearts, β–galactosidase expression was evident for up to 6 mo *(192)*. Expression of erythropoietin, at levels sufficient to elevate hematocrits of mice, has been detected for greater than 30 wk *(57,191)*. Therapeutic effects of human factor IX (hF.IX), delivered to a dog model of hemophilia B, have been detected at 1 wk postinjection, but could not be sustained because of host humoral response to this nonautologous protein *(120)*. However, immunohistochemical analysis at 10 wk demonstrate that expression of hF.IX persisted, despite circulating antibodies to the transgene product *(120)*.

Integration of rAAV into the host genome is one possible mechanism for stable transgene expression in muscle, but this issue has not been adequately addressed. Several factors ,such as association of the transgene with high-mol-wt DNA and head-tail arrangement of concatamerized rAAV, indicate integration had occurred *(116,118)*, but cloning and sequencing of vector cellular junctions will provide definitive proof. With the exception of delivery of nonautologous secreted products, no immune responses, generalized systemic problems *(119,120)*, nor transduction-related toxicity has been attributed to rAAV infection *(116,118,192)*. Co-infection of rAAV with helper virus (Ad) did not result in levels of transduction, which exceeded that of infection with rAAV alone, and was associated with substantial inflammation *(116,118)*. The effects of regeneration on skeletal muscle transduction has also been investigated. As with co-infection with Ad, gene transfer by rAAV was not facilitated by regeneration, and inflammatory responses resulted in elimination of transduced fibers by 8 wk postinfection *(191)*. Further studies will be required to determine whether inflammation was stimulated by experimental procedures alone, and how this may impact rAAV transduction of dystrophic muscle.

8. AAV-Based Therapeutics: Can Insulin Be Made in Skeletal Muscle?

Production of a circulating hormone, such as insulin from skeletal muscle, would have important consequences to children with juvenile or type I Diabetes mellitis. Studies aimed at using an AAV-based plasmid to produce insulin in skeletal muscle in vivo have been initiated, beginning with the production of proinsulin using a human muscle creatine kinase (hCKM) promoter *(6)*. In **Fig. 2A**, a diagram depicts the assembled pCKM-INS plasmid containing hCKM promoter and human insulin genomic DNA flanked by AAV-ITRs. Using a single transdermal injection of naked pCKM-INS DNA into the gastrocnemius muscle, released proinsulin was measured in peripheral blood of experimentally induced diabetic Lewis or BB/WOR rats, and was found to persist for over 3 mo at high levels (*see* **Fig. 3A**). Although significant measurable levels of proinsulin were found in these animals, the blood glucose levels showed no detectable evidence of change in response to the human prohormone *(6)*.

This expected reduced response to the prohormone prompted assembly of a second-generation bicistronic vector, pFurinsulin (*see* **Fig. 2B**), containing an engineered point mutation that produced a consensus recognition site for the endoprotease furin via substitution of arginine for leucine in the C/A peptide junction *(7)*. In addition, using an IRES sequence *(7,172)*, mouse furin cDNA was joined downstream from the stop codon of the insulin gene, to produce a bicistronic construct that would have the potential for immediate posttranslation removal of the C-peptide from proinsulin by the nascent synthesized

---

Fig. 2. *(opposite page)* Insulin-expression plasmids. Plasmid vectors are derived from the SSV-9 plasmid *(84)*, used as described *(18)*. Note that, in each, the entire expression cassette is flanked by the AAV ITR elements. (**A**) Diagram of the pCKM-INS plasmid. The hCKM promoter and a portion of the first exon (white arrow) are joined to a PCR fragment containing the human insulin gene beginning just before the first intron and ending with the stop codon. Thus, there are two native insulin gene introns contained within this segment, which should enhance expression of insulin mRNA sequences from this vector in vivo. (**B**) pFurinsulin plasmid. The components in pCKM-INS are augmented in pFurinsulin by the addition of an IRES sequence *(7,172)* to permit translation of two different peptides from a single mRNA. The first cistron is the genomic insulin segment, as seen in panel A. The second cistron is mouse furin cDNA *(198)*, which begins immediately after the IRES. In addition, at the indicated site, overlapping PCR primers were used to introduce a point mutation producing a leu-to-arg missense, which creates a consensus furin site *(7)*.

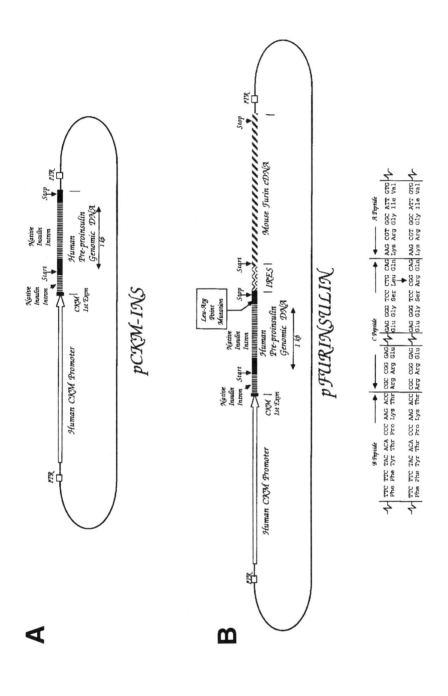

A

pCKM-INS

B

pFURINSULIN

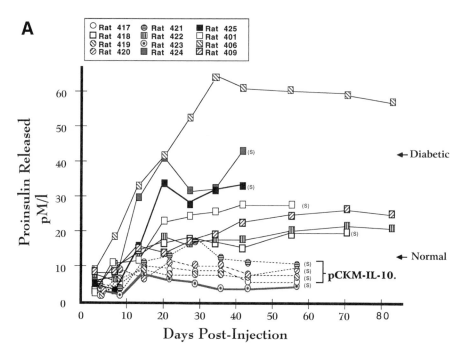

A

Legend:
- ○ Rat 417
- ⊟ Rat 418
- ◈ Rat 419
- ⬨ Rat 420
- ⊖ Rat 421
- ⊪ Rat 422
- ⊙ Rat 423
- ◪ Rat 424
- ■ Rat 425
- ▫ Rat 401
- ▨ Rat 406
- ▨ Rat 409

Y-axis: Proinsulin Released pM/l

X-axis: Days Post-Injection

← Diabetic

← Normal

] pCKM-IL-10.

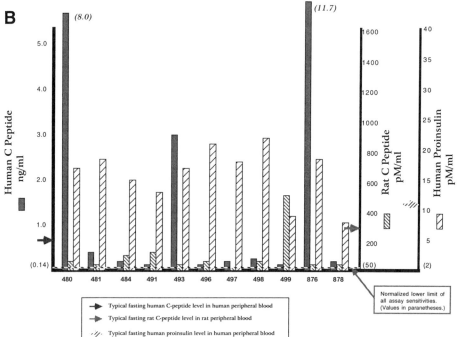

B

Y-axis (left): Human C Peptide ng/ml

(8.0)   (11.7)

Y-axis: Rat C Peptide pM/ml

Y-axis (right): Human Proinsulin pM/ml

X-axis labels: 480 481 484 491 493 496 497 498 499 876 878

Normalized lower limit of all assay sensitivities. (Values in paranetheses.)

- ➤ Typical fasting human C-peptide level in human peripheral blood
- ➤ Typical fasting rat C-peptide level in rat peripheral blood
- ⫶⫶⫶ Typical fasting human proinsulin level in human peripheral blood

mouse furin. Injection of this construct into skeletal muscle of diabetic animals produced significant release of human C-peptide into peripheral blood (*see* **Fig. 3B**), but little or no insulin, nor modification of blood glucose *(7)*. Histochemical analysis of the injected tissue, using an antibody specific for human insulin, revealed large vesicular structures that stained positive for insulin (**Fig. 4**), suggesting that the processed protein was present, but was not capable of being secreted. There are a number of possible explanations for the discrepancy between released C-peptide and insulin, which should be present in equimolar amounts. One would be that the nascent insulin might exist in this muscle in a polymerized state. During processing of proinsulin to insulin in secretory granules of β-cells, high levels of zinc (Zn) are present and required for stability of the secretory response *(196)*. Removal of Zn from preparations of insulin via chelation causes insulin to precipitate. Muscle cells have moderate levels of Zn, and therefore, without a mechanism for Zn accumulation, nascently synthesized insulin may have polymerized in muscle. In addition, the lack of secretory mechanism, and associated accessory proteins, might prevent release of accumulated insulin. A second explanation might be that insulin-binding protein may be upregulated in muscle in response to intracellular expression of insulin *(197)*, and this might prevent release and lead to rapid turnover of the

---

Fig. 3. *(opposite page)* Radioimmunoassay (RIA) values for human proinsulin, insulin and C-peptide released from muscle. (**A**) Graph illustrating RIA values for human proinsulin found in peripheral blood serum from diabetic rats injected with pCKM-INS (squares) and a control plasmid, pCKM-IL-10, (circles) after the indicated intervals of time. Arrows to the right of the graph indicate values for control samples provided with the RIA kit by the supplier (Linco, St. Louis, MO). The lower arrow is the normal level of proinsulin in human serum; the upper arrow marks the proinsulin level of a hyperinsulinemic sample known to have high circulating levels of proinsulin because of insulin insensitivity characteristic of type 2 diabetes. (**B**) Histogram of circulating hormones from experimentally induced (streptozotocin) diabetic Lewis rats injected with pFurinsulin plasmid *(7)*. Values for each indicated RIA are the normalized lower limit of sensitivity (basal values in parentheses). Human C-peptide (solid bars), rat C-peptide (fine hashed bars), and human proinsulin (course hashed bars) assays were run on serum collected from each animal at 10 d postinjection using commercial kits (Linco). The standards for the human and rat C-peptide assays were exchanged as a control experiment to rule out crossreactivity of the two antigens, and were found not to crossreact (data not shown), as indicated by the supplier. For animals 480 and 876, the human C-peptide values are not to scale, but are indicated in italics next to the bars. Arrows next to each *y*-axis indicate the normal circulating level of each antigen. Thus, animals 480, 493, and 876 had values ranging from 11 to 23.4× normal levels of circulating human C-peptide.

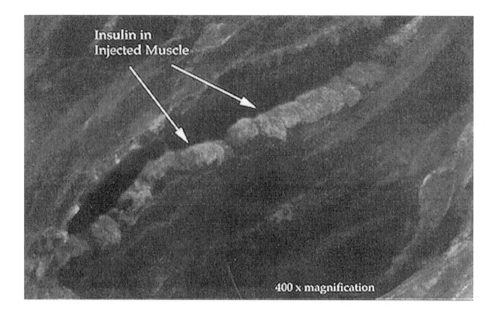

Fig. 4. Immunocytochemistry of human insulin in rat muscle. A frozen section from a muscle injected from rat 480 **(Fig. 3B)** with pFurinsulin plasmid from a rat with high circulating human C-peptide. Sections were treated with a mouse monoclonal antibody specific to human insulin (clone 10-I30, Fitzgerald) and goat anti-mouse secondary conjugated with FITC (Jackson Immunoresearch). Microscopy used a Leitz Fluorvert epifluorescent microscope and Kodak 400 ASA Ektachrome film. Notice the bag-like accumulation of insulin, as indicated. Control sections from the contralateral uninjected leg were negative (data not shown).

insulin. Last, the endoprotease site on the B/C junction may require remodeling to a more effective furin site, and thus partial cleavage, with furin producing the des 64,65 product, might explain the aborted release of insulin from the muscle *(198)*. Clearly, additional studies will be required to address these questions, but the high levels of proinsulin and C-peptide release in these studies indicate that overcoming these hurdles could potentially provide an adjunctive treatment for type 1 diabetes via sustained basal levels of insulin from muscle injection.

9. Looking Into the Crystal Ball

The future of rAAV-based gene therapies for targeting muscle is bright. Current methods in rAAV packaging, which provide rAAV stocks free from wild-type V or contaminating Ad *(51–56),* need only be optimized for consistent, high tranducing particle titers. The potential for repeated administration of rAAV, of either the same transgene or subsequent infection with different transgenes, should be explored further, to increase the utility of rAAV vectors in treating complex chronic disorders. Two safety issues remain to be fully addressed. First is the rare possibility of in vivo co-infection of genetically corrected cells with wild-type AAV and helper virus (Ad, HSV), leading to rescue, replication, and potential spread of infectious rAAV. Second, the desirability of utilizing Rep proteins to induce site-specific integration of rAAV is unclear. The inhibitory effects of Rep on cell growth have been well documented *(141,142)*. Only transient Rep expression, designed to mimic wild-type AAV infection, has been proposed in current strategies, but strict control of such expression cassettes is essential. Further, the possibility of deleterious effects of wild-type AAV, most notably on fetal development, are emerging *(69)*, and may be attributed to Rep protein functions. Consequences of disruption of the ORF at AAVS1 *(97)* with transgene integration are even less well understood.

Each of these issues can be avoided altogether, with the use of AAV-based plasmids. The mechanism of ITR-mediated stability of gene expression warrants further investigation to optimize their use in both plasmid and hybrid vectors. Muscle can be efficiently transduced by rAAV to provide stable transgene expression, and is one of the most attractive tissues to target for gene therapy for treatment of a variety of disorders. The time has come to intensify these studies: Intramuscular delivery of relevant gene product in large animal models of disease is imperative for the establishment of human clinical trials for AAV based gene therapy in skeletal muscle.

References

1. Wolff, J. A., Malone, R. W., Williams, P., Chong, W., Acsadi, G., Jani, A., and Felgner, P. L. (1990) Direct gene transfer into mouse muscle in vivo. *Science* **247,** 1465–1468.
2. Wolff, J. A., Ludtke, J. J., Acsadi, G., Williams, P., and Jani, A. (1992) Long-term persistence of plasmid DNA and foreign gene expression in mouse muscle. *Hum. Mol. Genet.* **1,** 363–369.
3. Jiao, S., Williams, P., Berg, R. K., Hodgeman, B. A., Liu, L., Repetto, G., and Wolff, J. A. (1992) Direct gene transfer into nonhuman primate myofibers in vivo. *Hum. Gene Ther.* **3,** 21–33.
4. Ma, J. X., Yang, Z., Chao, J., and Chao, L. (1995) Intramuscular delivery of rat kallikrein-binding protein gene reverses hypotension in transgenic mice expressing human tissue kallikrein. *J. Biol. Chem.* **270,** 451–455.
5. Mumper, R. J., Duguid, J. G., Anwer, K., Barron, M. K., Nitta, H., and Rolland, A. P. (1996) Polyvinyl derivatives as novel interactive polymers for controlled gene delivery to muscle. *Pharm. Res.* **13,** 701–709.
6. Bartlett, R. J., Secore, S. L., Denis, M., Fernandez, L., Tzakis, A., Alejandro, R., and Ricordi, C. (1997) Toward the biologic release of human insulin from skeletal muscle. *Transplant Proc.* **29,** 2199–2200.

7. Bartlett, R. J., Denis, M., Secore, S. L., Alejandro, R., and Ricordi, C. (1998) Toward engineering skeletal muscle to release peptide hormone from the human pre-proinsulin gene. *Transplant Proc.* **30,** 451–452.

8. Dhawan, J., Pan, L. C., Pavlath, G. K., Travis, M. A., Lanctot, A. M., and Blau, H. M. (1991) Systemic delivery of human growth hormone by injection of genetically engineered myoblasts. *Science* **254,** 1509–1512.

9. Dai, Y., Roman, M., Naviaux, R. K., and Verma, I. M. (1992) Gene therapy via primary myoblasts: long-term expression of factor IX protein following transplantation in vivo. *Proc. Natl. Acad. Sci. USA* **89,** 10,892–10,895.

10. Yao, S. N. and Kurachi, K. (1992) Expression of human factor IX in mice after injection of genetically modified myoblasts. *Proc. Natl. Acad. Sci. USA* **89,** 3357–3361.

11. Lozier, J. N. and Brinkhous, K. M. (1994) Gene therapy and the hemophilias. *JAMA* **271,** 47–51.

12. Tripathy, S. K., Svensson, E. C., Black, H. B., Goldwasser, E., Margalith, M., Hobart, P. M., and Leiden, J. M. (1996) Long-term expression of erythropoietin in the systemic circulation of mice after intramuscular injection of a plasmid DNA vector. *Proc. Natl. Acad. Sci. USA* **93,** 10,876–10,880.

13. Ledley, F. D. (1996) Pharmaceutical approach to somatic gene therapy. *Pharm. Res.* **13,** 1595–1614.

14. Lee, C. C., Pons, F., Jones, P. G., Bies, R. D., Schlang, A. M., Leger, J. J., and Caskey, C. T. (1993) Mdx transgenic mouse: restoration of recombinant dystrophin to the dystrophic muscle. *Hum. Gene Ther.* **4,** 273–281.

15. Davis, H. L., Whalen, R. G., and Demeneix, B. A. (1993) Direct gene transfer into skeletal muscle in vivo: factors affecting efficiency of transfer and stability of expression. *Hum. Gene Ther.* **4,** 151–159.

16. Davis, H. L., Michel, M. L., Mancini, M., Schleef, M., and Whalen, R. G. (1994) Direct gene transfer in skeletal muscle: plasmid DNA-based immunization against the hepatitis B virus surface antigen. *Vaccine* **12,** 1503–1509.

17. Manthorpe, M., Cornefert-Jensen, F., Hartikka, J., Felgner, J., Rundell, A., Margalith, M., and Dwarki, V. (1993) Gene therapy by intramuscular injection of plasmid DNA: studies on firefly luciferase gene expression in mice. *Hum. Gene Ther.* **4,** 419–431.

18. Bartlett, R. J., Secore, S. L., Singer, J. T., Bodo, M., Sharma, K., and Ricordi, C. (1996) Long-term expression of a fluorescent reporter gene via direct injection of plasmid vector into mouse skeletal muscle: comparison of human creatine kinase and CMV promoter expression levels in vivo. *Cell Transplant* **5,** 411–419.

19. Dunckley, M. G., Wells, D. J., Walsh, F. S., and Dickson, G. (1993) Direct retroviral-mediated transfer of a dystrophin minigene into mdx mouse muscle in vivo. *Hum. Mol. Genet.* **2,** 717–723.

20. Ragot, T., Vincent, N., Chafey, P., Vigne, E., Gilgenkrantz, H., Couton, D., et al. (1993) Efficient adenovirus-mediated transfer of a human mini-dystrophin gene to skeletal muscle of mdx mice. *Nature* **361,** 647–650.

21. Vincent, N., Ragot, T., Gilgenkrantz, H., Couton, D., Chafey, P., Gregoire, A., et al. (1993) Long-term correction of mouse dystrophic degeneration by

adenovirus-mediated transfer of a minidystrophin gene. *Nature Genet.* **5,** 130–134.

22. Morishita, R., Gibbons, G. H., Kaneda, Y., Ogihara, T., and Dzau, V. J. (1993) Novel and effective gene transfer technique for study of vascular renin angiotensin system. *J. Clin. Invest.* **91,** 2580–2585.

23. Kaneda, Y., Iwai, K., and Uchida, T. (1989) Introduction and expression of the human insulin gene in adult rat liver. *J. Biol. Chem.* **264,** 12,126–12,129.

24. Kaneda, Y., Iwai, K., and Uchida, T. (1989) Increased expression of DNA cointroduced with nuclear protein in adult rat liver. *Science* **243,** 375–378.

25. Felgner, P. L., Gadek, T. R., Holm, M., Roman, R., Chan, H. W., Wenz, M., et al. (1987) Lipofection: a highly efficient, lipid-mediated DNA-transfection procedure. *Proc. Natl. Acad. Sci. USA* **84,** 7413–7417.

26. Nabel, E. G., Gordon, D., Yang, Z. Y., Xu, L., San, H., Plautz, G. E., et al. (1992) Gene transfer in vivo with DNA-liposome complexes: lack of autoimmunity and gonadal localization. *Hum. Gene Ther.* **3,** 649–656.

27. San, H., Yang, Z. Y., Pompili, V. J., Jaffe, M. L., Plautz, G. E., Xu, L., Felgner, J. H., Wheeler, C. J., et al. (1993) Safety and short-term toxicity of a novel cationic lipid formulation for human gene therapy. *Hum. Gene Ther.* **4,** 781–788.

28. Levy, M. Y., Barron, L. G., Meyer, K. B., and Szoka, F. C., Jr. (1996) Characterization of plasmid DNA transfer into mouse skeletal muscle: evaluation of uptake mechanism, expression and secretion of gene products into blood. *Gene Ther.* **3,** 201–211.

29. Nabel, E. G., Plautz, G., Boyce, F. M., Stanley, J. C., and Nabel, G. J. (1989) Recombinant gene expression in vivo within endothelial cells of the arterial wall. *Science* **244,** 1342–1344.

30. Nelson, D. L., Ledbetter, S. A., Corbo, L., Victoria, M. F., Ramirez-Solis, R., Webster, T. D., Ledbetter, D. H., and Caskey, C. T. (1989) Alu polymerase chain reaction: a method for rapid isolation of human-specific sequences from complex DNA sources. *Proc. Natl. Acad. Sci. USA* **86,** 6686–6690.

31. Hock, R. A. and Miller, A. D. (1986) Retrovirus-mediated transfer and expression of drug resistance genes in human haematopoietic progenitor cells. *Nature* **320,** 275–277.

32. Cone, R. D. and Mulligan, R. C. (1984) High-efficiency gene transfer into mammalian cells: generation of helper-free recombinant retrovirus with broad mammalian host range. *Proc. Natl. Acad. Sci. USA* **81,** 6349–6353.

33. Naldini, L., Blomer, U., Gallay, P., Ory, D., Mulligan, R., Gage, F. H., Verma, I. M., and Trono, D. (1996) In vivo gene delivery and stable transduction of nondividing cells by a lentiviral vector. *Science* **272,** 263–267.

34. Dai, Y., Schwarz, E. M., Gu, D., Zhang, W. W., Sarvetnick, N., and Verma, I. M. (1995) Cellular and humoral immune responses to adenoviral vectors containing factor IX gene: tolerization of factor IX and vector antigens allows for long-term expression. *Proc. Natl. Acad. Sci. USA* **92,** 1401–1405.

35. Yang, Y., Nunes, F. A., Berencsi, K., Furth, E. E., Gonczol, E., and Wilson, J. M. (1994) Cellular immunity to viral antigens limits E1-deleted adenoviruses for gene therapy. *Proc. Natl. Acad. Sci. USA* **91,** 4407–4411.

36. Muzyczka, N. (1992) Use of adeno-associated virus as a general transduction vector for mammalian cells. *Curr. Top. Microbiol. Immunol.* **158,** 97–129.

37. Flotte, T. R. and Carter, B. J. (1995) Adeno-associated virus vectors for gene therapy. *Gene Ther.* **2,** 357–362.

38. Xiao, X., Li, J., McCown, T. J., and Samulski, R. J. (1997) Gene transfer by adeno-associated virus vectors into the central nervous system. *Exp. Neurol.* **144,** 113–124.

39. Kaplitt, M. G. and Makimura, H. (1997) Defective viral vectors as agents for gene transfer in the nervous system. *J. Neurosci. Methods* **71,** 125–132.

40. Wagner, J. A. and Gardner, P. (1997) Toward cystic fibrosis gene therapy. *Annu. Rev. Med.* **48,** 203–216.

41. Xiao, X., deVlamink, W., and Monahan, J. (1993) Adeno-associated virus (AAV) vectors for gene transfer. *Adv. Drug Deliv. Rev.* **12,** 201–215.

42. Flotte, T. R., Afione, S. A., and Zeitlin, P. L. (1994) Adeno-associated virus vector gene expression occurs in nondividing cells in the absence of vector DNA integration. *Am. J. Respir. Cell Mol. Biol.* **11,** 517–521.

43. Podsakoff, G., Wong, K. K., Jr., and Chatterjee, S. (1994) Efficient gene transfer into nondividing cells by adeno-associated virus-based vectors. *J. Virol.* **68,** 5656–5666.

44. Russell, D. W., Miller, A. D., and Alexander, I. E. (1994) Adeno-associated virus vectors preferentially transduce cells in S phase. *Proc. Natl. Acad. Sci. USA* **91,** 8915–8919.

45. Halbert, C. L., Alexander, I. E., Wolgamot, G. M., and Miller, A. D. (1995) Adeno-associated virus vectors transduce primary cells much less efficiently than immortalized cells. *J. Virol.* **69,** 1473–1479.

46. Blacklow, N. R., Hoggan, M. D., and Rowe, W. P. (1968) Serologic evidence for human infection with adenovirus-associated viruses. *J. Natl. Cancer Inst.* **40,** 319–327.

47. Berns, K. I. and Bohenzky, R. A. (1987) Adeno-associated viruses: an update. *Adv. Virus Res.* **32,** 243–306.

48. Berns, K. I. and Linden, R. M. (1995) Cryptic life style of adeno-associated virus. *Bioessays* **17,** 237–245.

49. Walz, C. and Schlehofer, J. R. (1992) Modification of some biological properties of HeLa cells containing adeno-associated virus DNA integrated into chromosome 19. *J. Virol.* **66,** 2990–3002.

50. Flotte, T. R., Solow, R., Owens, R. A., Afione, S., Zeitlin, P. L., and Carter, B. J. (1992) Gene expression from adeno-associated virus vectors in airway epithelial cells. *Am. J. Respir. Cell Mol. Biol.* **7,** 349–356.

51. Tamayose, K., Hirai, Y., and Shimada, T. (1996) New strategy for large-scale preparation of high-titer recombinant adeno-associated virus vectors by using packaging cell lines and sulfonated cellulose column chromatography. *Hum. Gene Ther.* **7,** 507–513.

52. Inoue, N. and Russell, D. W. (1998) Packaging cells based on inducible gene amplification for the production of adeno-associated virus vectors. *J. Virol.* **72,** 7024–7031.

53. Salvetti, A., Oreve, S., Chadeuf, G., Favre, D., Cherel, Y., Champion-Arnaud, P., David-Ameline, J., and Moullier, P. (1998) Factors influencing recombinant adeno-associated virus production. *Hum. Gene Ther.* **9**, 695–706.

54. Ding, L., Lu, S., and Munshi, N. C. (1997) In vitro packaging of an infectious recombinant adeno-associated virus 2. *Gene Ther.* **4**, 1167–1172.

55. Conway, J. E., Zolotukhin, S., Muzyczka, N., Hayward, G. S., and Byrne, B. J. (1997) Recombinant adeno-associated virus type 2 replication and packaging is entirely supported by a herpes simplex virus type 1 amplicon expressing Rep and Cap. *J. Virol.* **71**, 8780–8789.

56. Xiao, X., Li, J., and Samulski, R. J. (1998) Production of high-titer recombinant adeno-associated virus vectors in the absence of helper adenovirus. *J. Virol.* **72**, 2224–2232.

57. Kessler, P. D., Podsakoff, G. M., Chen, X., McQuiston, S. A., Colosi, P. C., Matelis, L. A., Kurtzman, G. J., and Byrne, B. J. (1996) Gene delivery to skeletal muscle results in sustained expression and systemic delivery of a therapeutic protein. *Proc. Natl. Acad. Sci. USA* **93**, 14,082–14,087.

58. McLaughlin, S. K., Collis, P., Hermonat, P. L., and Muzyczka, N. (1988) Adeno-associated virus general transduction vectors: analysis of proviral structures. *J. Virol.* **62**, 1963–1973.

59. Samulski, R. J., Chang, L. S., and Shenk, T. (1989) Helper-free stocks of recombinant adeno-associated viruses: normal integration does not require viral gene expression. *J. Virol.* **63**, 3822–3828.

60. Siegl, G., Bates, R. C., Berns, K. I., Carter, B. J., Kelly, D. C., Kurstak, E., and Tattersall, P. (1985) Characteristics and taxonomy of Parvoviridae. *Intervirology* **23**, 61–73.

61. Berns, K. I. (1990) Parvovirus replication. *Microbiol. Rev.* **54**, 316–329.

62. Atchinson, R. W., Casto, B. C., and Hammond, W. M. (1965) Adeno-associated defective virus particles. *Science* **149**, 754–756.

63. Hoggan, M. D., Blacklow, N. R., and Rowe, W. P. (1966) Studies of small DNA viruses found in various adenovirus preparations: physical, biological, and immunological characteristics. *Proc. Natl. Acad. Sci. USA* **55**, 1467–1474.

64. Handa, H., Shiroki, K., and Shimojo, H. (1977) Establishment and characterization of KB cell lines latently infected with adeno-associated virus type 1. *Virology* **82**, 84–92.

65. Cheung, A. K., Hoggan, M. D., Hauswirth, W. W., and Berns, K. I. (1980) Integration of the adeno-associated virus genome into cellular DNA in latently infected human Detroit 6 cells. *J. Virol.* **33**, 739–748.

66. Yakinoglu, A. O., Heilbronn, R., Burkle, A., Schlehofer, J. R., and zur Hausen, H. (1988) DNA amplification of adeno-associated virus as a response to cellular genotoxic stress. *Cancer Res.* **48**, 3123–3129.

67. Yakobson, B., Koch, T., and Winocour, E. (1987) Replication of adeno-associated virus in synchronized cells without the addition of a helper virus. *J. Virol.* **61**, 972–981.

68. Yakobson, B., Hrynko, T. A., Peak, M. J., and Winocour, E. (1989) Replication of adeno-associated virus in cells irradiated with UV light at 254 nm. *J. Virol.* **63**, 1023–1030.

69. Walz, C., Schlehofer, J. R., Flentje, M., Rudat, V., and zur Hausen, H. (1992) Adeno-associated virus sensitizes HeLa cell tumors to gamma rays. *J. Virol.* **66,** 5651–5657.
70. Rutledge, E. A., Halbert, C. L., and Russell, D. W. (1998) Infectious clones and vectors derived from adeno-associated virus (AAV) serotypes other than AAV type 2. *J. Virol.* **72,** 309–319.
71. Summerford, C. and Samulski, R. J. (1998) Membrane-associated heparan sulfate proteoglycan is a receptor for adeno-associated virus type 2 virions. *J. Virol.* **72,** 1438–1445.
72. Srivastava, A., Lusby, E. W., and Berns, K. I. (1983) Nucleotide sequence and organization of the adeno-associated virus 2 genome. *J. Virol.* **45,** 555–564.
73. Cassinotti, P., Weitz, M., and Tratschin, J. D. (1988) Organization of the adeno-associated virus (AAV) capsid gene: mapping of a minor spliced mRNA coding for virus capsid protein 1. *Virology* **167,** 176–184.
74. Becerra, S. P., Koczot, F., Fabisch, P., and Rose, J. A. (1988) Synthesis of adeno-associated virus structural proteins requires both alternative mRNA splicing and alternative initiations from a single transcript. *J. Virol.* **62,** 2745–2754.
75. Muralidhar, S., Becerra, S. P., and Rose, J. A. (1994) Site-directed mutagenesis of adeno-associated virus type 2 structural protein initiation codons: effects on regulation of synthesis and biological activity. *J. Virol.* **68,** 170–176.
76. Mendelson, E., Trempe, J. P., and Carter, B. J. (1986) Identification of the *trans*-acting Rep proteins of adeno-associated virus by antibodies to a synthetic oligopeptide. *J. Virol.* **60,** 823–832.
77. Tratschin, J. D., Miller, I. L., and Carter, B. J. (1984) Genetic analysis of adeno-associated virus: properties of deletion mutants constructed in vitro and evidence for an adeno-associated virus replication function. *J. Virol.* **51,** 611–619.
78. Owens, R. A. and Carter, B. J. (1992) In vitro resolution of adeno-associated virus DNA hairpin termini by wild-type Rep protein is inhibited by a dominant-negative mutant of rep. *J. Virol.* **66,** 1236–1240.
79. Hermonat, P. L., Labow, M. A., Wright, R., Berns, K. I., and Muzyczka, N. (1984) Genetics of adeno-associated virus: isolation and preliminary characterization of adeno-associated virus type 2 mutants. *J. Virol.* **51,** 329–339.
80. Senapathy, P., Tratschin, J. D., and Carter, B. J. (1984) Replication of adeno-associated virus DNA. Complementation of naturally occurring rep- mutants by a wild-type genome or an ori- mutant and correction of terminal palindrome deletions. *J. Mol. Biol.* **179,** 1–20.
81. Gottlieb, J. and Muzyczka, N. (1988) In vitro excision of adeno-associated virus DNA from recombinant plasmids: isolation of an enzyme fraction from HeLa cells that cleaves DNA at poly(G) sequences. *Mol. Cell Biol.* **8,** 2513–2522.
82. Hong, G., Ward, P., and Berns, K. I. (1992) In vitro replication of adeno-associated virus DNA. *Proc. Natl. Acad. Sci. USA* **89,** 4673–4677.
83. Hong, G., Ward, P., and Berns, K. I. (1994) Intermediates of adeno-associated virus DNA replication in vitro. *J. Virol.* **68,** 2011–2015.

84. Samulski, R. J., Berns, K. I., Tan, M., and Muzyczka, N. (1982) Cloning of adeno-associated virus into pBR322: rescue of intact virus from the recombinant plasmid in human cells. *Proc. Natl. Acad. Sci. USA* **79**, 2077–2081.

85. Samulski, R. J., Srivastava, A., Berns, K. I., and Muzyczka, N. (1983) Rescue of adeno-associated virus from recombinant plasmids: gene correction within the terminal repeats of AAV. *Cell* **33**, 135–143.

86. Lusby, E., Fife, K. H., and Berns, K. I. (1980) Nucleotide sequence of the inverted terminal repetition in adeno-associated virus DNA. *J. Virol.* **34**, 402–409.

87. Ni, T. H., Zhou, X., McCarty, D. M., Zolotukhin, I., and Muzyczka, N. (1994) In vitro replication of adeno-associated virus DNA. *J. Virol.* **68**, 1128–1138.

88. Srivastava A (1987) Replication of the adeno-associated virus DNA termini in vitro. *Intervirology* **27**, 138–147.

89. Wang, X. S. and Srivastava, A. (1998) Rescue and autonomous replication of adeno-associated virus type 2 genomes containing Rep binding site mutations in the viral p5 promoter. *J. Virol.* **72**, 4811–4818.

90. Qing, K., Khuntirat, B., Mah, C., Kube, D. M., Wang, X. S., Ponnazhagan, S., et al. (1998) Adeno-associated virus type 2-mediated gene transfer: correlation of tyrosine phosphorylation of the cellular single-stranded D sequence-binding protein with transgene expression in human cells in vitro and murine tissues in vivo. *J. Virol.* **72**, 1593–1599.

91. Qing, K., Wang, X. S., Kube, D. M., Ponnazhagan, S., Bajpai, A., and Srivastava, A. (1997) Role of tyrosine phosphorylation of a cellular protein in adeno-associated virus 2-mediated transgene expression. *Proc. Natl. Acad. Sci. USA* **94**, 10,879–10,884.

92. Im, D. S. and Muzyczka, N. (1990) AAV origin binding protein Rep68 is an ATP-dependent site-specific endonuclease with DNA helicase activity. *Cell* **61**, 447–457.

93. Leonard, C. J. and Berns, K. I. (1994) Adeno-associated virus type 2: a latent life cycle. *Prog. Nucleic Acid Res. Mol. Biol.* **48**, 29–52.

94. Labow, M. A. and Berns, K. I. (1988) Adeno-associated virus rep gene inhibits replication of an adeno-associated virus/simian virus 40 hybrid genome in cos-7 cells. *J. Virol.* **62**, 1705–1712.

95. Berns, K. I., Kotin, R. M., and Labow, M. A. (1988) Regulation of adeno-associated virus DNA replication. *Biochim. Biophys. Acta.* **951**, 425–429.

96. Beaton, A., Palumbo, P., and Berns, K. I. (1989) Expression from the adeno-associated virus p5 and p19 promoters is negatively regulated in trans by the rep protein. *J. Virol.* **63**, 4450–4454.

97. Linden, R. M., Ward, P., Giraud, C., Winocour, E., and Berns, K. I. (1996) Site-specific integration by adeno-associated virus. *Proc. Natl. Acad. Sci. USA* **93**, 11,288–11,294.

98. Kotin, R. M. and Berns, K. I. (1989) Organization of adeno-associated virus DNA in latently infected Detroit 6 cells. *Virology* **170**, 460–467.

99. Kotin, R. M., Menninger, J. C., Ward, D. C., and Berns, K. I. (1991) Mapping and direct visualization of a region-specific viral DNA integration site on chromosome 19q13-qter. *Genomics* **10**, 831–834.

100. Kotin, R. M., Siniscalco, M., Samulski, R. J., Zhu, X. D., Hunter, L., Laughlin, C. A., et al. (1990) Site-specific integration by adeno-associated virus. *Proc. Natl. Acad. Sci. USA* **87,** 2211–2215.

101. Laughlin, C. A., Cardellichio, C. B., and Coon, H. C. (1986) Latent infection of KB cells with adeno-associated virus type 2. *J. Virol.* **60,** 515–524.

102. Samulski, R. J., Zhu, X., Xiao, X., Brook, J. D., Housman, D. E., Epstein, N., and Hunter, L. A. (1991) Targeted integration of adeno-associated virus (AAV) into human chromosome 19. *EMBO J.* **10,** 3941–3950.

103. Buller, R. M., Janik, J. E., Sebring, E. D., and Rose, J. A. (1981) Herpes simplex virus types 1 and 2 completely help adenovirus-associated virus replication. *J. Virol.* **40,** 241–247.

104. Schlehofer, J. R., Ehrbar, M., and zur Hausen, H. (1986) Vaccinia virus, herpes simplex virus, and carcinogens induce DNA amplification in a human cell line and support replication of a helpervirus dependent parvovirus. *Virology* **152,** 110–117.

105. Chiorini, J. A., Wiener, S. M., Yang, L., Smith, R. H., Safer, B., Kilcoin, N. P., et al. (1996) Roles of AAV Rep proteins in gene expression and targeted integration. *Curr. Top. Microbiol. Immunol.* **218,** 25–33.

106. Wang, X. S. and Srivastava, A. (1997) A novel terminal resolution-like site in the adeno-associated virus type 2 genome. *J. Virol.* **71,** 1140–1146.

107. Ni, T. H., McDonald, W. F., Zolotukhin, I., Melendy, T., Waga, S., Stillman, B., and Muzyczka, N. (1998) Cellular proteins required for adeno-associated virus DNA replication in the absence of adenovirus coinfection. *J. Virol.* **72,** 2777–2787.

108. Kotin, R. M., Linden, R. M., and Berns, K. I. (1992) Characterization of a preferred site on human chromosome 19q for integration of adeno-associated virus DNA by non-homologous recombination. *EMBO J.* **11,** 5071–5078.

109. Giraud, C., Winocour, E., and Berns, K. I. (1994) Site-specific integration by adeno-associated virus is directed by a cellular DNA sequence. *Proc. Natl. Acad. Sci. USA* **91,** 10,039–10,043.

110. Weitzman, M. D., Kyostio, S. R., Kotin, R. M., and Owens, R. A. (1994) Adeno-associated virus (AAV) Rep proteins mediate complex formation between AAV DNA and its integration site in human DNA. *Proc. Natl. Acad. Sci. USA* **91,** 5808–5812.

111. Chiorini, J. A., Wiener, S. M., Owens, R. A., Kyostio, S. R., Kotin, R. M., and Safer, B. (1994) Sequence requirements for stable binding and function of Rep68 on the adeno-associated virus type 2 inverted terminal repeats. *J. Virol.* **68,** 7448–7457.

112. Snyder, R. O., Im, D. S., Ni, T., Xiao, X., Samulski, R. J., and Muzyczka, N. (1993) Features of the adeno-associated virus origin involved in substrate recognition by the viral Rep protein. *J. Virol.* **67,** 6096–6104.

113. Berns, K. I. (1996) in *Papoviridae: The Viruses and Their Replication,* vol. 2 (Fields, B. N., Knipe, D. M., and Howley, P. M., eds.), Lippincott-Raven, Philadelphia, pp. 2173–2220.

114. Wonderling, R. S. and Owens, R. A. (1997) Binding sites for adeno-associated virus Rep proteins within the human genome. *J. Virol.* **71,** 2528–2534.

115. Surosky, R. T., Urabe, M., Godwin, S. G., McQuiston, S. A., Kurtzman, G. J., Ozawa, K., and Natsoulis, G. (1997) Adeno-associated virus Rep proteins target DNA sequences to a unique locus in the human genome. *J. Virol.* **71,** 7951–7959.

116. Xiao, X., Li, J., and Samulski, R. J. (1996) Efficient long-term gene transfer into muscle tissue of immunocompetent mice by adeno-associated virus vector. *J. Virol.* **70,** 8098–8108.

117. Clark, K. R., Sferra, T. J., and Johnson, P. R. (1997) Recombinant adeno-associated viral vectors mediate long-term transgene expression in muscle. *Hum. Gene Ther.* **8,** 659–669.

118. Fisher, K. J., Jooss, K., Alston, J., Yang, Y., Haecker, S. E., High, K., Pathak, R., Raper, S. E., and Wilson, J. M. (1997) Recombinant adeno-associated virus for muscle directed gene therapy. *Nature Med.* **3,** 306–312.

119. Herzog, R. W., Hagstrom, J. N., Kung, S. H., Tai, S. J., Wilson, J. M., Fisher, K. J., and High, K. A. (1997) Stable gene transfer and expression of human blood coagulation factor IX after intramuscular injection of recombinant adeno-associated virus. *Proc. Natl. Acad. Sci. USA* **94,** 5804–5809.

120. Monahan, P. E., Samulski, R. J., Tazelaar, J., Xiao, X., Nichols, T. C., Bellinger, D. A., Read, M. S., and Walsh, C. E. (1998) Direct intramuscular injection with recombinant AAV vectors results in sustained expression in a dog model of hemophilia. *Gene Ther.* **5,** 40–49.

121. Kaplitt, M. G., Leone, P., Samulski, R. J., Xiao, X., Pfaff, D. W., O'Malley, K. L., and During, M. J. (1994) Long-term gene expression and phenotypic correction using adeno-associated virus vectors in the mammalian brain. *Nature Genet.* **8,** 148–154.

122. McCown, T. J., Xiao, X., Li, J., Breese, G. R., and Samulski, R. J. (1996) Differential and persistent expression patterns of CNS gene transfer by an adeno-associated virus (AAV) vector. *Brain Res.* **713,** 99–107.

123. Kaplitt, M. G. and Pfaff, D. W. (1996) Viral vectors for gene delivery and expression in the CNS. *Methods* **10,** 343–350.

124. Flannery, J. G., Zolotukhin, S., Vaquero, M. I., LaVail, M. M., Muzyczka, N., and Hauswirth, W. W. (1997) Efficient photoreceptor-targeted gene expression in vivo by recombinant adeno-associated virus. *Proc. Natl. Acad. Sci. USA* **94,** 6916–6921.

125. Flotte, T. R., Afione, S. A., Solow, R., Drumm, M. L., Markakis, D., Guggino, W. B., Zeitlin, P. L., and Carter, B. J. (1993) Expression of the cystic fibrosis transmembrane conductance regulator from a novel adeno-associated virus promoter. *J. Biol. Chem.* **268,** 3781–3790.

126. Afione, S. A., Conrad, C. K., Kearns, W. G., Chunduru, S., Adams, R., Reynolds, T. C., et al. (1996) In vivo model of adeno-associated virus vector persistence and rescue. *J. Virol.* **70,** 3235–3241.

127. Koeberl, D. D., Alexander, I. E., Halbert, C. L., Russell, D. W., and Miller, A. D. (1997) Persistent expression of human clotting factor IX from mouse liver after intravenous injection of adeno-associated virus vectors. *Proc. Natl. Acad. Sci. USA* **94,** 1426–1431.

128. Snyder, R. O., Miao, C. H., Patijn, G. A., Spratt, S. K., Danos, O., Nagy, D., Gown, A. M., Winther, B., Meuse, L., Cohen, L. K., Thompson, A. R., and Kay, M. A. (1997) Persistent and therapeutic concentrations of human factor IX in mice after hepatic gene transfer of recombinant AAV vectors. *Nature Genet.* **16**, 270–276.

129. Shaughnessy, E., Lu, D., Chatterjee, S., and Wong, K. K. (1996) Parvoviral vectors for the gene therapy of cancer. *Semin. Oncol.* **23**, 159–171.

130. Wong, K. K., Jr. and Chatterjee, S. (1996) Adeno-associated virus based vectors as antivirals. *Curr. Top. Microbiol. Immunol.* **218**, 145–170.

131. Russell, D. W. and Hirata, R. K. (1998) Human gene targeting by viral vectors. *Nature Genet.* **18**, 325–330.

132. Xiao, X., Xiao, W., Li, J., and Samulski, R. J. (1997) Novel 165-base-pair terminal repeat sequence is the sole *cis* requirement for the adeno-associated virus life cycle. *J. Virol.* **71**, 941–948.

133. Bowers, W. J., Howard, D. F., and Federoff, H. J. (1997) Gene therapeutic strategies for neuroprotection: implications for Parkinson's disease. *Exp. Neurol.* **144**, 58–68.

134. Kohn, D. B. (1997) Gene therapy for haematopoietic and lymphoid disorders. *Clin Exp Immunol.* **107(Suppl 1)**, 54–57.

135. Duan, D., Fisher, K. J., Burda, J. F., and Engelhardt, J. F. (1997) Structural and functional heterogeneity of integrated recombinant AAV genomes. *Virus Res.* **48**, 41–56.

136. Samulski, R. J. (1993) Adeno-associated virus: integration at a specific chromosomal locus. *Curr. Opin. Genet. Dev.* **3**, 74–80.

137. Walsh, C. E., Liu, J. M., Xiao, X., Young, N. S., Nienhuis, A. W., and Samulski, R. J. (1992) Regulated high level expression of a human gamma-globin gene introduced into erythroid cells by an adeno-associated virus vector. *Proc. Natl. Acad. Sci. USA.* **89**, 7257–7261.

138. Rutledge, E. A. and Russell, D. W. (1997) Adeno-associated virus vector integration junctions. *J. Virol.* **71**, 8429–8436.

139. Wu, P., Phillips, M. I., Bui, J., and Terwilliger, E. F. (1998) Adeno-associated virus vector-mediated transgene integration into neurons and other nondividing cell targets. *J. Virol.* **72**, 5919–5926.

140. Minami, M., Poussin, K., Brechot, C., and Paterlini, P. (1995) Novel PCR technique using Alu-specific primers to identify unknown flanking sequences from the human genome. *Genomics* **29**, 403–408.

141. Kube, D. M., Ponnazhagan, S., and Srivastava, A. (1997) Encapsidation of adeno-associated virus type 2 Rep proteins in wild-type and recombinant progeny virions: Rep-mediated growth inhibition of primary human cells. *J. Virol.* **71**, 7361–7371.

142. Prasad, K. M. and Trempe, J. P. (1995) Adeno-associated virus Rep78 protein is covalently linked to viral DNA in a preformed virion. *Virology* **214**, 360–370.

143. Ferrari, F. K., Samulski, T., Shenk, T., and Samulski, R. J. (1996) Second-strand synthesis is a rate-limiting step for efficient transduction by recombinant adeno-associated virus vectors. *J. Virol.* **70**, 3227–3234.

144. Fisher, K. J., Gao, G. P., Weitzman, M. D., DeMatteo, R., Burda, J. F., and Wilson, J. M. (1996) Transduction with recombinant adeno-associated virus for gene therapy is limited by leading-strand synthesis. *J. Virol.* **70**, 520–532.

145. Alexander, I. E., Russell, D. W., and Miller, A. D. (1994) DNA-damaging agents greatly increase the transduction of nondividing cells by adeno-associated virus vectors. *J. Virol.* **68**, 8282–8287.

146. Alexander, I. E., Russell, D. W., Spence, A. M., and Miller, A. D. (1996) Effects of gamma irradiation on the transduction of dividing and nondividing cells in brain and muscle of rats by adeno-associated virus vectors. *Hum. Gene Ther.* **7**, 841–850.

147. Fisher, K. J., Kelley, W. M., Burda, J. F., and Wilson, J. M. (1996) Novel adenovirus-adeno-associated virus hybrid vector that displays efficient rescue and delivery of the AAV genome. *Hum. Gene Ther.* **7**, 2079–2087.

148. Wilson, J. M., Birinyi, L. K., Salomon, R. N., Libby, P., Callow, A. D., and Mulligan, R. C. (1989) Implantation of vascular grafts lined with genetically modified endothelial cells. *Science* **244**, 1344–1346.

149. Crystal, R. G. (1995) Transfer of genes to humans: early lessons and obstacles to success. *Science* **270**, 404–410.

150. Ertl, H. C. and Xiang, Z. (1996) Novel vaccine approaches. *J. Immunol.* **156**, 3579–3582.

151. Descamps, V., Duffour, M. T., Mathieu, M. C., Fernandez, N., Cordier, L., Abina, M. A., et al. (1996) Strategies for cancer gene therapy using adenoviral vectors. *J. Mol. Med.* **74**, 183–189.

152. Lew, D., Parker, S. E., Latimer, T., Abai, A. M., Kuwahara-Rundell, A., Doh, S. G., et al. (1995) Cancer gene therapy using plasmid DNA: pharmacokinetic study of DNA following injection in mice. *Hum. Gene Ther.* **6**, 553–564.

153. Mullen, C. A. and Blaese, R. M. (1996) Gene therapy of cancer. *Cancer Chemother. Biol. Response Modif.* **16**, 285–294.

154. Parker, S. E., Vahlsing, H. L., Serfilippi, L. M., Franklin, C. L., Doh, S. G., Gromkowski, S. H., et al. (1995) Cancer gene therapy using plasmid DNA: safety evaluation in rodents and non-human primates. *Hum. Gene Ther.* **6**, 575–590.

155. Ulmer, J. B., Donnelly, J. J., Parker, S. E., Rhodes, G. H., Felgner, P. L., Dwarki, V. J., et al. (1993) Heterologous protection against influenza by injection of DNA encoding a viral protein. *Science* **259**, 1745–1749.

156. Kohn, D. B. and Sarver, N. (1996) Gene therapy for HIV-1 infection. *Adv. Exp. Med. Biol.* **394**, 421–428.

157. Van Ginkel, F. W., Liu, C., Simecka, J. W., Dong, J. Y., Greenway, T., Frizzell, R. A., et al. (1995) Intratracheal gene delivery with adenoviral vector induces elevated systemic IgG and mucosal IgA antibodies to adenovirus and beta-galactosidase. *Hum. Gene Ther.* **6**, 895–903.

158. Gao, G. P., Yang, Y., and Wilson, J. M. (1996) Biology of adenovirus vectors with E1 and E4 deletions for liver-directed gene therapy. *J. Virol.* **70**, 8934–8943.

159. Yang, Y., Greenough, K., and Wilson, J. M. (1996) Transient immune blockade prevents formation of neutralizing antibody to recombinant adenovirus and allows repeated gene transfer to mouse liver. *Gene Ther.* **3**, 412–420.

160. Barr, D., Tubb, J., Ferguson, D., Scaria, A., Lieber, A., Wilson, C., Perkins, J., and Kay, M. A. (1995) Strain related variations in adenovirally mediated transgene expression from mouse hepatocytes in vivo: comparisons between immunocompetent and immunodeficient inbred strains. *Gene Ther.* **2**, 151–155.
161. Acsadi, G., Lochmuller, H., Jani, A., Huard, J., Massie, B., Prescott, S., et al. (1996) Dystrophin expression in muscles of mdx mice after adenovirus-mediated in vivo gene transfer. *Hum. Gene Ther.* **7**, 129–140.
162. Yang, Y., Jooss, K. U., Su, Q., Ertl, H. C., and Wilson, J. M. (1996) Immune responses to viral antigens versus transgene product in the elimination of recombinant adenovirus-infected hepatocytes in vivo. *Gene Ther.* **3**, 137–144.
163. McCoy, R. D., Davidson, B. L., Roessler, B. J., Huffnagle, G. B., Janich, S. L., Laing, T. J., and Simon, R. H. (1995) Pulmonary inflammation induced by incomplete or inactivated adenoviral particles. *Hum. Gene Ther.* **6**, 1553–1560.
164. Kotin, R. M. (1994) Prospects for the use of adeno-associated virus as a vector for human gene therapy. *Hum. Gene Ther.* **5**, 793–801.
165. Jooss, K., Yang, Y., Fisher, K. J., and Wilson, J. M. (1998) Transduction of dendritic cells by DNA viral vectors directs the immune response to transgene products in muscle fibers. *J. Virol.* **72**, 4212–4223.
166. Manning, W. C., Zhou, S., Bland, M. P., Escobedo, J. A., and Dwarki, V. (1998) Transient immunosuppression allows transgene expression following readministration of adeno associated viral vectors. *Hum. Gene Ther.* **9**, 477–485.
167. Flotte, T. R., Afione, S. A., Solow, R., Drumm, M. L., Markakis, D., Guggino, W. B., Zeitlin, P. L., and Carter, B. J. (1993) Expression of the cystic fibrosis transmembrane conductance regulator from a novel adeno associated virus promoter. *J. Biol. Chem.* **268**, 3781–3790.
168. Baudard, M., Flotte, T. R., Aran, J. M., Thierry, A. R., Pastan, I., Pang, M. G., Kearns, W. G., and Gottesman, M. M. (1996) Expression of the human multidrug resistance and glucocerebrosidase cDNAs from adeno-associated vectors: efficient promoter activity of AAV sequences and in vivo delivery via liposomes. *Hum. Gene Ther.* **7**, 1309–1322.
169. Chang, L. S., Shi, Y., and Shenk, T. (1989) Adeno-associated virus P5 promoter contains an adenovirus E1A-inducible element and a binding site for the major late transcription factor. *J. Virol.* **63**, 3479–3488.
170. Shi, Y., Seto, E., Chang, L. S., and Shenk, T. (1991) Transcriptional repression by YY1, a human GLI-Kruppel-related protein, and relief of repression by adenovirus E1A protein. *Cell* **67**, 377–388.
171. Smale, S. T. and Baltimore, D. (1989) "Initiator" as a transcription control element. *Cell* **57**, 103–113.
172. Urabe, M., Hasumi, Y., Ogasawara, Y., Matsushita, T., Kamoshita, N., Nomoto, A., et al. (1997) Novel dicistronic AAV vector using a short IRES segment derived from hepatitis C virus genome. *Gene* **200**, 157–162.
173. Mizuno, M. and Yoshida, J. (1998) Improvement of transduction efficiency of recombinant adeno-associated virus vector by entrapment in multilamellar liposomes. *Jpn. J. Cancer Res.* **89**, 352–354.

174. Doll, R. F., Crandall, J. E., Dyer, C. A., Aucoin, J. M., and Smith, F. I. (1996) Comparison of promoter strengths on gene delivery into mammalian brain cells using AAV vectors. *Gene Ther.* **3**, 437–447.

175. Philip, R., Brunette, E., Kilinski, L., Murugesh, D., McNally, M. A., Ucar, K., et al. (1994) Efficient and sustained gene expression in primary T lymphocytes and primary and cultured tumor cells mediated by adeno-associated virusplasmid DNA complexed to cationic liposomes. *Mol. Cell Biol.* **14**, 2411–2418.

176. Fu, Y., Wang, Y., and Evans, S. M. (1998) Viral sequences enable efficient and tissue-specific expression of transgenes in *Xenopus. Nat. Biotechnol.* **16**, 253–257.

177. Fisher, K. J., Kelley, W. M., Burda, J. F., and Wilson, J. M. (1996) Novel adenovirus-adeno-associated virus hybrid vector that displays efficient rescue and delivery of the AAV genome. *Hum. Gene Ther.* **7**, 2079–2087.

178. Flotte, T. R. and Carter, B. J. (1997) In vivo gene therapy with adeno-associated virus vectors for cystic fibrosis. *Adv. Pharmacol.* **40**, 85–101.

179. Johnston, K. M., Jacoby, D., Pechan, P. A., Fraefel, C., Borghesani, P., Schuback, D., et al. (1997) HSV/AAV hybrid amplicon vectors extend transgene expression in human glioma cells. *Hum. Gene Ther.* **8**, 359–370.

180. Fraefel, C., Jacoby, D. R., Lage, C., Hilderbrand, H., Chou, J. Y., Alt, F. W., Breakefield, X. O., and Majzoub, J. A. (1997) Gene transfer into hepatocytes mediated by helper virus-free HSV/AAV hybrid vectors. *Mol. Med.* **3**, 813–825.

181. Palombo, F., Monciotti, A., Recchia, A., Cortese, R., Ciliberto, G., and La Monica, N. (1998) Site-specific integration in mammalian cells mediated by a new hybrid baculovirus-adeno associated virus vector. *J. Virol.* **72**, 5025–5034.

182. Miller, J. L., Donahue, R. E., Sellers, S. E., Samulski, R. J., Young, N. S., and Nienhuis, A. W. (1994) Recombinant adeno-associated virus (rAAV)-mediated expression of a human gamma-globin gene in human progenitor-derived erythroid cells. *Proc. Natl. Acad. Sci. USA* **91**, 10,183–10,187.

183. Ponnazhagan, S., Mukherjee, P., Wang, X. S., Qing, K., Kube, D. M., Mah, C., et al. (1997) Adeno-associated virus type 2-mediated transduction in primary human bone marrow-derived CD34+ hematopoietic progenitor cells: donor variation and correlation of transgene expression with cellular differentiation. *J. Virol.* **71**, 8262–2867.

184. Walsh, C. E., Nienhuis, A. W., Samulski, R. J., Brown, M. G., Miller, J. L., Young, N. S., and Liu, J. M. (1994) Phenotypic correction of Fanconi anemia in human hematopoietic cells with a recombinant adeno associated virus vector. *J. Clin. Invest.* **94**, 1440–1448.

185. Blau, H. M. and Springer, M. L. (1995) Muscle-mediated gene therapy. *N. Engl. J. Med.* **333**, 1554–1556.

186. Miller, J. B. and Boyce, F. M. (1995) Gene therapy by and for muscle cells. *Trends Genet.* **11**, 163–165.

187. Xing, Z., Ohkawara, Y., Jordana, M., Graham, F. L., and Gauldie, J. (1997) Adenoviral vector-mediated interleukin-10 expression in vivo: intramuscular gene transfer inhibits cytokin responses in endotoxemia. *Gene Ther.* **4**, 140–149.

188. Miller, G., Steinbrecher, R. A., Murdock, P. J., Tuddenham, E. G., Lee, C. A., Pasi, K. J., and Goldspink, G. (1995) Expression of factor VII by muscle cells in vitro and in vivo following direct gene transfer: modelling gene therapy for haemophilia. *Gene Ther.* **2,** 736–742.

189. Goldman, M. J. and Wilson, J. M. (1995) Expression of alpha v beta 5 integrin is necessary for efficient adenovirus-mediated gene transfer in the human airway. *J. Virol.* **69,** 5951–5958.

190. Huard, J., Lochmuller, H., Acsadi, G., Jani, A., Holland, P., Guerin, C., Massie, B., and Karpati, G. (1995) Differential short-term transduction efficiency of adult versus newborn mouse tissues by adenoviral recombinants. *Exp. Mol. Pathol.* **62,** 131–143.

191. Snyder, R. O., Spratt, S. K., Lagarde, C., Bohl, D., Kaspar, B., Sloan, B., Cohen, L. K., and Danos, O. (1997) Efficient and stable adeno-associated virus-mediated transduction in the skeletal muscle of adult immunocompetent mice. *Hum. Gene Ther.* **8,** 1891–1900.

192. Kaplitt, M. G., Xiao, X., Samulski, R. J., Li, J., Ojamaa, K., Klein, I. L., et al. (1996) Long-term gene transfer in porcine myocardium after coronary infusion of an adeno-associated virus vector. *Ann. Thorac. Surg.* **62,** 1669–1676.

193. Rolling, F., Nong, Z., Pisvin, S., and Collen, D. (1997) Adeno-associated virus-mediated gene transfer into rat carotid arteries. *Gene Ther.* **4,** 757–761.

194. Maeda, Y., Ikeda, U., Ogasawara, Y., Urabe, M., Takizawa, T., Saito, T., Colosi, P., Kurtzman, G., Shimada, K., and Ozawa, K. (1997) Gene transfer into vascular cells using adeno-associated virus (AAV) vectors. *Cardiovasc. Res.* **35,** 514–521.

195. Halbert, C. L., Alexander, I. E., Wolgamot, G. M., and Miller, A. D. (1995) Adeno-associated virus vectors transduce primary cells much less efficiently than immortalized cells. *J. Virol.* **69,** 1473–1479.

196. Brange, J., Hallund, O., and Sorensen, E. (1992) Chemical stability of insulin. Isolation, charac-terization and identification of insulin transformation products. *Acta Pharm. Nord.* **4,** 223–232.

197. Kuo, W. L. and Montag, A. G., Rosner, M. R. (1993) Insulin-degrading enzyme is differentially expressed and developmentally regulated in various rat tissues. *Endocrinology* **132,** 604S–611S.

198. Kaufmann, J. E., Irminger, J. C., Mungall, J., Halban, P. A. (1997) Proinsulin conversion in GH3 cells after coexpression of human proinsulin with the endoproteases PC2 and/or PC3. *Diabetes* **46,** 978–82.

11

Rapid Establishment of Myeloma Cell Lines Expressing Fab(Tac)-Protamine, a Targetable Protein Vector, Directed Against High-Affinity α-Chain of Human Interleukin-2 Receptor

Sun U. Song and Wayne A. Marasco

1. Introduction

A recombinant bifunctional fusion protein, consisting of a recombinant antibody and a DNA-binding protein, can be used as a nonviral gene delivery vector (**Fig. 1**). In this lab, such a fusion protein, composed of a human antibody Fab(105) moiety against the envelope glycoprotein of HIV-1, gp120, and a human DNA-binding moiety (protamine), was developed (*1*). Chen et al. (*1*) showed that the bifunctional fusion protein complexed with plasmid DNA, encoding the catalytic subunit of *Pseudomonas* exotoxin, a complex known as a genetic immunotoxin, and was specifically transferred into HIV-1-infected cells by receptor-mediated endocytosis, resulting in selective killing of the target cells. However, the low level of Fab(105)-protamine fusion protein secreted from the stably transduced COS cells has been a limiting factor for experiments requiring large amounts of the fusion protein.

Myeloma cell lines have been used to express recombinant antibodies in high levels, using a glutamine synthetase (GS) gene as an amplifiable selectable marker (*2*). The same protocol was used for the production of a fusion protein consisting of Fab against human interleukin-2 receptor α-chain (IL-2Rα, Tac, CD25) and human protamine. The authors found that the selection and amplification steps using a GS marker were lengthy, and the surviving myeloma cells after amplification with methionine sulfoximine (MSX), which is an inhibitor of GS, were not stable when they were expanded. Therefore, a modified selection method, in which 5 μM MSX is added to the glutamine-free

From: *Methods in Molecular Biology, vol. 133: Gene Targeting Protocols*
Edited by: E. Kmiec © Humana Press Inc., Totowa, NJ

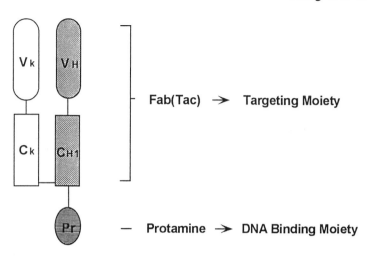

Fig. 1. Schematic diagram of Fab(Tac)-protamine fusion protein. Recombinant Fab(Tac) antibody is composed of Fd fragment (V_H and C_{H1}), and κ chain (V_L and C_L) which are connected by a disulfide bond. Protamine protein is fused with the carboxyl end of Fd.

selection medium, was tested. This method allowed establishment of stable myeloma cell lines expressing the fusion protein in 5–7 wk compared to 10–12 wk by the conventional method.

High-affinity IL-2R is a heterotrimer composed of α–, β– and λ–chains *(3)*. The β– and λ–chains (IL-2Rβ and $λ_c$) form a receptor of intermediate affinity, which is present on resting T-cells *(4)*. Expression of the 55-kDa α-chain, and hence the high-affinity receptor, occurs only transiently following engagement of the T-cell antigen receptor, and is a key point of regulation in the T-cell response to antigen.

The upregulation of IL-2Rα, in association with T-cell activation, has made this receptor chain a natural target for suppressive immunotherapy. Strategies based on blockage of the high-affinity receptor by monoclonal antibodies directed against IL-2Rα have been used to dampen a variety of undesirable T-cell-mediated reactions, including allograft rejection, graft-vs-host disease, and some forms of autoimmunity *(5)*. Furthermore, the constitutive upregulation of IL-2Rα in certain T- and B-cell malignancies has made this surface molecule a target for cytotoxic therapy. For example, one of the phenotypic hallmarks of leukemic cells from patients with adult T-cell leukemia (ATL), an aggressive and rapidly fatal T-cell malignancy associated with Human T-Cell leukemia virus (HTLV)-I infections, and T cells immortalized by HTLV-I in vitro, is the constitutive, high-level expression of IL-2Rα. Immunotoxins consisting of IL-2Rα antibody (either monoclonal or recombinant antibody) fused with toxin protein moiety, such as ricin A chain and *Pseudomonas* exotoxin, have been used to kill leukemic T-cells in ATL patients. This killing occurs as the result of endocytosis of the recombinant toxin moiety that is initiated by the binding of IL-2Rα antibody to the receptor *(5,6)*. However, directing protein immunotoxins to the IL-2Rα chain has met with limited success, because of the immunogenicity of the toxin protein moiety. The utilization of humanized murine or human antibodies has, to a great extent, solved the immunogenicity problem of the targeting moiety. Indeed, humanized antibodies to IL-2Rα have been made, and were shown to be less immunogenic than the murine version, when administered to monkeys *(7)*. However, for the highly immunogenic toxin moiety, the problem still remains.

The expression system described below will aid in determining if recombinant human Fab-protamine fusion proteins can be produced in adequate amounts to perform in vivo gene transfer studies to deliver a therapeutic gene(s) to target cells in small animals. This chapter explains the construction of Fab(Tac)-protamine-GS expression vector DNA and establishment of myeloma cell lines expressing Fab(Tac)-protamine fusion protein. The overall procedures for the production of Fab(Tac)-protamine fusion protein are shown in **Fig. 2**.

2. Materials

2.1. Construction of Fab(Tac)-Protamine-GS Expression DNA

1. Chinese hamster ovary (CHO) cells (obtained from American type culture collection ATCC).
2. RiboClone cDNA synthesis system (Promega, cat. no. C1630): oligo (dT) primer, Molloney murine leukemia virus MMLV reverse transcriptase, reaction buffers, ribonuclease inhibitor.
3. Primers for cloning of GS gene: forward (5'-TCT TAC TGG CGC GCC ACC ATG GCC ACC TCA GCA AGT TCC CAC TTG AAC AAA AAC-3') and reverse (5'-TAT TGC GGC CGC TTA TTA GTT TTT GTA TTG GAA GGG CTC GTC GCC AGT CTC-3').
4. Polymerase chain reaction (PCR) apparatus.
5. Cytomegalovirus (CMV) Promoter driving eukaryotic expression vector (pRC/CMV), (Invitrogen, Carlsbad, CA). (pRC/CMV) expression vector (Invitrogen, Carlsbad, CA).
6. In vitro transcription and translation-coupled (TNT) reaction system (Promega, cat. no. L4610): rabbit reticulocyte lysate, T7 RNA polymerase, amino acid mixture (minus cysteine), reaction buffer.
7. Restriction enzymes: *Asc*I, *Not*I, *Xba*I, *Nhe*I, and *Pac*I.
8. T4 DNA ligase.
9. Hybridoma cells producing anti-Tac monoclonal antibodies.
10. Primers for cloning of Fd and κ-chains of Fab(Tac): forward for Fd (5'-TTT TGG CGC GCC ACC ATG GAA AGG CAC TGG ATC-3') and reverse for Fd (5'-TTT TCT AGA AGG ACA GGG CTT GAT TGT-3'), forward for κ (5'-TTT

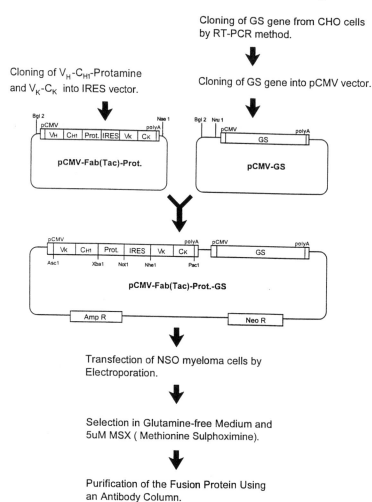

Fig. 2. Schematic representation of overall procedures for the production of Fab(Tac)-protamine fusion protein in NSO myeloma cells. GS gene is cloned from CHO cells using a set of primers made from the 5' end and 3' ends of GS coding sequence by PCR. GS gene was cloned into pRC/CMV expression vector. Fd and κ–chains are recovered by PCR from the hybridoma cells expressing anti-Tac monoclonal antibodies, and then cloned into IRES vector, which already contains the protamine sequence. pCMV-Fab(Tac)-protamine DNA is transferred to pCMV-GS vector to construct pCMV-Fab(Tac)-protamine-GS expression DNA. This construct is transfected into NSO myeloma cells. These myeloma cells are selected in glutamine-free plus 5 μM MSX, and then survived colonies are screened by FACS. The fusion protein is purified using an anti-body-affinity column.

GCT AGC ACC ATG CAT TTT CAA GTG CAG-3') and reverse for κ (5'-ACT GTT AAT TAA CTA CTA ACA CTC ATT CCT GTT GAA-3').

11. Internal ribosome entry site (IRES) vector (available in the lab): IRES sequence was transferred from pCITE2a (Novagene) into pRC/CMV vector.

2.2. Establishment of Myeloma Cell Lines Expressing Fab(Tac)-Protamine Fusion Protein

1. Culture medium for C8166 cells: RPMI 1640, 10% FBS.
2. Phosphate-buffered saline (PBS) (1X).
3. Linearized pCMV-Fab(Tac)-protamine-GS expression plasmid DNA (40 μg per transfection).
4. Gene pulser apparatus (Bio-Rad).
5. Cuvets for electroporation (Bio-Rad).
6. Ice.
7. 96-well tissue culture plates.
8. 24-well tissue culture plates.
9. Six-well tissue culture plates.
10. Eight-tip pipetor.
11. NSO mouse myeloma cell line (obtained from MRC).
12. MSX (Sigma, cat. no. M5379).
13. Selection medium (Gibco-BRL): RPMI 1640 (without L-glutamine), 10% calf serum (dialyzed), 10% NCTC-109, and minimum essential medium nonessential amino acids.
14. Fluorescent-activated cell sorting (FACS) solution: 1% FBS and 0.1% sodium azide in PBS.
15. Microcentrifuge and benchtop centrifuge.
16. Secondary antibodies (Boehringer Mannheim, Indianapolis, IN): goat antimouse IgG-fluorescein isothiocyanate (FITC)-labeled (cat. no. 60529) and goat antimouse IgG-Horse Radish Peroxidase (HRP)-conjugated (cat. no. 60530).
17. 4% Formaldehyde in PBS.
18. FACS tubes (Falcon, cat. no. 2052).

3. Methods

3.1. Construction of Fab(Tac)-Protamine-GS Expression DNA

3.1.1. Cloning of Glutamine Synthetase Gene

1. Total RNA is extracted from CHO cells using the guanidine thiocyanate method.
2. This RNA is used to synthesize cDNA using an oligo dT primer with RiboClone cDNA synthesis system (Promega).
3. Using a set of primers made from the 5' and 3' end of GS coding sequence *(8)*, the GS gene is amplified by PCR reaction.
4. The PCR products were cut with *Asc*I and *Not*I restriction enzymes and cloned into pRC/CMV expression vector, which was also cut with the same enzymes.
5. After cloning into the vector, GS gene was verified by DNA sequencing and in vitro TNT reaction system (Promega).

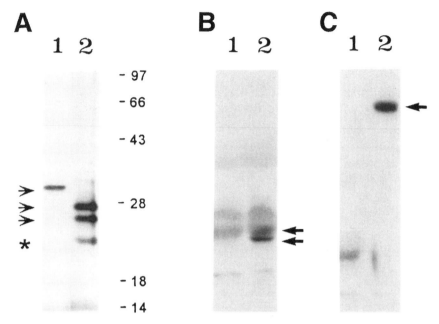

Fig. 3. In vitro TNT products of pCMV-Fab(Tac)-protamine construction and Western blot analysis of the concentrated supernatant from a FACS-screened positive clone. **(A)** The protein products from a TNT reaction of pCMV-Fab(Tac)-protamine construction. Lane 1, single-chain antibody against p17 of HIV-1. Lane 2, Fd-protamine and κ–chains of anti-Tac. Asterisk shows a prematurely terminated product. **(B)** SDS-PAGE gel under reducing conditions. Lane 1, fivefold concentrated culture medium. Lane 2, fivefold concentrated supernatant from a positive clone. Arrows show the denatured Fd-protamine and κ–chains. **(C)** SDS-PAGE gel under nonreducing conditions. Lane 1 and lane 2 are the same as in Panel B. The arrow shows the nondenatured Fab(Tac)-protamine protein.

3.1.2. Cloning of Fd and κ Chain of Fab(Tac)

Synthesis of cDNA, using total RNA from hybridoma cells producing monoclonal antibodies against Tac protein, was done with the same method described above. Using two different sets of primers, Fd and κ-chains were amplified by separate PCR reactions. These PCR fragments were digested with *Asc*I and *Xba*I for Fd fragments and *Nhe*I and *Pac*I for κ fragments, and then cloned into the IRES expression vector **(Fig. 2)**. The Fd coding sequence was cloned in-frame, with the coding sequence of protamine in the IRES vector. The sizes of Fd-protamine and κ-chains were also conformed by TNT reaction **(Fig. 3A)**.

3.1.3. Construction of pCMV-Fab(Tac)-Protamine-GS Expression DNA

To construct Fab(Tac)-protamine-GS expression DNA, as shown in **Fig. 2**, the *Bgl*II-*Nae*I DNA fragments of pCMV-Fab(Tac)-protamine vector were cloned into the pCMV-GS plasmid DNA cut with *Bgl*II and *Nru*I.

3.2. Establishment of Myeloma Cell Lines Expressing Fab(Tac)-Protamine Fusion Protein

3.2.1. Transfection of pCMV-Fab(Tac)-Protamine-GS Expression DNA into NSO Myeloma Cells

NSO mouse myeloma cells are harvested by centrifugation at 1,000 rpm for 5 min from cultures in exponential growth phase, washed once in PBS, and resuspended at 1×10^7 cells/mL in fresh PBS. Linearized pCMV-Fab(Tac)-protamine-GS plasmid DNA (40 µg in 0.1–0.2 mL H_2O or restriction enzyme buffer) with *Sma*I restriction enzyme, is added to 1×10^7 cells (*see* **Note 1**). The cells and DNA are then transferred into a cuvet and kept on ice for 5 min. This cuvet is then subjected to two pulses of 1500 V at a capacitance of 3 µF, using a Bio-Rad gene pulser. Cells are put back to ice for 5 min, and plated in 50 µL nonselective medium per well on a 96-well culture plate.

3.2.2. Selection in Glutamine-Free Medium and 5 µM Methionine Sulphoxiomine

On the day after transfection, 100 µL of selection medium (glutamine-free medium plus 5 µ*M* methionine sulphoximine) is added to each well of the 96-well plate, without replacing the nonselective medium. Plates are then incubated for 3–4 wk, until surviving colonies appear and become large enough to be transferred to 24-well plates, in completely glutamine-free medium (*see* **Note 2**). In the middle of this incubation period, usually 2 wk after the beginning of the selection, 50 µL fresh selection medium is added.

3.2.3. Screening of Selected Clones by Fluorescence Activated Cell Sorting

Once cells are confluent in a well of the 24-well plate, collect 100–200 µL culture medium from 1 mL culture, and use it as a primary antibody protein for FACS analysis.

1. Pellet the 1×10^6 C8166 cells, which is an HTLV-I immortalized T-cell line derived by in vitro infection of human cord blood and expresses high levels of Tac protein, by 20-s pulse in a microcentrifuge.
2. Discard the supernatant, and resuspend the cells in 1 mL cold FACS solution.
3. Pellet the cells again, and resuspend in 100–200 µL collected culture medium from a 24-well plate.
4. Incubate on ice for 1 h.
5. Add 1 mL cold FACS solution, and pellet the cells by centrifugation for 20 s.
6. Wash the cells once more with 1 mL cold FACS solution.
7. Prepare a 1:20 dilution of goat antimouse IgG-FITC-labeled secondary antibody in FACS solution.
8. Resuspend the cells in 50 µL of the secondary antibody.
9. Incubate on ice for 45 min in the dark, e.g., covered with foil.

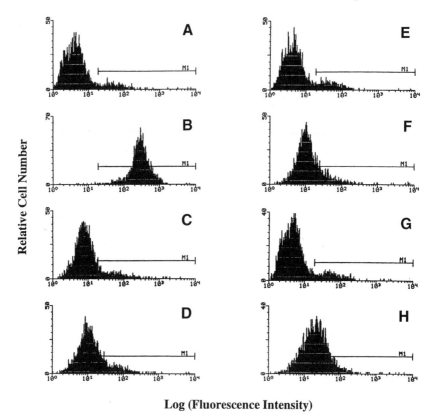

Log (Fluorescence Intensity)

Fig. 4. Examples of primary screening of Fab(Tac)-protamine producing clones by FACS analysis using Tac-expressing cells (C8166) on the cell surface. Supernatants from selected clones were incubated with C8166 cells, and Fab(Tac)-protamine protein was detected by antimouse IgG F(ab)′₂ conjugated with FITC. Binding was then analyzed by FACS. **(A)** Straight culture medium (negative control). **(B)** Supernatant from hybridoma cells expressing anti-Tac monoclonal antibodies (positive control). **(C–H)** Supernatants from six different selected clones.

10. Wash the cells twice with 1 mL cold FACS solution.
11. Resuspend the cells in 0.4 mL 4% formaldehyde in PBS and transfer to FACS tubes.
12. Store the tubes in the dark at 4°C until analyzed.

(Examples of the results of FACS analysis are shown in **Fig. 4.**)

4. Notes

1. When the number of selected clones from transfections, using either deproteinated DNA in H₂O after linearization with a restriction enzyme or DNA in restriction buffer, were compared, there was no difference between the types of DNA used

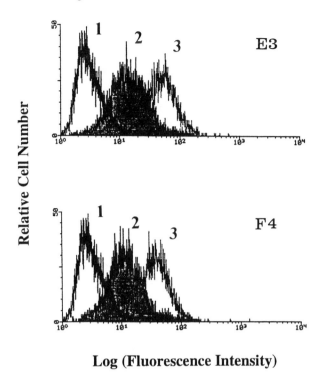

Log (Fluorescence Intensity)

Fig. 5. FACS analysis using the concentrated supernatants of two different positive clones. FACS analysis was done as described in **Fig. 4**. About fivefold concentrated supernatants of two positive clones (E3 and F4) were tested. Peak 1, fivefold concentrated culture medium (negative control). Peak 2, nonconcentrated supernatant of the positive clone. Peak 3, fivefold concentrated supernatant of the positive clone.

for transfection. However, a difference was observed in the number of selected clones between the blunt-ended, linearized DNA and stagger-ended DNA. The linearized DNA containing blunt ends generated about 4–5× as many clones as that with DNA with staggered ends.

2. About 20% of the selected clones in glutamine-free medium plus 5 μ*M* MSX died after they were transferred to a 24-well plate from a 96-well plate. All the surviving clones in the 24-well plates have been stable, and the expression of the fusion protein has not been changed for at least 4 mo. These selected cell lines have been kept in selection medium. Another advantage of this selection method is that most selected clones in a 96-well plate are single clones per well, so that a limiting dilution is not necessary for further subcloning.

3. There could be more binding of the fusion proteins to target cells, as shown in **Fig. 5**, when the supernatant concentrated from the positive clones using a protein concentrator (Amicon).

4. An affinity column of antimouse IgG coupled Sepharose has been shown to be the best way to purify this type of fusion protein. Binding was shown to be too tight to be eluted off a DNA-cellulose column. For details of the construction of fusion protein-DNA complexes, *see* Chen et al. *(1)*.

References

1. Chen, S.-Y., Zani, C., Khouri, Y. F., and Marasco, W. A. (1995) Design of a genetic immunotoxin to eliminate toxin immunogenicity. *Gene Ther.* **2,** 116–123.
2. Bebbington, C. R., Renner, G., Thomson, D., King, D., Abrams, D., and Yarranton, G. T. (1992) High-level expression of a recombinant antibody from myeloma cells using a glutamine synthetase gene as an amplifiable selectable marker. *Bio/Technology* **10,** 169–175.
3. Takeshita, T., Asao, H., Ohtani, K., Ishii, N., Kumaki, S., Tanaka, N., et al. (1992) Cloning of the r chain of the human IL-2 receptor. *Science* **257,** 379–382.
4. Bich-Thuy, L. T., Dukovich, M., Peffer N. J., Fauci, A. S., Kehrl, J. H., and Greene, W. C. (1987) Direct activation of human resting T cells by IL-2: the role of an IL-2 receptor distinct from the Tac protein. *J. Immunol.* **139,** 1550–1556.
5. Waldmann, T. A. (1994) Anti-IL-2 receptor monoclonal antibody (Anti-Tac) treatment of T-cell lymphoma. *Important Adv. Oncol.* 131–141.
6. Ramilo, O., Bell, K. D., Uhr, J. W., and Vitetta, E. S. (1993) Role of CD25+ and CD25- T cells in acute HIV infection in vitro. *J. Immunol.* **150,** 5202–5208.
7. Queen, C., Schneider, W. P., Selick, H. E., Payne, P. W., Landolfi, N. F., Duncan, J. F., et al. (1989) Humanized antibody that binds to the interleukin-2 receptor. *Proc. Natl. Acad. Sci. USA* **86,** 10,029–10,033.
8. Hayward, B. E., Hussain, A., Wilson, R. H., Lyons, A., Woodcock, V., McIntosh, B., and Harris, T. J. R. (1986) Cloning and nucleotide sequence of cDNA for an amplified glutamine synthetase gene from the Chinese hamster. *Nucleic Acid Res.* **14,** 999–1008.

12

EBV-Derived Episomes to Probe Chromatin Structure and Gene Expression in Human Cells

Juliette Fivaz, M. Chiara Bassi, Stéphane Pinaud, Larry Richman, Melanie Price, and Jovan Mirkovitch

1. Introduction

Gene therapy necessitates the controlled expression of the transferred gene. The expression of the most genes is regulated at the level of transcription initiation. Research in the past two decades has provided a wealth of information about the mechanisms of transcriptional control in human cells. The analysis of the promoter and enhancer DNA elements, and of the corresponding DNA-binding proteins, has provided an understanding of the basic mechanisms of transcription initiation *(1)*. This information is now used to devise gene expression cassettes for gene therapy.

However, It has become clear that the precise regulation of transcription by promoters and enhancers is dependent on still poorly characterized structures and sequences present in the genomic DNA when compacted into cell nuclei. Chromatin, the ill-defined cellular structure formed by the genomic DNA and its associated proteins *(2)*, is now considered a key player in gene expression. The maintenance of active or repressed transcriptional states, the stable inheritance of transcriptional expression patterns, and the homogeneous expression of a gene in a cell population, implicate regulation by DNA elements that are not part of the now-classical promoter-enhancer elements, and are controlled by proteins that are not simple transcription factors *(3,4)*. The goal of this chapter is to describe how to reconstitute in living cells such complex chromatin structures on defined DNA templates, which are placed on Epstein-Barr virus (EBV)-derived episomes.

The major protein constituents of chromatin are the core histone proteins, which, in the presence of DNA, assemble into nucleosomes. This basic structure

From: *Methods in Molecular Biology, vol. 133: Gene Targeting Protocols*
Edited by: E. Kmiec © Humana Press Inc., Totowa, NJ

of chromatin has been proposed to mediate both activation and repression of transcription for diverse genes by diverse mechanisms *(5,6)*. Higher-order structure of chromatin has been proposed to create independent expression domains in the genome *(7,8,9)*. In this case, boundary elements define a domain where expression is stable and independent of neighboring transcriptional units. These sequence elements, known as insulators, are of great interest for gene therapy, which requires the stable expression of transferred genes, independent of the local chromosomal context.

Because chromatin is a complex structure, the characterization of the respective roles of its diverse components has been a major challenge in understanding transcription regulation. In vitro studies, using reconstituted nucleosomes, have been instrumental in defining the problems the cell must solve, to regulate the transcription of its genes. On the other hand, the study of resident genes in intact cells or isolated nuclei, although technically challenging, is very informative, because the analyzed structures are assembled and maintained by the living cell. Unfortunately, in mammalian cells, the genomic DNA cannot be easily modified by homologous recombination, to test the role of various DNA sequences on chromatin structure and gene expression. In order to bypass that limitation, the authors have characterized a gene transfer system that can faithfully reproduce the regulation and chromatin structure found on original genes.

Most gene transfer systems, such as transient transfection or selection of stably integrated transformants, do not provide the homogeneous population required for the study of DNA protein structures. In transient transfection, usually most cells do not incorporate the template DNA, and, in those transfected cells, most of the template DNA does not participate in transcription because it is found in a large excess. The significance of studies conducted on stable transformants suffers from the clonal variation caused by the influence of neighboring sequence on the integrated construct. The EBV-derived episomes have been described as vectors for gene transfer *(10)*. The authors, and others, *(11,12)* have found that various gene-control elements are accurately regulated when placed on these templates, and reconstitute tissue-specific nucleosomal patterns. The use of EBV-derived episomes therefore constitutes a relatively simple procedure to obtain homogeneous structures on designed templates to probe the role of various chromatin components on gene expression. The contribution of various chromatin structures found on gene therapy expression cassettes can then be assessed in functional assays.

2. Materials

2.1. Cell Culture

Jurkat, Raji, and Daudi cells are grown in RPMI 1640 supplemented with 10% fetal calf serum (FCS). HeLa, 293, and U87MG cells are grown in

Dulbocco's modified Eagle's medium supplemented with 10% FCS. All cells are grown at 37°C in the presence of 5% CO_2. Cells are grown either in Sarstedt bacterial Petri dishes (Jurkat, Daudi, and Raji) or in Nunc tissue culture Petris or flasks (HeLa, 293, and U87MG).

2.2. Plasmids

Various episomal vectors can be obtained from Invitrogen, Carlsbad, CA. Plasmids pRcEBNA1, pHERL, and pHERG can be obtained from this laboratory. Plasmids are grown in DH5α or XL1-blue cells, and purified using Qiagen, Hilden, Germany midiprep kits.

2.3. Electroporation and Selection of Cells

The authors routinely use the Bio-Rad, Hercles, CA Gene Pulser with 0.4-cm Bio-Rad cuvets. Cells are selected with hygromycin (Boehringer Mannheim, Indianapolis, IN) at different concentrations for different cell lines.

2.4. Isolation of Nuclei

2.4.1. Stock Solutions to Keep at –20°C

1. A10x: 150 mM Tris-HCl, pH 7.4, 2 mM spermine, 5 mM spermidine, 20 mM K-EDTA, pH 7.4, 800 mM KCl.
2. A10x: 150 mM Tris-HCl, pH 7.4, 2 mM spermine, 5 mM spermidine, 800 mM KCl.
3. Spermine tetrahydrochloride (Sigma, St. Louis): 0.139 g/10 mL is 40 mM.
4. Spermidine trihydrochloride (Sigma): 0.255 g/10 mL is 100 mM.
5. Dithiothreitol (DTT): Dissolve in water at 1 M. Store aliquots at –20°C.
6. Thiodiglycol: from Fluka, Milwaukee, WI or Pierce, Rockford, IL, store at 4°C.
7. Proteinase K: Dissolve at 10 mg/mL in H_2O. Store aliquots at –20°C.
8. DNaseI (Boehringer Mannheim): Dissolve at 20 U/μL in 10 mM Tris-HCl, pH 7.4, 5 mM MgCl2, 5 mM CaCl2, 1 mM DTT, 50% glycerol. Stable at –20°C for a year.
9. Micrococcal nuclease (MN) (Worthington, Lakewood, NJ): Dissolve at 50 U/μL in 50 mM Tris-HCl, pH 8.0, 0.05 mM $CaCl_2$, 20% glycerol. Aliquots of 20 μL are stored at –70°C. Note that $CaCl_2$ is essential for MN activity.

2.4.2. Protease Inhibitors

A cocktail of phenylmethanesulfonyl fluoride (PMSF), aprotinin, leupeptin, and pepstatin is usually used. 5,5'-Dithio*bis* (2-nitrobenzoic acid) (3,3'-6) (Fluka, cat. no. 43760) (DTNB), benzamidine, and NaF can be used in addition, but may inhibit some enzymatic reactions.

1. PMSF: Dissolve at 0.1 or 0.2 M in EtOH. Store at 4°C (serine proteases inhibitor).
2. Aprotinin: Dissolve at 3 mg/mL in H_2O. Store aliquots at –20°C (serine proteases inhibitor).
3. Leupeptin: Dissolve at 1 mg/mL in H_2O. Store aliquots at –20°C (serine and thiol proteases inhibitor).

4. Pepstatin: Dissolve at 2 mg/mL in methanol. Store at –20°C (aspartic proteases inhibitor). DTNB: (Fluka 43760). Dissolve in water, neutralize with KOH. Use at 0.5 m*M*. (thiol proteases inhibitor).
5. Benzamidine: Dissolve at 1 *M* in water. Use at 1 m*M* (serine proteases inhibitor). NaF: Dissolve at 1 *M* in water. Use at 5 m*M* (inhibits phosphatases and some proteases).

2.4.3. Nuclei Isolation Solutions

The following solutions are prepared just before use, and kept on ice (*see* **Note 1**):

1. Solution 1: A10X diluted 40× (final 37.5 m*M* Tris-HCl, pH 7.4, 0.05 m*M* spermine, 0.125 m*M* spermidine, 0.5 m*M* K-EDTA, pH 7.4, 20 m*M* KCl), 0.5 m*M* K-EDTA additional, 1% thiodiglycol, 1 m*M* DTT, 0.2 m*M* PMSF, 3 µg/mL aprotinin, 0.5 µg/mL leupeptin, 1 µg/mL pepstatin.
2. Solution 2: A10X diluted 40× (final 37.5 m*M* Tris-HCl, pH 7.4, 0.05 m*M* spermine, 0.125 m*M* spermidine, 0.5 m*M* K-EDTA, pH 7.4, 20 m*M* KCl), 20% glycerol, 1% thiodiglycol, 1 m*M* DTT, 0.2 m*M* PMSF, 3 µg/mL aprotinin, 0.5 µg/mL leupeptin, 1 µg/mL pepstatin.
3. W: A10X diluted 40× (final 37.5 m*M* Tris-HCl, pH 7.4, 0.05 m*M* spermine, 0.125 m*M* spermidine, 0.5 m*M* K-EDTA, pH 7.4, 20 m*M* KCl), 5% glycerol, 1% thiodiglycol, 1 m*M* DTT, 0.2 m*M* PMSF, 3 µg/mL aprotinin, 0.5 µg/mL leupeptin, 1 µg/mL pepstatin.
4. DB1/2: A10X-EDTA diluted 20× (final 75 m*M* Tris-HCl, pH 7.4, 0.1 m*M* spermine, 0.25 m*M* spermidine, 40 m*M* KCl), 5% glycerol, 1% thiodiglycol, 1 m*M* DTT, 0.2 m*M* PMSF, 3 µg/mL aprotinin, 0.5 µg/mL leupeptin, 1 µg/mL pepstatin, 0.1 m*M* $CaCl_2$, 5 m*M* $MgCl_2$.
5. TENSK: 25 m*M* Tris-HCl, pH 8.0, 10 m*M* NaEDTA, 200 m*M* NaCl, 0.4% SDS, with 0.1 mg/mL proteinase K added just before use.

3. Methods
3.1. Isolation of Cell Clones that Express EBNA1 Protein

EBNA1 is a virally encoded protein that is necessary for the maintenance of the EBV genome in infected cells, as well as for the replication of EBV-derived episomes. Commercially available EBV-derived vectors contain an EBNA1-coding sequence, which is most often just a piece of the EBV genome. Although no promoter is present, transcription of EBNA1 in these vectors is mediated by some nonspecific initiation from pUC-derived sequences. The authors and others (*13*) have found that expression of EBNA1 in cells prior to gene transfer greatly increases transfection efficiency and the stability of the transferred episomes (*see* **Note 2**). The authors have therefore made an expression construct using the RcCMV vector (Invitrogen; opened *Hin*dIII-*Xba*I and sites were filled with Klenow enzyme), in which were placed the EBNA1 coding sequence obtained from the pREP4 episomal vector (Invitrogen; fragment *Cla*I-*Nsi*I blunted with T4 DNA polymerase). The resulting construct was called RcEBNA1. A 6-kb *Sal*I fragment isolated from RcEBNA1 contains the EBNA1 and neomycin resistance expression cassettes, with very little extra sequences. An alternative is to use the plasmid pCMV-EBNA (Invitrogen or Clontech) co-transfected with a selectable marker.

Transfection of the 6 kb *Sal*I fragment of RcEBNA1 results in cells expressing EBNA1. Stable transformant clones are isolated by G418 selection. Clones that express EBNA1 can be identified either by transfection of an EBV-derived vector or by Western blot analysis (*see* **Note 3**). The authors experience is that, when a cell line can tolerate the EBNA1 protein (*see* **Note 4**), most clones obtained using the Rc/EBNA1 vector express the protein. However, the functionality of the transferred EBNA1 must be verified. In this case, transfection of an EBV plasmid carrying a selectable marker should result in the rapid identification of a resistant population, when compared to the EBNA1-negative original cell line. The episomal status of the transferred plasmid should then be verified by Southern analysis (*see* **Note 5**). If the episomal DNA must be recovered, purification can be carried out either by Hirt extraction or by simpler alkaline-lysis types of procedures (*see* **Note 6**).

3.2. EBV-Derived Vectors for Analysis of Gene Expression and Chromatin Structure

The authors have modified the commercially available pREP4 vector from Invitrogen *(14)* by introducing an expression cassette to measure luciferase or green fluorescent protein (GFP) activities. The aim was to place the cassette as far as possible from the *oriP* region, which has been shown to be an EBNA1-dependent enhancer of transcription in transient and stable transfections *(15,16)*. However, such an enhancer role for *oriP* has not been demonstrated on episomes in which that sequence has to function primarily as a replication origin. In order to analyze the structure of active genes, the authors decided to create an expression cassette with either luciferase or GFP, so that the activity of test promoters can be easily measured (*see* **Note 7**).

Briefly, to construct such vectors, the authors first removed the original expression/polylinker, found close to the *oriP*, by a *Sal*I digestion and religation of pREP4. To construct the vector, hygromycin-EBNA-replication-luciferase (pHERL; *see* **Fig. 1**), the *Cla*I site found between the EBNA1 coding sequence and the pUC sequences was used to introduce a cassette containing the bovine growth hormone polyadenylation signal (*Sac*I-*Xho*I fragment from Rc/CMV), followed by part of the polylinker and the luciferase and polyadenylation signal of the vector pGL2-Basic (Promega, Madison, WI). The bovine polyadenylation signal minimizes nonspecific transcription-initiated upstream.

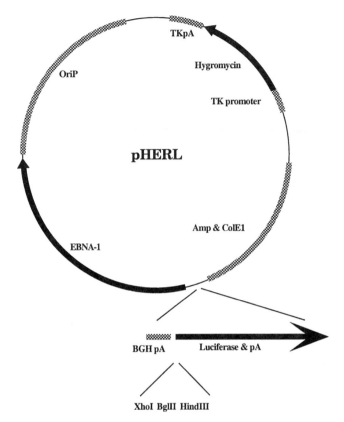

Fig. 1. Shuttle vector pHERL. pHERL was constructed as described in the text. A similar vector, called pHERG, carries the green fluorescent protein (eGFP; Clontech) in place of the luciferase coding sequence (from the pGL2-Basic of Promega).

The restriction sites for *Xho*I, *Bgl*II, and *Hind*III, derived from the pGL2-Basic polylinker are unique and are placed just upstream of the luciferase coding sequence. The authors also made the vector hygromycin-EBNA-replication-GFP (pHERG), in which the GFP coding sequence obtained by PCR as a *Hind*III-*Xba*I fragment from the vector pEGFP-C1 (Clontech), followed by the *Xba*I-*Bam*HI polyadenylation of pGL3-Basic (Promega), replaces the luciferase and polyadenylation site of pGL2-Basic (*Hind*III-*Bam*HI deletion) in pHERL.

3.3. Electroporation of Jurkat Cells and Selection of Population that Stably Maintain EBV-Derived Episomes

The authors have made the cell line J3EB1 by isolating a G418-resistant clone expressing EBNA1 from Jurkat cells electroporated with the *Sal*I fragment of RcEBNA1. EBV episomes can be easily maintained in this cell line. This subheading describes how to electroporate this cell line, and how to select a population that carries such episomes. A similar procedure can be used for Raji or Daudi cells, as well as for 293 or HeLa cells that express EBNA1 (*see* **Subheading 3.5.**).

J3EB1 cells are maintained between 2 and 10×10^5 cells/mL in RPMI 1640 supplemented with 10% FCS at 37°C in the presence of 5% CO_2 and 500 µg/mL G418. For electroporation of episomal plasmids, about 10^6 cells are pelleted for 5 min at 400g and resuspended in 350 µL of RPMI 1640 without serum at room temperature (RT). The cells are placed in a 0.4-cm-wide electroporation cuvet, and 1 µL plasmid DNA at 1 µg/µL is added (*see* **Note 8**). The expression per episome is optimal using low DNA amounts (*see* **Note 9**). Electroporation is rapidly performed at 260 V with a capacitance of 960 µF. The electroporated cells are immediately diluted in 15 mL RPMI 1640 with 10% FCS preheated at 37°C. Selection of hygromycin-resistant cells carrying episomes is started 2 d after electroporation by the addition of 100 µg/mL hygromycin. At this concentration, hygromycin is not very toxic to J3EB1 cells, but cells carrying episomes have a growth advantage (*see* **Note 10**). A control plate consists of cells electroporated in the absence of an episome. Electroporated cells are grown for 2–3 wk, until the negative control plate does not present any live cells. During this selection, cells are diluted about four fold when reaching a concentration of about 1.5×10^6 cells/mL as the medium turns yellow. Expression from the episomes can be measured by luciferase assays (pHERL) or GFP expression (pHERG). In this latter case, the selection of positive cells can be followed by fluorescent-activated cell sorting (FACS) analysis, if a strong promoter is placed upstream of the GFP sequence (*see* **Note 11**).

3.4. Electroporation of Raji and Daudi Cells

Raji and Daudi cells are B-cell lymphomas which are infected by EBV. Therefore, they express the EBNA1 protein, and can be easily transfected by EBV-derived episomes. A procedure identical to that described above for Jurkat cells can be used, except that selection is carried out at 200 µg/mL, of hygromycin. An alternative, which works well for Raji and Daudi cells, is to carry the electroporation in ice-cold PBS. Such a procedure can also be used for Jurkat cells, although lower levels of expression are obtained (*see* **Note 8**).

Raji and Daudi cells are maintained between 30 and 100×10^4 cell/mL in RPMI 1640 supplemented with 10% FCS at 37°C in the presence of 5% CO_2. For electroporation of episomal plasmids, about 3×10^5 cells are pelleted for 5 min at 400g, and are resuspended in 700 µL ice-cold PBS. The cells are placed in a 0.4-cm-wide prechilled electroporation cuvet, and 1 µL plasmid DNA at 1 µg/µL is added. Electroporation is rapidly performed at 280 V, with a capacitance of 960 µF. The electroporated cells are then left in the cuvet placed on ice for an additional 5 min before being diluted in 15 mL RPMI 1640 with 10% FCS preheated at 37°C. Selection of hygromycin-resistant cells carrying episomes is started 2 d after electroporation, by the addition of 200 µg/mL hygromycin.

3.5. HeLa, 293, and U87MG Cells

Episomes can be easily placed in various cell lines growing on plates that express EBNA1. 293 cells expressing EBNA1 can be obtained either from Invitrogen or by transfection of the *Sal*I fragment of RcEBNA1 (*see* **Subheading 3.1.**). HeLa cells expressing EBNA1 were obtained from Eric Gilson (Ecole Normale Supérieure, Lyon, France). Clones expressing EBNA1 were obtained from the glioblastoma line U87MG by transfection of the *Sal*I fragment of RcEBNA1. EBV-derived episomes can be very easily placed into the cells by common calcium-phosphate transfection and selection in the presence of 50 µg/mL (U87MG) or 200 (293 and HeLa) µg/mL hygromycin. However, if structural studies on chromatin must be performed, electroporation is preferred, and is carried out as described in **Subheading 3.3.** for Jurkat cells (*see* **Note 12**). In this case, the average number of episomes per cell can be controlled by the amount of DNA present during electroporation (*see* **Notes 8** and **9**).

3.6. Isolation of Nuclei and Nuclease Digestion

Examples are for one 150 cm^2 dish (about 2×10^7 HeLa cells; about 0.5×10^7 of other lines that grow to lower densities). One diploid mouse or human cell contains 6 pg of DNA in G1 (that is, 6×10^{-12}g). The same volumes can be used for cells that grow in spinner (*see* **Note 13**). Up to 20 dishes can be done at the same time, if two or three people can be mobilized for the washing and scraping of the plates, the rest of the manipulation can easily be carried out by a single person. All solutions are prepared in advance. Centrifuges and all materials are cooled to 4°C, or are chilled on ice. Once cells are taken out of the incubator, the procedure should be carried out without delay. The first part, up to the first dounce step, is done in the cold room.

3.6.1. No-detergent, Intact Nuclear Membrane Nuclei

1. Aspirate medium. Put 10 mL ice-cold PBS over cells. Shake the plate a little, aspirate PBS.
2. Leave plate tilted for 1 min to drain off a maximum of PBS (important, in order to have hypotonic conditions in next step).
3. Add 4 mL (or more) solution 1, and disperse well over cell layer carefully. Leave plate in cold room, on a horizontal surface, for 5 min, to swell the cells.
4. Scrape the cells with a silicon rubber policeman and place in a dounce. Most cells are already broken after scraping. Lyse cells with 5–10 strokes of a B-fitting pestle on ice. Put the nuclei in a 15- or 50-mL Falcon tube.

5. Spin for 5 min at 1000*g* at 4°C, with low or no brake. Aspirate supernatant.
6. Resuspend in 2.5 mL solution 2 with glass pipet. Put in dounce and do three strokes of a B pestle.
7. Spin for 5 min at 1000*g* at 4°C, with low or no brake. Aspirate supernatant.
8. Resuspend pellet with Gilson P1000 in adequate amount of specific buffer (such as W if EDTA is needed, or DB1/2 for nuclease digestion). Additional treatments should be carried out immediately.

3.6.2. Mild Detergents, Solubilized Nuclear Membrane Nuclei

1. The procedure is similar to the hypotonic procedure, but the swelling step is omitted. Also, the stock solution A10X is diluted only 10×, instead of 40×. Once nuclei are extracted with detergent, they must be kept in the presence of detergents; otherwise, they will stick to plastic and glassware. Detergents are usually either 0.1% Triton X-100 or 0.05% NP40. These two detergents produce free radicals when stored for extended periods as diluted aqueous solutions (typically, 10 or 20%). 0.1% digitonin (no free radicals, but expensive and difficult to solubilize) can be used, but may be inhibitory to some enzymatic reactions.
2. Aspirate medium. Put 10 mL ice-cold PBS over cells. Shake plate a little, aspirate PBS.
3. Add 4 mL or more solution 1 + detergent, and disperse over cell layer carefully. Scrape the cells with a silicon rubber policeman, and place in a dounce homogenizer. Dounce with 5–10 strokes of a B fitting pestle. Put the nuclei in a 15- or 50-mL Falcon tube.
4. Spin for 5 min at 1000*g* at 4°C, with low or no brake (very important if using a 50-mL tube). Aspirate supernatant.
5. Resuspend in 2.5 mL solution 2 + detergent with glass pipet. Put in dounce and disperse with three strokes of a B pestle.
6. Spin for 5 min at 1000*g* at 4°C, with low or no brake. Aspirate supernatant.
7. Resuspend pellet with Gilson P1000 in adequate amount of specific buffer (W + detergent, if EDTA is needed, or DB1/2 + detergent, for nuclease digestion). Additional treatments should be carried out immediately.

3.6.3. Nuclease Treatments

1. Resuspend about 10^7 nuclei in 200 μL buffer DB1/2.
2. Heat up at 25°C for 2–3 min.
3. Add DNase I 1–100 μg/mL (stock at 5 mg/mL in 50% glycerol); appropriate concentrations differ between cell types and genes. Vortex well.
4. After 1 min, quench with 10 m*M* NaEDTA and 400 μL of TENSK, and shake to mix. This can be left overnight at 37°C or 1–2 h at 50°C. At this stage, appropriate digestion can be assessed by briefly shaking the tubes. Because increasing concentrations of nuclease decrease viscosity, one should observe increasing foaming between samples as nuclease concentration is increased.
5. Alternatively, DNase I treatment could be done for 10 min on ice. Also, the presence of 0.1 m*M* Ca^{2+} may increase DNase I activity: For example, the enzyme

may prefer to cut close to a previous cut. This could be of advantage if DNase I hypersensitivity sites are to be mapped.

6. The procedure is the same for MN, except that the concentration of $CaCl_2$ is increased to 1 mM, and the digestion is done for 5 min at 25°C. Concentrations of MN, ranging from 10 to 3000 U/mL, can be adapted for different cell types and genes.

3.6.4. Isolation of Genomic DNA

1. Samples of genomic DNA are left in SDS-proteinase K buffer overnight at 37°C, or for 2–4 h at 50°C. Not much care should be taken about shearing if genomic DNA is to be used for indirect end-labeling.

2. Samples are extracted 3× with phenol:chloroform:isoamylalcohol (PCI, 25:24:1) at RT. This is most conveniently done in screw-capped tubes of 15- or 50-mL polypropylene tubes (Falcon or Corning) in which the aqueous and phenol phases can be vigorously mixed. All PCI extractions are first heated for a few minutes at 37°C, to warm the PCI that has been stored at 4°C, followed by mixing and centrifugation at RT. The limited DNA shearing resulting from the vigorous mixing will not interfere with indirect end-labeling. Polypropylene tubes with PCI can be safely centrifuged at 2,000g to separate the phases, and the PCI is removed with a pipet. If a large interphase forms, it can be recovered in microtubes for a 5 min spin. In this case, the interphase is smaller, and more aqueous phase can be recovered.

3. DNA is recovered after precipitation with 2.5 vol of ethanol, usually in Falcon 15-mL snap-cap polypropylene tubes. Alternatively, 1 vol of 2-propanol can be used. The aqueous phase of the last PCI is transferred to a new tube, which contains either ethanol or isopropanol. For large genomic DNA, it is important to mix the aqueous phase well in ethanol, by shaking vigorously. Because the aqueous phase is viscous, a precipitate may form around a small volume of aqueous DNA, and prevent ethanol from reaching these parts, if not mixed enough. This will result in problems during resuspension. If the genomic DNA is fragmented (as after nuclease treatments of nuclei), the samples are left for 2 h or overnight at –20°C, and the DNA is recovered after a 20 min 5000g centrifugation (e.g., Sorvall SS34 or HB4 types of rotors).

4. After centrifugation, genomic DNA precipitates are dried under vacuum. Samples are then resuspended in 5 mM Tris-HCl, pH 8.0, 0.1 mM NaEDTA. The DNA should dissolve in 1–2 h at RT with gentle mixing and occasional vigorous shaking.

4. Notes

1. Solution 1 and solution 2 are made of A1/4, which is relatively low salt and low polyamine concentrations. This swells nuclei that may be fragile. For some cell lines, this results in lysis of nuclei. In this case, the concentration of polyamines can be increased two- to fourfold to stabilize nuclei. Triton X-100 and NP40 from 10 or 20% aqueous stocks can be added to 0.1 and 0.05% final, respectively. In this case, stock solutions A10X and A10X-EDTA are diluted only 10×,

instead of 40× in solution 1, solution 2, and W. For DNase I digestion, Ca^{2+} may affect the result in two ways. First, DNase I activity is four- to 10-fold higher in the presence of Ca^{2+} than in the presence of ethyleneglyed-bis-ominoethylether tetra acetic acid (EGTA). In the absence of both added calcium and EGTA, DNase I seems to work as if the stock solution were made up with $CaCl_2$. However, EGTA treatment of nuclei may change some nuclear structures dependent on Ca^{2+}, which were not titrated with EDTA during isolation, because EDTA has a weaker affinity for Ca^{2+} than EGTA. Thiodiglycol (TDG) may be optional, particularly if no detergent is used. Glycerol is a weak free radical scavenger.

2. Most studies involving EBV-derived episomes have been conducted on Raji and Daudi cells, B-cell lymphomas infected by EBV, which produce EBNA1 from the viral genome. On the other hand, EBNA1 expression may not be sufficient for stable maintenance of the episomes, as has been described for A431 cells *(17)*.

3. EBNA1 antiserum can be obtained from humans by screening human samples. A positive-control protein extract for the EBNA1 Western analysis can be obtained by making a transient transfection of 293 cells with the RcEBNA1 plasmid. The EBNA1 protein encoded by RcEBNA1 has an approximate mol wt of 56 kDa.

4. EBNA1 is a pleiotropic protein with a complex structure *(18)*. EBNA1 is also a putative oncogene *(19)*. It is probable that various parts of cell physiology are changed by the presence of EBNA1. It is important to note that some cell types may not tolerate EBNA1. For example, the authors were not successful in obtaining U937 or HL60 cells stably expressing EBNA1.

5. The episomal status of the transferred episomal plasmids can be verified in a number of ways. One rapid approach is to isolate total DNA from the resistant cell population, and to run it on a Southern blot after digestion of genomic DNA with a restriction enzyme that does not cut into the episome. In that case, one should expect a single band that runs as the uncut original plasmid. Extra bands originate either from partial nicking (verified by running the uncut original plasmid on the same gel), or, in some cases, by integration of the transferred plasmid. As described in **Notes 10** and **12**, various parameters can lead to integration.

6. To obtain cellular DNA enriched in episomes, Hirt extracts can be performed *(20)*. Alternatively, an easier alkaline lysis procedure can be used *(21)*. The insert placed on the episome can be very large, because special YACS can be placed on such episomes *(22)*.

7. The luciferase or GFP expression cassettes can also be placed between the *oriP* and the hygromycin cassette, in either orientation. Regulated transcription has still been obtained from various promoters (mouse c-*fos* and human interferon-inducible ISG54) placed in that position, despite the close presence of the *oriP* region (unpublished data).

8. The concentration of DNA during electroporation is critical, and will determine the average number of episomes in cells. **Figure 2** shows that the number of episomes taken by the cells increase with the DNA amount present at electroporation. Moreover, for J3EB1 cells, the electroporation conditions described in **Subheading 3.3.** (medium at RT) appear more

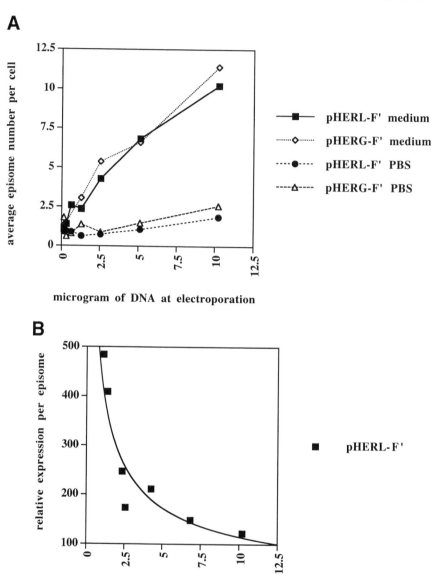

Fig. 2. DNA concentration at electroporation determines copy number and levels of expression per template. The EBNA1-positive Jurkat line J3EB1 was electroporated as described in the text, with the episomes pHERL and pHERG carrying the mouse c-*fos* promoter (from –474 to +151, relative to the transcriptional start site). (**A**) increasing amounts of plasmid DNA were present when electroporation was conducted, either in medium at RT (*see* **Subheading 3.3.**), or in ice-cold PBS (*see* **Subheading 3.4.**). The average number of episomes per cell was determined by Southern analysis, using stan-

efficient than the conditions described for Raji and Daudi cells in **Subheading 3.4.** (ice-cold PBS).

9. In the authors' experience, the expression per episome is maximal when the average copy per cell is kept low. Figure 2B presents the expression of the luciferase reporter gene from the pHERL-F' plasmid electroporated in medium samples presented in **Fig. 2A.** The c-*fos* promoter was induced with phorbol-12-myristate-13-acetate (PMA), and luciferase activities normalized to the average number of episomes per cell. It is clear that increasing the number of episomes in a cell results in a lower expression per episome. The authors suppose that only one or a few episomes remain in an actively transcribing state; the others get into a repressed configuration. Supporting this hypothesis is the observation that increasing the average number of episomes per cell eliminates the specific footprint observed by DNase I digestion of isolated nuclei (unpublished data).

10. In order to prevent the episomes from integrating into the genome, it is essential to use only a low selective pressure during hygromycin selection. The authors usually use concentrations that kill slowly, and selection is mostly the result of the growth advantage of the cells that have incorporated episomes. **Figure 3** presents a Southern of two independent electroporations of J3EB1 cells that have been selected either at 100 µg/mL or 200 µg/mL hygromycin. Clearly, at higher hygromycin concentration, a number of high-mol-wt bands appear in a Southern analysis corresponding to various integration events in the population.

11. The homogeneity of expression of GFP can be easily assayed by FACS. J3EB1 cells growing in medium can be directly analyzed. As presented in **Fig. 4,** the absence of a negative peak indicates that all resistant cells express GFP, although in various amounts. The strong Rous Sarcoma Virus (RSV) promoter shows a large peak distinct from the control vector (the latter overlaps with untransfected cells, data not shown), when the weaker c-*fos* promoter results in a peak that partially overlaps the negative cells. Because GFP activity is rather stable, a transient induction of the c-*fos* promoter by PMA does not dramatically change the overall aspect of the FACS pattern (data not shown). However, the luciferase activity obtained from the pHERL vector has a rather short half-life, and permits the analysis of transiently inducible promoters in cells stably transfected with episomes.

12. The authors observed that the calcium phosphate procedure results in a high average of episomes per cell for 293, HeLa, and U87MG cells. Increasing the number of episomes favors structural heterogeneity, transcriptional repression, and integration from part of the episomes (unpublished data). The average number of episomes per cell can be best controlled by the concentration of DNA during electroporation, as described in Note 8.

---

dard amounts of plasmid DNA and quantification by phosphorimager. (**B**) The luciferase expression after PMA induction in the cell populations presented in panel A (pHERL-Fos, medium) was normalized to the average number of episomes per cell, and plotted against that number.

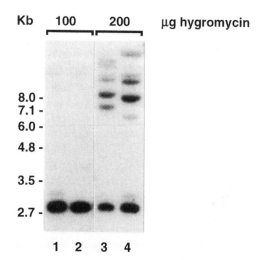

Fig. 3. Strong selection favors episome integration. J3EB1 cells were electroporated with the episome pHERL, as described in **Subheading 3.2.** In two independent electroporations, cells carrying episomes were selected either at 100 µg/mL (lanes 1 and 2) or at 200 µg/mL (lanes 3 and 4) of hygromycin. Total cellular DNA was digested with *Xho*I and *Bam*HI, and probed with luciferase sequences to reveal the expression cassette.

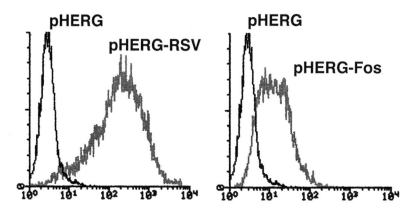

Fig. 4. FACS analysis of cells carrying GFP-coding episomes. J3EB1 cells were electroporated with the vector pHERG, as well as with derivatives carrying either the strong RSV promoter or the mouse c-*fos* promoter (from –375 to +9). Cell populations resistant to hygromycin were selected and analyzed by FACS for GFP expression.

13. For the analysis of genomic DNA, it is best to isolate nuclei in the presence of EDTA, to inhibit endogenous nucleases. EDTA also inhibits metalloproteases that may digest nuclear proteins. Isolation of nuclei in the presence of EDTA is most easily done in the presence of polyamines, which stabilize nuclei. Isolation,

in the absence of polyamines or divalent cations, often results in the lysis of nuclei. At all stages of the procedure, nuclei can be observed with the phase microscope, to visually assess their purity. Nuclei can be observed in the presence of 1 μg/mL 4',6-Diamidine-2-phenylindol-dihydrochloride (DAPI) in UV fluorescence to assess possible nuclei lysis. Lysed nuclei will appear as fibrous structures that light up with DAPI.

Acknowledgments

We would like to thank Eric Gilson (Ecole Normale Supérieure, Lyon, France) for the EBNA1-positive HeLa cells, and Ernst Winocour (Weizmann Institute, Rehovot, Israel) for the 293-EBNA1 cells. This work was made possible by grants from the Swiss Federal Office for Public Health, the Swiss National Foundation for Scientific Research, and the Swiss Research against Cancer, and by support from ISREC.

References

1. Latchman, D. (1995) *Eukaryotic Transcription Factors*. Academic Press, London.
2. Wolffe, A. (1995) *Chromatin*. Academic Press, London.
3. Bonifer, C., Huber, M. C., Jagle, U., Faust, N., and Sippel, A. E. (1996) Prerequisites for tissue specific and position independent expression of a gene locus in transgenic mice. *J. Mol. Med.* **74,** 663–71.
4. Lewin, B. (1998) Mystique of epigenetics. *Cell* **93,** 301–303.
5. Owen-Hughes, T. A. and Workman, J. L. (1994) Experimental analysis of chromatin function in transcription control. *Crit. Rev. Eukaryotic Gene Expression* **4,** 403–441.
6. Felsenfeld, G. (1996) Chromatin unfolds. *Cell* **86,** 13–19.
7. Felsenfeld, G., Boyes, J., Chung, J., Clark, D., and Studitsky, V. (1996) Chromatin structure and gene expression. *Proc. Natl. Acad. Sci. USA* **93,** 9384938–8.
8. Kamakaka, R. T. (1997) Silencers and locus control regions: opposite sides of the same coin. *Trends Biochem. Sci.* **22,** 124–128.
9. Mirkovitch, J. (1998) A few lances at the function of chromatin and nuclear higher-order structure in transcription regulation, in *Gene Therapy* (Xanthopoulos, K. G., ed.), vol. H105, Springer Verlag, Berlin, pp. 1–16.
10. Margolskee, R. F. (1992) Epstein-Barr virus based expression vectors. *Curr. Top. Microbiol. Immunol.* **158,** 67–95.
11. Gong, Q. H., McDowell, J. C., and Dean, A. (1996) Essential role of NF-E2 in remodeling of chromatin structure and transcriptional activation of the epsilon-globin gene in vivo by 5' hypersensitive site 2 of the beta-globin locus control region. *Mol. Cell. Biol.* **16,** 6055–6064.
12. Albert, T., Mautner, J., Funk, J. O., Hörtnagel, K., Pullner, A., and Eick, D. (1997) Nucleosomal structures of c-*myc* promoters with transcriptionally engaged RNA polymerase II. *Mol. Cell. Biol.* **17,** 4363–4371.
13. Cachianes, G., Ho, C., Weber, R. F., Williams, S. R., Goeddel, D. V., and Leung, D. W. (1993) Epstein-Barr virus-derived vectors for transient and stable expression of recombinant proteins. *BioTechniques* **15,** 255–259.

14. Groger, R. K., Morrow, D. M., and Tykocinski, M. L. (1989) Directional antisense and sense cDNA cloning using Epstein-Barr virus episomal expression vectors. *Gene* **81,** 285–294.

15. Reisman, D. and Sugden, B. (1986) *trans* activation of an Epstein-Barr viral transcriptional enhancer by the Epstein-Barr viral nuclear antigen 1. *Mol. Cell.Biol.* **11,** 3838–3846.

16. Wysokenski, D. A. and Yates, J. L. (1989) Multiple EBNA1–binding sites are required to form an EBNA1–dependen enhancer and to activate a minimal replicative origin within *oriP* of Epstein-Barr virus. *J. Virol.* **63,** 2657–2666.

17. Vidal, M., Wrighton, C., Eccles, S., Burke, J., and Grosveld, F. (1990) Differences in human cell lines to support stable replication of Epstein-Barr virus-based vectors. *Biochem. Biophy. Acta* 1**048,** 171–177.

18. Ambinder, R. F., Mullen, M., Chang, Y.-N., Hayward, G. S., and Hayward, S. D. (1991) Functional domains of Epstein-Barr virus nucleat antigen EBNA-1. *J. Virol.* **65,** 1466–1478.

19. Wilson, J. B., Bell, J. L., and Levine, A. J. (1996) Expression of Epstein-Bar virus nuclear antigen-1 induces B-cell neoplasia in transgenic mice. *EMBO J.* **15,** 3117–3126.

20. Hirt, B. (1967) Selective extraction of polyoma DNA from infected mouse cell cultures *J. Mol. Biol.* **26,** 365–369.

21. Kioussis, D., Wilson, F., Daniels, C., Leveton, C., Taverne, J. and Playfair, J., H. (1987) Expression and rescuing of a cloned human tumour necrosis factor gene using an EBV-based shuttle cosmid vector *EMBO J.* **6,** 355–61.

22. Simpson, K., McGuigan, A., and Huxley, C. (1996) Stable episomal maintenance of yeast artificial chromosomes in human cells. *Mol. Cell. Biol.* **16,** 5117–5126.

13

Triplex-Directed Site-Specific Genome Modification

Karen M. Vasquez and John H. Wilson

1. Introduction

The ability to target and manipulate specific mammalian genes has been a long sought goal in biotechnology and biomedicine. The realization of this goal has only recently become feasible, with advances in genetic engineering. Through the use of gene targeting strategies, it is possible to replace genetic information on the chromosome, delete sequences from the chromosome, create transgenic mice, and develop new approaches to gene therapy of human genetic diseases *(1)*.

Targeted homologous recombination has proven a valuable tool in biotechnology, and in studies of gene function and chromosomal dynamics *(2–5)*. The potential of gene targeting in gene therapeutic applications is promising, but there are several limitations to the technology currently available. One major limitation is the extremely low rate of homologous recombination in mammalian cells, typically 10^{-8}–10^{-5} per cell per generation (reviewed in **ref. 6**). Low rates of recombination generally limit the frequency of targeted recombination to less than one recombinant in 10^4–10^7 treated cells. In mammalian cells, there is an additional complication, in that random integration of transfected DNA is, on average, 1000-fold higher than targeted recombination *(7,8)*.

Triplex technology offers an alternative approach to site-specific modification in mammalian cells as a means of manipulating the human genome *(9)*. Triplex formation involves specific recognition of a purine-rich stretch of duplex DNA by a single strand oligonucleotide. The triplex-forming oligonucleotide (TFO) binds in the major groove of such a duplex segment by forming specific hydrogen bonds between bases in the TFO and the purine bases in the underlying duplex *(9)*. Two types of triplex can be formed, depending on the arrangement of the TFO in the major groove: parallel triplexes, in which

From: *Methods in Molecular Biology, vol. 133: Gene Targeting Protocols*
Edited by: E. Kmiec © Humana Press Inc., Totowa, NJ

the TFO has the same 5'-to-3' orientation as the purine-rich strand of the duplex, and antiparallel triplexes, in which the TFO has the opposite orientation relative to the purine-rich strand. Antiparallel triplexes are formed by purine (GA) or mixed (GT) TFOs, which form canonical G:G-C, A:A-T, and T:A-T triplets through reverse Hoogsteen hydrogen bonds. Pyrimidine TFOs form parallel triplexes with canonical C+:G-C (C+ represents protonation of N3 of C) and T:A-T triplets resulting from Hoogsteen hydrogen bonds *(10,11)*. Purine or mixed TFOs are advantageous for applications in cells, because, unlike pyrimidine TFOs, they form stable triplexes at physiological pH, without modification *(12)*.

Triplex formation in a gene can inhibit transcription and, therefore, directly inactivate the targeted gene. Additionally, by incorporating a damaging agent on the oligonucleotide, site-specific DNA damage can be achieved. Because DNA damage is thought to stimulate homologous recombination, triplex technology offers a potential strategy for stimulating targeted recombination in a gene-specific manner. Here are reviewed methods commonly used in forming and characterizing triple helices, and two test systems are described for assessing mutation and recombination using triplex technology.

1.1. Identification of Potential Triplex-Forming Sites

A computer search can identify potential triplex-forming target sites in genes of interest. Sequences are scanned for those containing a minimum of 80% purines (or 80% pyrimidines) over a 15-bp stretch. The potential triplex-forming sites can be screened by synthesizing target duplexes and corresponding TFOs designed to bind in either parallel or antiparallel orientations. In designing TFOs, the triplets discussed above, and listed in **Table 1**, should be used (a parallel triplex refers to one formed with a pyrimidine TFO and an antiparallel triplex to one formed with a purine or mixed [GT] TFO). If the purine-rich stretch of the duplex target site is interrupted by a pyrimidine (a mismatch), then several choices can be made for the corresponding TFO base, including modified bases or base analogs. **Table 1** lists the unmodified base of choice at any site in the target duplex, based on data obtained by nuclear magnetic resonance (NMR), thermal melting, and binding analysis *(13)*. As an initial screen, band-shift analysis or plasmid-fragment binding can be used to detect TFO binding to its target duplex (*see* **Subheadings 4.2.** and **4.3.**). For use in cells, TFOs should be synthesized with a 3'-propanolamine to protect against the prevalent 3' exonucleases in cells *(14,15*; available as CPG, Glen Research, Sterling, VA).

2. Materials

1. DNase I buffer: 10 mM Tris-HCl, pH 7.5, 10 mM CaCl$_2$, 10 mM MgCl$_2$, 50% glycerol (v:v).
2. DMS reaction buffer: 50 mM sodium cacodylate, pH 7.0, 1 mM EDTA, pH 8.0.

Table 1
Unmodified TFO Bases for Binding
to Purine-Rich Strand of Target Duplex

Base in target duplex	Base in TFO	
Purine (canonical)	Parallel triplex	Antiparallel triplex
G	C	G
A	T	T/A
Pyrimidine (mismatch)[a]		
T	G	C
C	T/C	T

[a]A mismatch may reduce binding by a factor of 10–100 or more, depending on the sequence context of the mismatch *(13)*.

3. DMS stop solution: 1.5 *M* sodium acetate, pH 7.0, 1 *M* β-mercaptoethanol.
4. Polyacrylamide native gel loading dye: 20% sucrose, 0.2% bromphenol blue/xylene cyanole (w/v).
5. Polyacrylamide denaturing gel loading dye: bromphenol blue and xylene cyanole 0.2% (w/v) of each dye in formamide.
6. Triplex-binding buffer (TBB) (5X): 50% sucrose, 50 m*M* MgCl$_2$, 5 m*M* spermine, 50 m*M* Tris-HCl pH 7.8.
7. TBE: 89 m*M* Tris-HCl, 89 m*M* boric acid, 2 m*M* EDTA.
8. TBM: 89 m*M* Tris-HCl, 89 m*M* boric acid, 10 m*M* MgCl$_2$.
9. TE: 10 m*M* Tris-HCl, pH 7.8, 1 m*M* EDTA, pH 8.0.

3. Methods

The most useful methods available for purification of oligonucleotides include reverse-phase high-pressure liquid chromatography (HPLC), polyacrylamide gel electrophoresis (PAGE), and size-exclusion chromatography. Reverse-phase HPLC should be employed following synthesis of oligonucleotides to separate full-length material from failure sequences, and PAGE purification is recommended as an additional step to ensure a high level of purity. Size-exclusion columns are useful for removing salts and exchanging buffers prior to and following purification, and prior to storage.

3.1. HPLC (Reverse-Phase) Purification

1. Following deprotection, purify oligos by HPLC, using a C18 column and a linear gradient of acetonitrile (0–50%) in 0.1 *M* triethylammonium acetate, pH 7.3.
2. Detritylate oligos in 80% aqueous acetic acid at 22°C ~1 h.
3. Redissolve oligos in 100 m*M* NaCl, and desalt by size-exclusion chromatography.

3.2. Size-Exclusion Chromatography

Prepacked columns (e.g. NAP-5 column, Pharmacia LKB Biotechnology, Uppsala, Sweden) are very convenient; however, mini-columns can be easily prepared *(16)*.

1. Equilibrate size-exclusion column with TE, and apply the sample in a small volume, and run sample over column (≤500 µL for NAP-5).
2. Elute sample in TE (1 mL for NAP-5), and determine concentration by UV spectrophotometry.

3.3. PAGE Purification (for Oligos ~15–50-mers)

Oligos should be purified by size exclusion, as described above, before and after PAGE purification.

1. Add 1:1 (v/v) formamide/dye to oligo sample.
2. Heat sample at ≥90°C for 5 min prior to loading on the gel.
3. Load sample on preheated (50°C) polyacrylamide gel (10–15% acrylamide, 7 *M* urea, buffered in 1X TBE).
4. Run samples at 50–60°C at 60 W ~1–2 h, until there is sufficient separation to visualize full-length oligos from n-1 to a few nucleotides.
5. UV shadow to visualize DNA, cut out full-length product, and add gel fragment to 2–4 mL H$_2$O. DNA at >1 µg can be visualized in a gel by removing the gel from the plates, placing on a fluorescent surface (most white paper is adequate) and detecting the DNA by holding a UV lamp (254 nm) over the gel.
6. Incubate the gel fragment overnight at 55°C.
7. Spin sample to pellet acrylamide, remove H$_2$O containing DNA, concentrate by use of a Speed-Vac or Centricon filter unit (Amicon, Beverly, MA 3000 MWCO), and purify by size-exclusion chromatography, as described above. This step is essential to remove low-mol-wt contaminants eluted from the gel.

3.4. Detection and Specificity of Triplex Formation

Several methods for detecting triplex formation are described below. Specificity of TFO binding can also be determined by these methods, and, therefore, all binding assays should include a binding-specificity control TFO (a TFO with the same base composition as the specific TFO, but with a scrambled sequence). Although effects on gene function in cells have been demonstrated for triplexes with K_d <10^{-6} *M*, even higher affinities (K_d <10^{-8} *M*) are recommended.

3.4.1. Duplex Preparation for Band-Shift Analysis

1. Anneal single strands that correspond to the duplex region covering the potential triplex-binding site, plus ~10 bp on either side, by mixing a 1:1 molar ratio of strands (10^{-6} *M* final strand concentration) in 100 m*M* Tris, 10 m*M* MgCl$_2$.
2. Heat ≥90°C ~10 min and gradually cool to room temperature.

INTRON 1 SITE: Hamster APRT

```
5'-CTTGTGGGGTCTCCGCCCCCCTTTCCCCGGCCACCAGC-3'
3'-GAACACCCCAGAGGCGGGGGGAAAGGGGCCGGTGGTCG-5'
      5'-TGTGGTGGGGGGTTTGGGG-3'      2TAP
```

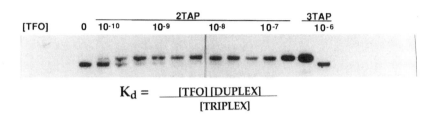

$$K_d = \frac{[TFO][DUPLEX]}{[TRIPLEX]}$$

Fig. 1. Triplex formation at the intron 1 site of APRT. The nucleotide sequences of the synthetic intron 1 APRT target site duplex and the specific TFO (2TAP) are shown. Band-shift analysis of triplex formation is demonstrated by incubating increasing concentrations of TFO with radiolabelled target duplex in TBB, and subjecting to PAGE. The control TFO (3TAP) has an identical base composition to 2TAP, but a scrambled sequence.

3. Radiolabel 5' ends of the duplex (1 μL of the duplex in a 10-μL reaction volume), using T4 polynucleotide kinase (according to supplier recommendations) and [γ-^{32}P]-ATP at 37°C for 1 h. Phenol:chloroform extract the duplex.
4. Add nondenaturing loading dye to sample. Load sample on 12% polyacrylamide gel (PAG) (native; buffered in 1X TBE). Run at 60 V ~3–4 h.
5. Expose the gel to autoradiographic film (<1 min), and develop film to detect the band of interest. (Following extraction of the band from the gel, another exposure should be taken to ensure the removal of the proper band).
6. Cut out radiolabelled full-length duplex from the gel and elute by using an electroeluter (1X TBE can be used as elution buffer).
7. Purify duplex by size-exclusion chromatography.
8. Store sample at 4°C at 10^{-10} M for band-shift assays.

3.4.2. Band-Shift Analysis

Band-shift analysis allows detection of triplex by a shift in electrophoretic mobility of radiolabelled duplex to a slower migrating band (triplex). This assay is useful for determining a K_d value (**Fig. 1**), and requires only small amounts of material. The K_d can be estimated as the concentration at which 50% of the radiolabel is in the duplex band and 50% is in the triplex band (the reaction should be carried out under pseudo-first-order conditions with duplex concentration $<10^{-10}$ M, and [TFO] = 10^{-10}–10^{-6} M.

1. In a 10 μL reaction, add 6 μL H$_2$O, 1 μL radiolabeled duplex at 10^{-10} M, 1 μL TFO (final concentration of 10^{-6} M through 10^{-10} M to determine concentration dependence of triplex formation), and 2 μL 5X TBB.

2. Incubate at 37°C until reaction is at equilibrium (as determined by time course analysis).
3. Add loading dye to reaction, and run on 12% native PAG (buffered with 1X TBM).
4. Dry gel and expose to film. For quantitation of a K_d, determine percent of triplex formed by counting radioactivity in duplex vs triplex, using a blot analyzer (e.g., PhosphorImager Molecular Dynamics, Sunnyvale, CA).
5. To calculate K_d, plot data points as percent triplex vs log (TFO concentration), and fit a binding curve to the points using a nonlinear least squares routine (e.g., in Sigma Plot, SPSS Inc., Chicago, IL or PSI-Plot Polysoftware International, Salt Lake City, UT).

3.4.3. TFO Plasmid Fragment Binding

If several potential TFO-binding sites are identified in a gene of interest, and the gene is contained in a plasmid, a useful method to determine triplex formation and specificity is by plasmid-fragment binding. To test TFO binding specificity, generate a series of restriction fragments by digestion of the plasmid DNA with restriction enzymes. Restriction enzymes should be selected to generate several fragments (without destroying the triplex-binding site) of sizes that are easily separated by agarose gel electrophoresis. Specificity is determined by TFO binding only to the fragment that contains the triplex-binding site.

1. Radiolabel purified TFOs using T4 polynucleotide kinase and [γ-^{32}P]-ATP, followed by phenol:chloroform extraction.
2. Column-purify or gel-purify labeled TFO, as described in **Subheadings 3.2.** and **3.3.**
3. Digest ~5 μg plasmid containing the target duplex site with restriction endonucleases of choice.
4. EtOH precipitate the plasmid DNA and resuspend in TE.
5. Add labeled TFO to the sample containing plasmid DNA (unlabeled) in 1X TBB.
6. Incubate at 37°C to allow triplex formation.
7. Subject samples to electrophoresis through a 1% agarose gel buffered with 1X TBM.
8. Restriction fragments can be visualized by ethidium bromide staining and triplexes can be detected by autoradiography.

3.4.4. DNase I Protection Assay (Preparation of Target Duplex)

In a DNase I protection assay, the triplex is formed first and then the duplex fragment is digested with DNase I. If triplex is formed, then the region bound by TFO will be protected from cleavage. This assay differs from those previously described, because the reaction is complete prior to subjecting the samples to PAGE. This method localizes the TFO binding site, and, therefore, is a test of binding specificity. The target DNA (synthetic duplex or a plasmid fragment) should be radiolabelled on the purine-rich strand only, for best results.

1. To generate a target duplex from a plasmid, digest the plasmid with a restriction enzyme that cleaves near the 5' end of the purine-rich strand of the TFO-binding site.

2. Remove 5' phosphate by incubating sample with calf intestinal alkaline phosphatase (CIP) at 37°C ~ 1 h.
3. Heat-inactivate the CIP, phenol:chloroform-extract the sample, and EtOH-precipitate the DNA.
4. Radiolabel 5' end of the purine-rich strand using T4 polynucleotide kinase and [γ-^{32}P]-ATP, followed by phenol:chloroform extraction.
5. Digest with another restriction enzyme to obtain fragment of desired size (preferably <300 bp).
6. Purify the labeled fragment (to separate from other labelled fragments) on a 5–10% native PAG (for fragments ~50–300 bp), as described in PAGE **Subheading 3.3.**

3.4.4.1. PREPARATION OF A G-LADDER

The radiolabeled target duplex should be treated with dimethyl sulfate (DMS) and piperidine to locate the Gs in the sequence, so that the triplex binding site can be easily identified on the gel.

3.4.4.1.1. DMS Reaction

1. Add 200 μL DMS reaction buffer and 1 μL DMS to 5 μL radiolabelled target duplex.
2. Incubate 5 min at 22°C.
3. Add 40 μL DMS stop solution, 1 μL tRNA at 10 mg/mL, and 0.6 mL 100% EtOH.
4. Incubate for 10 min in a solution of dry ice/EtOH.
5. Centrifuge for 10 min at 4°C, and collect supernatant.
6. Add 0.25 mL 0.3 *M* sodium acetate/1 m*M* EDTA on ice and 0.75 mL 100% EtOH to precipitate the DNA (repeat precipitation).
7. Wash in 70% EtOH, centrifuge for 10 min, remove supernatant, and air-dry 10 min.

3.4.4.1.2. Piperidine Reaction

1. Resuspend the pellet from the DMS reaction in 100 μL 1 *M* piperidine.
2. Heat at 90°C for 30 min.
3. Freeze in dry ice, and Speed-Vac sample.
4. Add 100 μL H$_2$O, freeze in dry ice, and Speed-Vac (repeat step 4).
5. Resuspend in formamide/dye for electrophoresis.

3.4.4.2. DNASE I PROTECTION ASSAY

1. Incubate radiolabeled target duplex with increasing concentrations of TFO in 1X TBB at 37°C in a final volume of 10 μL, to allow for triplex formation.
2. Add DNase I at 0.12 U/mL (dilute DNase I in DNase I buffer), and incubate at 37°C ~15 min.
3. Stop the reaction by adding 90 μL of a solution containing 500 m*M* Tris-HCl, pH 7.8, 20 m*M* EDTA, and 90 mg/mL calf thymus DNA.
4. EtOH-precipitate the DNA by addition of 300 μL EtOH, store on ice for 20 min, and centrifuge in an Eppendorf for 30 min at 4°C.
5. Collect the supernatant and dry samples in a Speed-Vac.

6. Redissolve the samples in 10 μL formamide/dye and heat at 90°C for 5 min prior to electrophoresis.
7. Subject samples (including the G-ladder) to PAGE on a high-resolution denaturing gel (10–15%, depending on the fragment length) buffered in 1X TBE at 60 W ~1–2 h (50–60°C).
8. Dry the gel and expose to film. The region protected from cleavage will indicate the TFO-binding site.

3.4.5. Protection from Restriction Digestion

If the potential triplex-forming site contains a restriction enzyme recognition site, triplex formation can be detected by first forming triplex, and then digesting with the restriction enzyme. If triplex is formed, it will afford protection from cleavage. This assay can be carried out on a synthetic target duplex (as described in **Subheading 3.4.2.**), or on a plasmid target (as described in **Subheading 3.4.3.**, but with the plasmid duplex labeled, rather than the TFO).

1. Add TFO to radiolabeled target duplex in 1X TBB, and incubate at 37°C.
2. Digest DNA by adding the restriction enzyme in buffer, and incubate according to supplier recommendations (buffers containing KCl may enhance triplex dissociation [17], and should be avoided; other buffer constituents may also have an effect on triplex dissociation, and should be tested prior to use).
3. Run sample on PAG (for synthetic target duplex) or agarose gel (for plasmid target duplex).
4. Dry gel, and expose to film to detect the fragment containing the triplex-binding site and the cleaved products.

3.4.6. Detection of Triplex Formation by Physical Techniques

Triplex formation has been detected by several physical methods (reviewed in **ref. 13**), including thermal melting, circular dichroism (CD) spectroscopy, NMR analysis, calorimetry measurements, and filter binding (18). In general, these methods are not useful for K_d analysis, except for filter binding, which can be used to determine a K_d value, with one caveat: G-rich TFOs tend to form secondary structures that do not pass through the filter, and, therefore, filter binding has been used successfully only with pyrimidine TFOs. Because pyrimidine TFOs require protonation of N3 on cytosine (19), these oligos are not recommended for use in cells without modification.

3.5. Triplex-Directed Photocrosslinking by Psoralen-TFOs In Vitro

Psoralen can be covalently linked to the 5' end of the TFO during synthesis (phosphoramidites modified with 4(-hydroxymethyl-4,5',8-trimethylpsoralen [HMT] are commercially available; Glen Research). Crosslinking is most efficient if one of the preferred psoralen crosslinking sites, 5'-TpA or 5'-ApT, is located immediately adjacent to the end of the triplex-binding site corresponding to the psoralen-tagged end of the TFO. The psoralen derivative is currently available with a 2-carbon or 6-carbon linker. If the psoralen reaction site is within a 1–2 bp range of the last base of the TFO, then a 2-carbon linker is sufficient, but if the reaction site is 2–3 bases from the TFO site, then the 6-carbon linker should be used *(20)*. If monoadducts are desired, only a T is required near the triplex-binding site (within a 3-bp range).

3.5.1. Characterization of Psoralen-Modified TFOs

Note that psoralen derivatives are very light-sensitive, and should be protected from light as much as possible during preparation and handling.

1. Following synthesis and HPLC purification, oligos should be PAGE- or column-purified, as described above, in **Subheadings 3.2.** and **3.3.**
2. Determine concentration of the psoralen-TFO by UV spectroscopy. HMT absorbs at 365 nm, but the extinction coefficient is low (~5000), and, therefore, it is difficult to quantitate psoralen at concentrations <20 μM.
3. Determine integrity of psoralen using fluorescence spectroscopy. This can be done in a semiquantitative fashion by recording the emission spectrum of a standard HMT sample of known concentration, and comparing it to the HMT-modified TFO. Spectra can be conveniently measured using solutions of HMT and HMT-modified psoralen at concentrations of >10^{-7} M. An emission spectrum is recorded using a scanning spectrofluorimeter, with a constant excitation wavelength of 365 nm. Identical instrumental settings (slit width, amplifier gain, and so on) should be used for both samples, in order for the intensities to be compared quantitatively. In addition to using the peak intensity values to estimate the amount of psoralen attached to the TFO, the shape of the spectrum is diagnostic for a chemically intact psoralen moiety *(21)*; altered spectral shape is indicative of degraded material. The photoreactivity can also be checked in the spectrofluorimeter by measuring the spectra before and after prolonged exposure to UV light from the instrument's lamp, or from a hand-held UV lamp.

3.5.2. Photochemistry Reactions (Irradiation Conditions)

1. Incubate psoralen-TFO with radiolabeled target duplex in 1X TBB at 37°C under dark conditions. Use of concentrations well above K_d, with the psoralen-TFO in excess, helps ensure quantitative triplex formation prior to irradiation.
2. Using a light source that emits at or near 365 nm, focus the light on the sample, and irradiate samples for times ranging from 0 to 60 min, to determine the appropriate conditions for maximal crosslinking. In general, 0.5–5 J/cm^2 is required. A filter should be used to eliminate infrared and UV <320 nm (e.g., a NaNO$_3$ solution filter), which can cause photoreversal of psoralen-DNA adducts.

3.5.3. Analysis of Photoadducts by Denaturing PAGE

1. Following irradiation of samples, add 1:1 (v:v) of formamide/dye to samples, and incubate at >90°C ~5 min.

2. Subject samples to denaturing PAGE (7 *M* urea in gel buffered with 1X TBE; 15% acrylamide for duplexes <50 bp) at 60°C (run at 60 W ~1–2 h).

3. Dry gel and visualize photoadducts by autoradiography. Monoadducts and crosslinks should have altered mobilities (monoadduct: one strand of the target duplex + psoralen-TFO; crosslink: both duplex strands + psoralen-TFO), and, as a first approach, photoproducts can be analyzed by migration patterns (**Fig. 2**). (The number and position of terminal phosphates on the duplex strands can affect the mobility of the crosslinked species, so that, if both strands are radiolabeled, multiple crosslink bands may be observed, unless both strands are exhaustively phosphorylated [*see 20*].)

4. To calculate percent and distribution of photoadducts, quantitate radioactivity in ssDNA, monoadducts, and crosslinks, using a blot analyzer (e.g., PhosphorImager).

3.6. Oligonucleotide Dye Modifications

In addition to psoralens, other dyes can be attached to TFOs to enhance binding affinity *(22–24)*, serve as spectroscopic reporter groups, or serve as alternative DNA-damaging agents. Amine reactive dyes can be readily attached to oligos that contain a 3'-propanolamine group, which can be added during synthesis. The propanolamine on the 3' end protects oligos from degradation by 3' exonucleases in cells *(25)*, and makes available a primary amine group, which facilitates attachment chemistry. A variety of amine reactive dyes (with DNA damaging potential) are commercially available as succinimidyl esters, iodoacetamides, and isothiocyanates.

3.6.1. Covalent Attachment of Photoreactive Dyes to Oligonucleotides

1. Gel- or column-purify oligos (as described in **Subheadings 3.2.** and **3.3.**) in H_2O (Tris contains amine groups that will compete with the oligo primary amine group in the reaction).

Fig. 2. *(opposite page)* Photoadduct formation with psorTFO1 at the intron 1 site of APRT. (Top) Schematic diagram of the proposed photochemical reactions with psorTFO1 containing a 4'-hydroxymethyl-4,5',8-trimethylpsoralen group on the 5' end, and a proposed psoralen reaction pathway for a 5'-TpA site. (Bottom) Electrophoretic analysis of photo adducts formed by psorTFO1 at the native APRT intron 1 site. End-labelled target duplex (5×10^{-8} *M*) was incubated for 2 h with either psorTFO1 or a control psoralen TFO (psorTFOC), at a concentration of 1×10^{-6} *M* in TBB. The control oligonucleotide, psorTFOC, has the same base composition as psorTFO1, but a scrambled sequence that does not bind the intron 1 site. The preformed triplex was irradiated for various times, as indicated, using a Xe/Hg arc lamp, and then subjected to denaturing PAGE and autoradiography. Positions on the gel are indicated for the labelled duplex strands and for the photoadducts whose mobilities correspond to monoadducts (two connected lines) or crosslinks (three connected lines). py, pyrimidine-rich strand of the target duplex; pu, purine-rich strand.

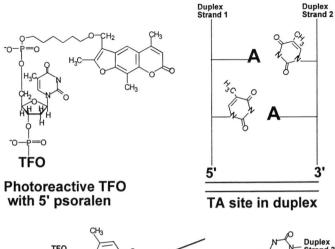

TFO

Photoreactive TFO with 5' psoralen

Duplex Strand 1

Duplex Strand 2

A

A

5'

3'

TA site in duplex

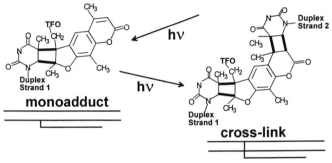

TFO

hν

Duplex Strand 1

monoadduct

hν

Duplex Strand 2

TFO

Duplex Strand 1

cross-link

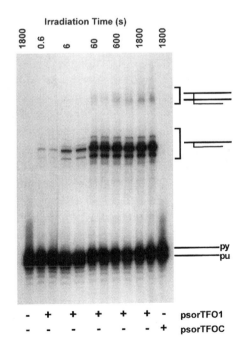

Irradiation Time (s)

1800 0.6 6 60 600 1800 1800

py
pu

| - | + | + | + | + | + | - | psorTFO1 |
| - | - | - | - | - | - | + | psorTFOC |

2. Dissolve the dye in dimethylformamide (DMF) at 20 mg/mL (the DMF should be dry, and the reaction carried out under dark conditions).
3. In a 100 µL total reaction volume, add 10 µL oligo (~10^{-5} M), 10 µL DMF, 10 µL dye (at 20 mg/mL) in DMF, and 2 µL 1 M NaHCO$_3$, pH 9.5.
4. Incubate on a shaker at 22°C for 2 h.

3.6.2. Column Purification

To separate free dye from TFO-conjugated dye, a size-exclusion column (e.g., NAP-5 column, Pharmacia) can be used as follows:

1. Stop the reaction by adding 0.4 mL 10 mM Tris-HCl, pH 7.8.
2. Equilibrate NAP-5 column in 10 mM Tris-HCl, pH 7.8.
3. Load sample (0.5 mL) on the column, and allow sample to flow into the matrix.
4. Elute sample by adding 1 mL 10 mM Tris, pH 7.8, to the column, and collect entire 1 mL fraction, which will contain both dye-modified and unmodified TFO.

Following column purification, spectroscopy can be used to determine the reaction yield by calculating the concentration ratio of oligo to dye (which should be 1:1). If the extinction coefficient of the dye is too low to detect a peak by UV or visible-light spectroscopy, then fluorescence can be used (*see* **Subheading 3.5.**).

3.7. Determination of Effects of TFOs on Mutation and Recombination in Cells

Mutation and recombination in mammalian cells have been assayed using extrachromosomal vectors and chromosomal targets (*9*). In general, genes are used whose function can be selected for, or against, or both. The most commonly used native genes are hypoxanthine-guanine phosphoribosyltransferase (HPRT) and adenine phosphoribosyltransferase (APRT), which are involved in nucleotide salvage pathways, and whose function can be selected for or against. Several different bacterial genes have been used in mutation and recombination studies. These include genes for antibiotic resistance, such as the neomycin (*neo*) and hygromycin (*hygro*) genes, which allow cell survival in the presence of the antibiotic: the herpesvirus thymidine kinase (TK) gene, which causes cell death in the presence of certain thymidine analogs (*26*), or allows survival of cells that are missing their own gene for thymidine kinase (*6*); and bacterial genes, such as *supF*, whose function can be detected by a color assay in certain strains of bacteria (*27–29*). Here the authors describe the use of the bacterial *supF* gene in an extrachromosomal assay of triplex-stimulated mutation and the APRT gene in a chromosomal assay of recombination.

3.7.1. Addition of TFOs to Cells

The uptake and stability of oligos in cells can vary, depending on a number of factors, including cell type and oligo modifications. Studies using oligos contain-

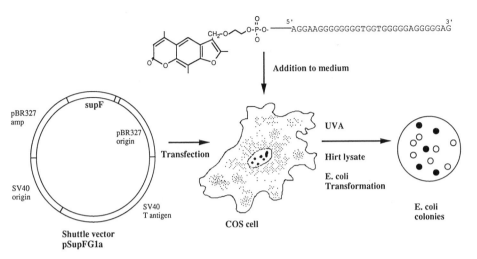

Fig. 3. Experimental strategy for targeted mutagenesis of SV40 DNA mediated by intracellular triple helix formation within COS cells. The SV40 shuttle vector DNA, pSupFG1, was transfected into COS cells by electroporation. Separately, the psoralen-conjugated oligonucleotides were subsequently added to the extracellular growth medium. After time was allowed for oligonucleotide entry into cells, and for possible intracellular triple helix formation, the cells were exposed to ultraviolet A (UVA) irradiation to photoactivate the psoralen and generate targeted adducts. Following vector replication, the cells were lysed, and the vector molecules were harvested for transformation into *E. coli* to allow genetic analysis of the *supF* gene. The structure of the psoralen (4'-hydroxymethyl-4,5',8-trimethylpsoralen attached at the 4' hydroxymethyl position via a two-carbon linker to the 5' phosphate of the oligonucleotide) is shown.

ing a phosphodiester backbone and a 3'-propanolamine group in cells, serum, and mice have demonstrated that oligos are taken up readily and are quite stable *(25,30)*.

1. Purify oligos by elution from a Sephadex column equilibrated in H$_2$O or TE (as described in **Subheading 3.2.**).
2. Concentrate oligos to ~mM concentration by use of a Centricon or Speed-Vac.
3. Add oligo to cell culture media to a final concentration of ~µM.
4. Incubate at 37°C in an incubator at least 2 h, to allow uptake of oligos into the nucleus. (Serum-free media should be used during the incubation period, to avoid oligo degradation).

3.7.2. SupF *Assay for Triplex-Stimulated Mutation*

The general strategy for targeted mutagenesis of the *supF* gene on an extra-chromosomal plasmid in monkey COS cells is shown in **Fig. 3 *(28)***. The plasmid is a simian virus-40 (SV40)-based shuttle vector, which can replicate in monkey cells by virtue of the SV40 origin of replication and the SV40 T-antigen gene, and can also replicate in bacterial cells by virtue of the pBR327 origin. Additionally, the shuttle vector contains the *amp* gene, to allow selection of bacterial cells that have taken up the plasmid. The *supF* gene encodes a tRNA that suppresses amber mutations; in bacterial strain SY204*lacZ125*(am), the encoded *supF* gene produces blue colonies on plates containing X-Gal and isopropyl-β-D-thiogalactopyranoside (IPTG); mutated versions produce white colonies.

1. Grow COS cells to about 70% confluence (2×10^6 cells per 10-cm dish) in Dulbecco's modified Eagle's Medium (DMEM), supplemented with 10% fetal calf serum (FCS).
2. Trypsinize cells by washing with PBS, and then incubating in trypsin for 5 min at 37°C.
3. Resuspend cells in DMEM at 10^7 cells per mL, add 3 µg plasmid DNA (pSupFG1) to 10^6 cells.
4. Transfect cells by electroporation (Bio-Rad, Hercules, CA; setting, 25 µF, 250 W, and 250 V; 0.4-cm-diameter cuvet). Store cells on ice for 10 min, and then dilute with DMEM and incubate at 37°C for 30 min.
5. Add TFOs to the cell suspension at a final concentration of 2 µM. Incubate ~2 h at 37°C, with agitation every 15 min. For psoralen-modified TFOs, avoid light.
6. Irradiate cells with 366 nm light by using a light source that can be evenly distributed over the entire cell sample (e.g., a hand-held UV-366 lamp) and filtered to omit ultraviolet B (UVB) and infrared light. Typically, 0.5–5 J/cm^2 is appropriate for maximal photoreaction.
7. Isolate the shuttle vector 48 h after addition of TFO by a modified alkaline lysis procedure *(28)*.
8. Transform *Escherichia coli* strain SY204 (*lacZ125*[am]) with 1 µL of the isolated shuttle vector sample by electroporation (Bio-Rad; setting, 2.5 µF, 250 W, and 1800 V; 0.1-cm-diameter cuvet).
9. Plate the transformed *E. coli* cells onto Luria-Bertani plates containing 50 µg ampicillin/mL, 100 µg X-Gal/mL, and 1 µM IPTG, and incubate at 37°C overnight.
10. Colonies containing a mutant *supF* gene, which is unable to suppress the amber mutation in the host cell β-galactosidase gene, are detected as white colonies among the wild-type blue ones.
11. Mutant *supF* genes can be characterized by extraction of the plasmid, followed by DNA sequencing.

These studies showed that a 30-nucleotide-long TFO that binds to the *supF* gene with a K_d of $2 \times 10^{-8} M$ stimulated mutation about 10-fold; a scrambled-sequence oligonucleotide of the same length did not stimulate mutation above background levels. The same TFO with an attached psoralen, which bound to the *supF* gene with a K_d of $3 \times 10^{-9} M$, stimulates mutation 50- to 100-fold. In the absence of psoralen, the analyzed mutations consisted mostly of point mutations that were clustered around the TFO-binding site. With psoralen and irradiation, the majority of mutations affected the 5'-ApT immediately adjacent to the TFO-binding site. Triplex-induced mutagenesis in the absence of psoralen was not detected in xeroderma pigmentosum group A cells nor in

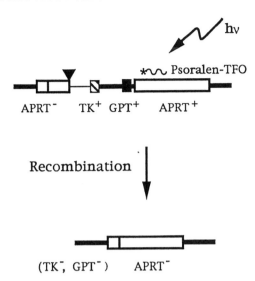

Fig. 4. *APRT* recombination assay. Chromosomal substrate for testing effect of a TFO on recombination. The upstream copy of the *APRT* gene contains a 3' deletion (indicated by the triangle) and a mutation in exon 2 (indicated by the bar); the downstream copy is wild-type. The expected genotype associated with a recombination event can be selected for by using drug selections for TK⁻, GPT⁻, and APRT⁻.

Cockayne's syndrome group B cells, indicating a requirement for excision repair and for transcription-coupled repair, respectively, in the process.

3.7.3. APRT Assay for Triplex-Stimulated Recombination

The general strategy for detecting chromosomal recombination at the APRT locus in Chinese hamster ovary (CHO) cells is shown in **Fig. 4**. This intra-chromosomal recombination substrate was created by a standard gene-targeting protocol using cell line ATS65tg, which contains a point mutation in the APRT gene and has been rendered HPRT⁻ by selection in 6-thioguanine. The recombination substrate in the targeted cell line, GSC4, comprises a 6.9-kb duplicated segment of the APRT gene. The upstream copy of the gene is APRT⁻ by virtue of a point mutation that eliminates an *Eco*RV restriction site; the downstream copy is APRT⁺. Two additional selectable markers, the herpesvirus TK gene and the bacterial guanine phosphoribosyltransferase (*GPT*) gene, are located between the duplicated APRT genes. Recombination (and mutation) are detected by loss of APRT gene function. Typically, gene conversion, in which the *Eco*RV mutation is transferred from the upstream copy to the downstream copy, occurs 5–10 × more frequently than crossovers (popouts), which eliminate one copy of the repeated DNA and the intervening plasmid DNA.

Cell lines and targeting vectors are available for creating the duplicated recombination substrate by FLP/FRT site-specific recombination *(31)*. Any TFO-binding site can be inserted into the polylinker adjacent to the FRT site in the vector and targeted rapidly to the APRT locus, in order to test the effects of TFO binding on recombination at a defined, well-studied chromosomal locus *(5)*.

1. Grow CHO cell line GSC4 to about 70% confluence in DMEM supplemented with 10% FCS and nonessential amino acids.
2. Add experimental or control (scrambled-sequence) TFOs, up to 10 µM, to media. Incubate cells at 37°C for 6 h to allow TFO uptake into nuclei.
3. Irradiate cells with 366 nm light, as described below:
   a. Use a light source that can be evenly distributed over the entire cell monolayer (e.g., a hand-held UV-366 lamp), and filtered to omit UVB and infrared light.
   b. Typically, 0.5–5 J/cm^2 is appropriate for maximal photoreaction. Following irradiation, allow 24 h for cells to recover prior to replating.
   c. Plate for cell survival, as well as for selected phenotype.
4. After 24 h, trypsinize cells, and replate at 2×10^5 cells per 10-cm plate in complete medium. For cell survival, replate at 2×10^2 and 2×10^3 cells per 10-cm plate in complete medium.
5. For APRT⁻ selection, after 5 d, replace medium with DMEM containing 10% FCS, and supplemented with 400 µM 8-azaadenine, which will kill cells that carry a functional APRT gene. (A 5-d waiting period is included before selection, to allow previously expressed APRT protein to decay.)
6. After ~ 14 d, APRT⁻ colonies can be isolated by standard procedures for further growth and characterization, or they can be stained for counting, using 50% methanol, 10% glacial acetic acid, and 0.4% (w:v) Coomassie blue.
7. For characterization of the mutant colonies, transfer isolated colonies to 24-well plates and grow until confluent, then transfer to two 10-cm plates. When confluent, isolate DNA from one plate, and use the other plate to prepare cell samples for storage at –80°C.
8. The status of the recombination substrate in the surviving APRT⁻ cells can be characterized by PCR or by Southern blotting: Crossovers have only one copy of the gene; gene convertants have two copies, with the *Eco*RV mutation in the downstream copy.

These studies showed no stimulation of intrachromosomal homologous recombination in the absence of UV irradiation by either the specific oligonucleotide with or without psoralen or the scrambled-sequence control oligonucleotide. In the presence of the specific TFO with an attached psoralen, a dose-dependent three-fold stimulation of recombination was observed. At the native site, which was used in these studies, only monoadduct formation was possible *(20)*.

References

1. Capecchi, M. R. (1989) Altering the genome by homologous recombination. *Science* **244,** 1288–1292.

2. Rothstein, R. (1983) One-step gene disruption in yeast. *Methods Enzymol.* **101,** 202–211.
3. Botstein, D. and Fink, G. (1988) Yeast: an experimental organism for modern biology. *Science* **240,** 1439–1443.
4. Mansour, S. L., Thomas, K. R., and Capecchi, M. R. (1988) Disruption of the proto-oncogene int-2 in mouse embryo-derived stem cells: a general strategy for targeting mutations to non-selectable genes. *Nature* **336,** 348–352.
5. Sargent, R. G., Merrihew, R. V., Nairn, R., Adair, G., Meuth, M., and Wilson, J. H. (1996) Influence of a (GT)29 microsatellite sequence on homologous recombination in the hamster adenine phosphoribosyltransferase gene. *Nucleic Acids Res.* **24,** 746–753.
6. Bollag, R. J., Waldman, A. S., and Liskay, R. M. (1989) Homologous recombination in mammalian cells. *Annu. Rev. Genet.* **23,** 199–225.
7. Roth, D. B. and Wilson, J. H. (1986) Nonhomologous recombination in mammalian cells: role for short sequence homologies in the joining reaction. *Mol. Cell. Biol.* **6,** 4295–4304.
8. Thomas, K. R. and Capecchi, M. R. (1987) Site-directed mutagenesis by gene targeting in mouse embryo-derived stem cells. *Cell* **51,** 503–512.
9. Vasquez, K. M. and Wilson, J. H. (1998) Triplex-directed modification of genes and genes activity. *Trends Biochem. Sci.* **23,** 4–9.
10. Cooney, M., Czernuszewicz, G., Postel, E. H., Flint, S. J., and Hogan, M. E. (1988) Site-specific oligonucleotide binding represses transcription of the human c-myc gene in vitro. *Science* **241,** 456–459.
11. Beal, P. A. and Dervan, P. B. (1991) Second structural motif for recognition of DNA by oligonucleotide-directed triple-helix formation. *Science* **251,** 1360–1363.
12. Rajagopal, P. and Feigon, J. (1989) Triple-strand formation in the homopurine: homopyrimidine DNA oligonucleotides d(G-A)4 and d(T-C)4. *Nature* **339,** 637–640.
13. Radhakrishnan, I. and Patel, D. J. (1994) DNA triplexes: solution structures, hydration sites, energetics, interactions, and function. *Biochemistry* **33,** 11405–11416.
14. Stein, C. A., Subasinghe, C., Shinozuka, K., and Cohen, J. S. (1988) Physico-chemical properties of phosphorothioate oligodeoxynucleotides. *Nucleic Acids Res.* **16,** 3209–3221.
15. Tidd, D. M. and Warenius, H. M. (1989) Partial protection against serum nuclease degradation using terminal methylphosphonate groups. *Br. J. Cancer* **60,** 343–350.
16. Sambrook, J., Fritsch, E. F., and Maniatis, T. (1989) *Molecular Cloning: A Laboratory Manual.* Cold Spring Harbor Laboratory Press, Cold Spring Harbor, NY.
17. Vasquez, K. M., Wensel, T. G., Hogan, M. E., and Wilson, J. H. (1995) High-affinity triple helix formation by synthetic oligonucleotides at a site within a selectable mammalian gene. *Biochemistry* **34,** 7243–7251.
18. Shindo, H., Torigoe, H., and Sarai, A. (1993) Thermodynamic and kinetic studies of DNA triplex formation of an oligohomopyrimidine and a matched duplex by filter binding assay. *Biochemistry* **32,** 8963–8969.
19. Lee, J. S., Johnson, D. A., and Morgan, A. R. (1979) Complexes formed by (pyrimidine)n.(purine)n DNAs on lowering the pH are three-stranded. *Nucleic Acids Res.* **6,** 3073–3091.

20. Vasquez, K. M., Wensel, T. G., Hogan, M. E., and Wilson, J. H. (1996) High-efficiency triple-helix-mediated photo-cross-linking at a targeted site within a selectable mammalian gene. *Biochemistry* **35,** 10,712–10,719.

21. Pieles, U. and Englisch, U. (1989) Psoralen covalently linked to oligodeoxyribonucleotides: synthesis, sequence specific recognition of DNA and photo-cross-linking to pyrimidine residues of DNA. *Nucleic Acids Res.* **17,** 285–299.

22. Sun, J. S., Francois, J. C., Montenay-Garestier, T., Saison-Behmoaras, T., Roig, V., Thuong, N. T., and Helene, C. (1989) Sequence-specific intercalating agents: intercalation at specific sequences on duplex DNA via major groove recognition by oligonucleotide-intercalator conjugates. *Proc. Natl. Acad. Sci. USA* **86,** 9198–9202.

23. Young, S. L., Krawczyk, S. H., Matteucci, M. D., and Toole, J. J. (1991) Triple helix formation inhibits transcription elongation in vitro. *Proc. Natl. Acad. Sci. USA* **88,** 10,023–10,026.

24. Cassidy, S. A., Strekowski, L., Wilson, W. D., and Fox, K. R. (1994) Effect of a triplex-binding ligand on parallel and antiparallel DNA triple helices using short unmodified and acridine-linked oligonucleotides. *Biochemistry* **33,** 15,338–15,347.

25. Nelson, P. S., Sherman-Gold, R., and Leon, R (1989) New and versatile reagent for incorporating multiple primary aliphatic amines into synthetic oligonucleotides. *Nucleic Acids Res.* **17,** 7179–7186.

26. Borreli, E., Heyman, R., Hsi, M., and Evans, R. M. (1988) Targeting of an inducible toxic phenotype in animal cells. *Proc. Natl. Acad. Sci. USA* **85,** 7572–7576.

27. Wang, G. and Glazer, P. M. (1995) Altered repair of targeted psoralen photoadducts in the context of an oligonucleotide-mediated triple helix. *J. Biol. Chem.* **270,** 22,595–22,601.

28. Wang, G., Levy, D. D., Seidman, M. M., and Glazer, P. M. (1995) Targeted mutagenesis in mammalian cells mediated by intracellular triple helix formation. *Mol. Cell. Biol.* **15,** 1759–1768.

29. Wang, G., Levy, D. D., Seidman, M. M., and Glazer, P. M. (1996) Mutagenesis in mammalian cells induced by triple helix formation and transcription-coupled repair. *Science* **271,** 802–805.

30. Zendegui, J. G., Vasquez, K. M., Tinsley, J. H., Kessler, D. J., and Hogan, M. E. (1992) In vitro stability and kinetics of absorption and disposition of 3' phosphopropyl amine oligonucleotides. *Nucleic Acids Res.* **20,** 307–314.

31. Merrihew, R. V., Sargent, R. G., and Wilson, J. H. (1995) Efficient modification of the APRT gene by FLP/FRT site-specific targeting. *Somatic Cell Mol. Genet.* **21,** 299–307.

14

Use of Quantitative Ligation-Mediated Polymerase Chain Reaction to Detect Gene Targeting by Alkylating Oligodeoxynucleotides

Howard B. Gamper, Irina Afonina, Evgeniy Belousov, Michael W. Reed, and Mikhail A. Podyminogin

1. Introduction

The authors describe the preparation and use of a unique class of reactive oligodeoxynucleotides (ODNs) that can sequence, specifically bind to, and alkylate complex genomic DNA under physiological conditions. The alkylating event, which is detected using a quantitative version of the ligation-mediated polymerase chain reaction (LM-PCR) *(1,2)* , acts as a marker for complex formation, and permits an estimation of the gene targeting frequency. Because alkylation of the DNA can take place within either a classical triple-stranded complex *(3)* or a recombinase-stabilized synaptic joint *(4)*, two different strategies for recognizing DNA can be directly compared. The ability to detect and quantify an early, perhaps rate limiting step, in genetic targeting should be useful in efforts to better understand and improve this important technique.

The alkylating ODNs described here are conjugated to chlorambucil, a clinically used nitrogen mustard. When an ODN–chlorambucil conjugate forms a triplex or a poststrand exchange synaptic complex with dsDNA, it can alkylate the *N*-7 position of nearby guanines in the host DNA with good efficiency and specificity. Following gene targeting, the recovered DNA is restricted upstream from the alkylation site and the adduct is converted to a nick by brief incubation at 95°C. The targeted gene segment is then amplified by quantitative LM-PCR, and the products are electrophoresed on a sequencing gel, along with a G-ladder. By comparing the relative amounts of amplified product attributable to heat-induced nicking vs restriction, the frequency of targeted alkylation can be determined.

From: *Methods in Molecular Biology, vol. 133: Gene Targeting Protocols*
Edited by: E. Kmiec © Humana Press Inc., Totowa, NJ

Using quantitative LM-PCR, the authors show that ODN–chlorambucil conjugates of sufficient length can bind to and efficiently alkylate a single-copy gene in purified human genomic DNA, using either of the two DNA recognition strategies. Triple-strand formation, with a homopurine run in the HLA DQβ1*0302 allele *(5)*, is demonstrated using a 21-nucleotide-long G/A-containing ODN, which is terminally conjugated to a chlorambucil group. Synaptic complex formation with a unique site in the same allele is achieved using 30- or 50-nucleotide-long ODNs in the presence of ReCA protein and adenosine 5'-O-(3-thiotriphosphate) (ATPγS). These ODNs contain all four bases, and are conjugated to a chlorambucil group through the 5-position of an internally placed aminopropyl dUTP. When similar gene targeting reactions take place in nuclei or cells, they can likewise be analyzed by quantitative LM-PCR following extraction and restriction of the modified DNA.

2. Materials
2.1. Synthesis and Purification of Chlorambucil-Modified ODNs

1. Reagents for introducing an amino group onto ODNs at the time of automated synthesis: aminohexyl controlled pore glass *(6)*, N-MMT-hexanolamine phosphoramidite linker (Glen Research, Sterling VA), and the 5'-(dimethoxytrityl) 3'-(cyanoethyl N,N-diisopropylphosphoramidite) of 5-(3-phthalimidopropyl)-2'-deoxyuridine *(7)*.
2. High pressure liquid chromatography (HPLC): A gradient HPLC system equipped with an ultraviolet (UV) detector (260 nm) is used. Triethylammonium (TEA) ion exchange of the ODNs is accomplished on a 7×250 mm PRP-1 column (Hamilton, Reno, NV). Purification and analysis of chlorambucil-ODNs is performed on a 4.6×250 mm C18 column (Rainin, Woburn, CA). For both column systems, solvent A = 0.1 M, pH 7.5, TEA acetate buffer, solvent B = acetonitrile.
3. Chlorambucil 2,3,5,6-tetrafluorophenyl ester (chlorambucil TFP ester): This compound is prepared from chlorambucil (Fluka, Milwaukee, WI) and tetrafluorophenyl trifluoroacetate, using standard conditions *(6)*. The chlorambucil TFP ester is a colorless syrup stored desiccated at 0–5°C.
4. Anhydrous dimethy sulfoxide (DMSO), ethyldiisopropylamine, 2% sodium perchlorate in acetone, 3 M sodium acetate, and butanol are used in conjugate synthesis and purification.
5. A Beckman (Fullerton, CA) GP centrifuge with a swinging bucket rotor is used for ODN precipitation.

2.2. Reaction of ODN$_T$ with Genomic DNA in a Triple-Strand Complex

1. Genomic DNA in 10 mM Tris-HCl, pH 7.5, 1 mM EDTA (TE); stored at 4°C.
2. 5X Triplex-forming buffer: 700 mM KCl, 50 mM MgCl$_2$, 100 mM HEPES-HCl, pH 7.0, 5 mM spermine; stored at 4°C.
3. 80 μM coralyne *(see* **Note 1**); stored at 4°C in the dark.

4. Chlorambucil–ODN$_T$: 100–500 μM stock; aliquots stored at –80°C; thaw on ice immediately before use (*see* **Note 2**).
5. 3 M Sodium acetate.
6. 70% Ethanol, kept at –20°C.

2.3. Reaction of ODN$_R$ with Genomic DNA in Synaptic Complex

1. Genomic DNA in TE buffer.
2. 10X Synaptic complex forming buffer: 100 mM Tris-acetate, pH 7.5, 500 mM NaOAc, 120 mM Mg(OAc)$_2$, 10 mM dithiothreitol (DTT), 50% glycerol; stored at –20°C.
3. 10 mM ATPγS: purchased as a 100-mM stock solution from Boehringer Mannheim and diluted 10-fold in water. (Cat. no. 1162306, Indianapolis, IN.)
4. RecA protein: 2 mg/mL (New England BioLabs, cat. no. 249L, Beverly, MA).
5. Chlorambucil–ODN$_R$: 100–500 μM stock; aliquots stored at –80°C; thaw on ice immediately before use (*see* **Note 2**).
6. TE buffer: 10 mM Tris-HCl, pH 7.5, 1 mM ethylenediamineterraucetic acid (EDTA).
7. 10% sodium dedecyl sulfate (SDS).
8. Proteinase K: 5 mg/mL (Sigma, cat. no. P-2308).
9. Phenol–chloroform: Add 24 mL chloroform and 1 mL isoamyl alcohol to 25 mL phenol saturated with 10 mM Tris-HCl, pH 8.0, 1 mM EDTA (Sigma, cat no. P-4557).
10. 3 M Sodium acetate.
11. 70% Ethanol, kept at –20°C.

2.4. Quantitative LM-PCR

1. Restriction endonuclease, selected according to the criteria outlined in Note 3, and the corresponding 10X restriction buffer.
2. 5X First-strand buffer: 200 mM NaCl, 50 mM Tris-HCl, pH 8.9, 25 mM MgSO$_4$, 0.05% gelatin (Sigma, cat. no. G-1393); store at –20°C.
3. 25 mM deoxynucleoside triphosphate (dNTP) mix, pH 7.0: Purchase individual 100 mM solutions of deoxyadenosine triphosphate (dATP), deoxythymidine triphosphate (dTTP), deoxyguanosine triphosphate (dGTP), and deoxycytosine triphosphate (dCTP) from Pharmacia LKB (Piscataway, NJ), and combine equal volumes; store at –20°C.
4. Primers 1, 2, and 3 (*see* **Note 4**): Each oligonucleotide primer is stored in a silanized tube at a concentration of at least 10 μM. Prior to use, primer 3 is freshly 5'-end-labeled to a specific activity of 4–9 × 10^6 cpm/pmol with T4 polynucleotide kinase and γ-^{32}P-ATP (3000 C$_i$mmol).
5. First-strand synthesis mix, 25 μL per reaction: 6.0 μL 5X first-strand buffer, 0.3 μL 1 pmol/μL primer 1, 0.24 μL 25 mM dNTP mix, pH 7.0, 18.2 μL water, 0.25 μL 2U/μL Thermococcus litoralis (Vent) DNA polymerase (New England Biolabs, cat. no. 254L). Prepare immediately before use. Mix all components except polymerase, chill on ice, and then add Vent polymerase.
6. Ligase dilution solution, 20 μL per reaction: 2.2 μL 1 M Tris-HCl, pH 7.5, 0.35 μL 1 M MgCl$_2$, 1.0 μL 1 M DTT, 0.25 μL 10 mg/mL bovine serum albumin (BSA;

DNase-free, Pharmacia LKB, no. 27-8915-01), 16.2 µL water. Prepare immediately before use and chill on ice.

7. Universal linker mix (*see* **Note 5**): 20 µ*M* linker (11-mer; 5'-GGTACTGGTCG), 20 µ*M* linker-primer (25-mer; 5'-CTCTTGATCCCGCTCGACCAGTACC), 250 m*M* Tris-HCl, pH 7.7. This mix is prepared in advance by adding stock solutions of the two ODNs, together with Tris-HCl buffer and water, to give the final concentrations indicated above. The solution is then heated 5 min at 95°C and cooled slowly to 4°C at which it is kept for 12 h. Aliquots are stored at –20°C and thawed on ice before use.

8. Ligase mix, 25 µL per reaction: 0.25 µL 1 *M* MgCl$_2$, 0.50 µL 1 *M* DTT, 0.75 µL 100 m*M* ATP, pH 7.0, 0.125 µL 10 mg/mL BSA, 17.4 µL water, 5.0 µL 20 µ*M* preannealed universal linker mix, 1.0 µL 3 Weiss U/µL T4 DNA ligase (Promega, cat. no. M1801, Madison, WI or Pharmacia LKB, cat. no. 27-0840-01). Prepare immediately before use.

9. 5X Taq buffer: 200 m*M* NaCl, 50 m*M* Tris-HCl, pH 8.9, 10 m*M* MgCl$_2$, 0.5% Triton X-100, 0.05% gelatin; store in aliquots at –20°C.

10. LM-PCR mix, 49.3 µL per reaction: 20 µL 5X Taq buffer, 0.8 µL 25 m*M* dNTP, 1 µL linker-primer (10 pmol/µL), 0.75 µL primer 2 (10 pmol/µL), 26.75 µL water.

11. Ampliwax beads (Perkin-Elmer, Norwalk, CT).

12. Taq polymerase: 5 U/µL (Promega, cat. no. M186A).

13. PCR stop solution: 250 µL 3 *M* NaOAc, pH 7.5, 25 µL 0.5 *M* EDTA, pH 8.0, 7 µL tRNA (10.3 µg/µL), and 940 µL water.

14. Gel loading buffer: 80% (v/v) formamide, 45 m*M* Tris base, 45 m*M* boric acid, 0.05% (w/v) bromphenol blue, 0.05% (w/v) xylene cyanol; store in aliquots at –20°C.

15. 3 *M* Sodium acetate.

16. 70% Ethanol, kept at –20°C.

17. Glycogen or tRNA carrier.

3. Methods

3.1. Synthesis and Purification of Chlorambucil-Modified ODNs

Guidelines for the design of chlorambucil-modified ODNs are described in **Note 6**. These ODNs are prepared by postsynthetic conjugation of a reactive chlorambucil derivative, with an alkylamino group present on the ODN.

1. ODNs that form a triple-stranded complex with DNA (ODN$_T$) are synthesized with a 5' or 3' aminohexyl group using *N*-MMT-hexanolamine phosphoramidite linker or aminohexyl controlled pore glass, respectively. ODNs that form a RecA protein-stabilized synaptic complex with DNA (ODN$_R$) are synthesized with an internal aminopropyl group, using the protected phosphoramidite of 5-(3-aminopropyl)-2'-deoxyuridine. The synthesis, HPLC purification, detritylation, and butanol precipitation of both types of ODNs are carried out using standard procedures, as previously described (**6**). Drying of the ODN solutions is performed under vacuum, using a centrifugal evaporator (Savant Speed-Vac).

2. TEA ion exchange of ODN_T (from a 2-μmol scale synthesis) is carried out by dissolving the ODN in 0.5 mL water and injecting it on a PRP-1 HPLC column. A gradient of 0–60% solvent B over 20 min (flow rate 2 mL/min) is run, and the ODN-containing peak (~16-min retention time for a 21-mer) is collected and dried overnight on a Speed-Vac (Savant, Holbrook, NY).

3. HPLC purified TEA ODN_T is dissolved in 0.5 mL water, and its concentration determined from the UV absorbance of a 1:100 dilution. Extinction coefficients for ODNs are determined using a nearest-neighbor model *(8)*. An aliquot containing 1 mg ODN_T is dried in a 1.7-mL Eppendorf tube on the Speed-Vac. The solid is dissolved in 0.2 mL anhydrous DMSO just prior to conjugation.

4. 10 μL ethyldiisopropylamine and 75 μL of a 20-mg/mL solution of chlorambucil TFP ester in DMSO (1.5 mg) is added to the ODN_T solution. The solution is shaken on a vortexer for 3 h, and the crude chlorambucil–ODN_T product is isolated by adding the reaction mix to 10 mL 2% sodium perchlorate in acetone. The precipitate is immediately pelleted by centrifugation at 3000*g* for 5 min. The pellet is vortexed with 2 mL acetone and recentrifuged. The washed pellet is dried for 10 min on a Speed-Vac, then stored at –80°C prior to HPLC purification.

5. The crude chlorambucil–ODN_T is dissolved in 0.25 mL water and injected on a C18 HPLC column. A gradient of 5–85% solvent B over 40 min (flow rate 1 mL/min) is run, and a ~2-mL-fraction containing the desired conjugate (20 min retention time for a 21-mer) is collected in a 14-mL polypropylene tube.

6. The pure product is immediately precipitated by adding 100 μL 3 M sodium acetate and 4 mL butanol for each mL of eluent collected. The precipitate is pelleted without delay by centrifugation at 3000*g* for 5 min, vortexed with 2 mL ethanol, and repelleted. The washed pellet is dried for 10 min on a Speed-Vac, dissolved in 0.2 mL water, and transferred to a 1.7-mL Eppendorf tube. After removing two 10-μL aliquots, the product is labeled and stored at –80°C.

7. One aliquot is used for concentration determination, as described in step 3 of this subheading (typical isolated yields of chlorambucil–ODN_T are 0.25–0.50 mg/mg of ODN_T).

8. The second aliquot is analyzed for purity by C18 HPLC, using a gradient of 5–85% solvent B over 40 min (typical purity is >90%). A 21-mer chlorambucil–ODN_T has a retention time of ~18 min, and hydrolyzed chlorambucil–ODN_T is detected as multiple peaks at 10–12 min.

9. The above procedure is applicable to the synthesis of chlorambucil–ODN_R conjugates. The retention time of a 30-mer chlorambucil-ODN_R is ~14 min on C18 HPLC, and yields are somewhat lower.

3.2. Reaction of ODN_T with Genomic DNA in Triple-Strand Complex

1. To a solution containing 2–10 μg of genomic DNA in TE, add 20 μL 5X triplex-forming buffer, 10 μL 80 μ*M* coralyne, and water, to give a final volume of 90 μL in a 1.7-mL Eppendorf tube.

2. Thaw an aliquot of stock chlorambucil–ODN$_T$ on ice and dilute with ice-cold water to 10X concentration. Add 10 μL to the reaction mixture, to give a final concentration of 10^{-5}–10^{-9} M chlorambucil–ODN$_T$.

3. Mix gently and incubate 1–6 hr at 37°C. The half-life for alkylation is ~45 min.

4. Add 10 μL 3 M NaOAc, pH 7.0, and 300 μL ice-cold 100% ethanol. Freeze in liquid nitrogen or on dry ice, and pellet the DNA by centrifugation at 12,000 rpm for 15 min in a microcentrifuge at 4°C. The pellet is washed with cold 70% ethanol, dried briefly in a Speed-Vac, and dissolved in 50 μL TE.

3.3. Reaction of ODN$_R$ with Genomic DNA in Synaptic Complex

1. To a solution of 2–10 μg genomic DNA in TE, add 10 μL 10X synaptic complex-forming buffer, 10 μL 10 mM ATPγS, and water, to give a final volume of 87 μL in a 1.7-mL Eppendorf tube. Keep on ice.

2. Thaw an aliquot of stock chlorambucil–ODN$_R$ on ice, dilute with ice-cold water to 1 μM, and add 10 μL to the reaction mixture.

3. Add 3 μL RecA protein solution, mix gently, and incubate the reaction mixture for 1–6 h at 37°C.

4. Add 82 μL TE, 10 μL 10% SDS, and 8 μL proteinase K, and incubate 30 min at 37°C.

5. Extract the reaction mixture with an equal volume of phenol–chloroform. Transfer the aqueous phase into a fresh 1.7-mL Eppendorf tube and extract 3× with ether, aspirating the organic layer.

6. Continue with subheading 3.2. step 4 using twice the volumes.

3.4. Quantitative LM-PCR

This quantitative LM-PCR protocol has been adapted from three comprehensive descriptions of the technique *(9–11)*. By incorporating a restriction step at the beginning of the protocol, and by adjusting the number of PCR cycles to remain within the exponential phase of amplification, the technique has been made quantitative. In each experiment, an aliquot of the genomic DNA is treated with dimethylsulfate and amplified, along with the rest of the samples, to provide a G-ladder *(9)*.

1. Restrict 2–10 μg control or alkylated genomic DNA to completion by incubating 3–6 h under optimal conditions with a threefold excess of restriction enzyme. When using a new restriction enzyme or amplifying a different sequence, complete restriction of the gene of interest should be verified by LM-PCR or Southern analysis. On a routine basis, an aliquot of the digested DNA should be analyzed by agarose electrophoresis to verify activity of the restriction endonuclease.

2. Adjust the volume to 100 μL with water, and ethanol-precipitate the DNA as described in **step 3.2.4.** Resuspend the pellet in TE to give a DNA concentration of ~0.5 μg/μL. Transfer 5 μL (2–2.5 μg DNA) to a 0.6-mL PCR tube, and chill on ice.

3. Prepare the first-strand synthesis mix (containing primer 1). Add 25 μL of this mix to the DNA.
4. Transfer PCR tubes into the pre-heated block (95°C) of a thermocycler, where the following program is carried out: 10 min at 95°C (cleavage of alkylated site[s] and denaturation of DNA [*see* **Note 7**]), 30 min at 60°C (primer annealing), 10 min at 76°C (first-strand synthesis). Transfer tubes to ice immediately after completion of the extension step.
5. Prepare ligase-dilution solution and ligase mix. Add universal linker mix and T4 DNA ligase to the ligase mix, upon completion of the extension step. Add 20 μL cold ligase-dilution solution and 25 μL cold ligase mix to each DNA sample, stirring gently with the pipet tip after each addition. Ligation is carried out overnight at 17°C.
6. Add 1 μL tRNA (5 μg/μL), 8.4 μL 3 *M* NaOAc, and 250 μL ethanol. Pellet and wash the DNA, as described in **Subheading 3.2., step 4.** Dissolve the DNA pellets in 50 μL water by letting the samples sit at room temperature for 30 min, with occasional vortexing, followed by brief centrifugation.
7. Add 49.3 μL LM-PCR mix and 1 Ampliwax bead to each tube. Mix with pipet tip.
8. Place tubes into the preheated block (94°C) of a thermocycler, and perform hot start by incubating the samples 3 min at 94°C, and then 5 min at 85°C. During the 85°C incubation, 0.7 μL Taq polymerase is added, with mixing.
9. Carry out 15 cycles of PCR using the following program (*see* **Note 8**): 1 min at 95°C (denaturation), 2 min at a temperature 0–2°C above the calculated melting temperature (T_m) of primer 2 (annealing), and 3 min at 76°C (extension).
10. After the last extension step, while incubating the samples at 85°C, add 2.5 μL ^{32}P-labeled primer 3 (1 pmol/μL) to each tube, and mix with a pipet.
11. Perform 13 more cycles of PCR, using the reaction profile in **step 9** of this **Subsection**, with the temperature of the annealing step adjusted for the T_m of primer 3. Allow the final extension to proceed 5 min, and then transfer the tubes to ice.
12. Transfer 95 μL of the PCR mixture to a 1.7-mL Eppendorf tube, and add 100 μL PCR stop solution and 450 μL ethanol. Pellet and wash the DNA as outlined in **Subheading 3.2., step 4**.
13. After brief drying in a Speed-Vac, dissolve each pellet in 2–3 μL gel-loading buffer.
14. Heat at 95°C for 2 min and quick-cool in ice.
15. Load samples onto a 40 cm long 8% polyacrylamide/7 *M* urea sequencing gel, and run at 50 W (50°C), until the xylene cyanol band has run two-thirds down the gel.
16. Transfer the gel onto Whatman 3MM paper, and dry in a gel dryer.
17. Expose the dried gel to a phosphorimager screen for several hours, and calculate the ratio of intensities for the restriction and alkylation-induced bands. This ratio represents the efficiency of targeted alkylation.

4. Notes

1. Coralyne is an aromatic heterocycle that can intercalate into triple-strand DNA *(12)*. Purine motif triplexes *(13)* are stabilized as much as 1000-fold in the presence of a saturating concentration of this agent *(14)*.

2. The stability of chlorambucil rapidly drops off as the temperature is raised. In aqueous solutions, this reagent is stable for months at $-80°C$, but at $37°C$ it has a half-life of only 45 min *(3)*. To maintain the integrity of chlorambucil–ODN conjugates, it is important to thaw stock solutions immediately prior to use and keep them ice-cold. By following these precautions, aliquots of the stock solution can be used repeatedly.

3. Selection of a restriction endonuclease for the quantitative LM-PCR protocol is based on the enzyme having a recognition site 50–200 nucleotides upstream from the alkylated base, and no recognition sites between that base and the downstream sequence complementary to the first primer.

4. There are three reverse primers used in LM-PCR, each complementary to the alkylated strand. Primer 1 should be located approx 150–300 nucleotides downstream from the alkylation site. Primers 2 and 3 should be closer to this site, and may partially overlap. The first-strand synthesis primer (primer 1) should form a hybrid with a T_m of $>60°C$. Primers 2 and 3 (the amplification and labeling primers, respectively) and the universal linker-primer should form hybrids with even higher T_ms. When selecting a primer, the T_m of the corresponding duplex is empirically calculated *(15)* and can be adjusted by altering the GC content and/or length of the primer.

5. At low temperature, the linker-primer normally used in LM-PCR *(1)* hybridizes to itself. This reaction competes with hybridization to the linker ODN, thereby decreasing the efficiency of ligation. By redesigning the linker-primer and linker ODNs to eliminate self-complementarity, the efficiency of the ligation reaction has been improved.

6. The design of chlorambucil–ODN conjugates is different for the two DNA recognition strategies. An ODN_T is typically 15–20 nucleotides in length, and is complementary in a Hoogsteen or reverse Hoogsteen sense to the targeted homopurine run in DNA *(13)*. Chlorambucil is conjugated to the 5' or 3' end of the ODN, so that, following triplex formation, the reactive group is positioned immediately adjacent to a guanine residue in the flanking duplex. The alkylation efficiency of this residue can range from 60 to 100%. By contrast, an ODN_R is homologous to the targeted sequence in DNA, and is at least 30 nucleotides long, and preferably 50 nucleotides long. Chlorambucil is conjugated to a 5-(aminopropyl)uracil base, centrally located in the ODN as part of a 5'-UpC sequence. Following strand exchange, chlorambucil reacts with the 5' neighboring G residue of the complementary DNA strand. Alkylation efficiency is dependent on the length of the ODN, ranging from 35–40% for a 30-mer to 55–60% for a 50-mer. **Figures 1** and **2** illustrate the use of the quantitative LM-PCR technique to detect targeted alkylation of the HLA DQβ1*0302 allele in human genomic DNA by chlorambucil–ODN_T and chlorambucil–ODN_R conjugates, respectively.

7. The authors have determined that *N*-7 guanine adducts, of the sort formed by dimethylsulfate or chlorambucil, can be quantitatively converted to nicks by incubating the DNA for 10 min at $95°C$ immediately prior to initiating first-strand synthesis. This eliminates the need to use piperidine and the accompanying DNA cleanup steps. The 5' end product is a substrate for T4 DNA ligase.

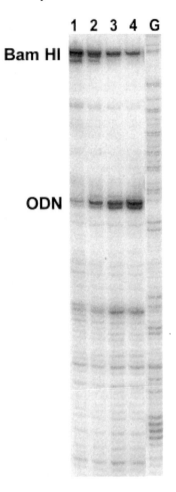

Fig. 1. Alkylation of the HLA DQβ1*0302 allele in human genomic DNA by a chloram-bucil–ODN$_T$ conjugate. A homopurine run in the first intron of this single-copy gene, present in DNA isolated from HT-29 cells, was targeted using a reactive 21-mer (5'-chlmb-AGGAGAAAGGAGAGGAGAGAG). Following incubation for 3 h at 37°C, the DNA was ethanol-precipitated and restricted with *Bam*HI. Quantitative LM-PCR was performed using the following primers (sense strand): 5'-CCATAATATTTAGTCCAGGC (primer 1), 5'-GTCTTGGGGCACGCCTAAATGACA (primer 2), and 5'-^{32}P-CTGCTGTGTCT CTGGAGAAATTCGTATCTTC (primer 3). Final concentrations of reactive ODN were: lane 1, 3.6 n*M*; lane 2, 18 n*M*; lane 3, 80 n*M*; and lane 4, 400 n*M*. Lane G, G-ladder.

8. To assure that the LM-PCR technique is quantitative, it is important to experi-
    mentally demonstrate that the amount of amplified product is a linear function of
    the input DNA. If necessary, LM-PCR conditions (cycle number, temperature,
    amount of DNA, and primers) are altered to achieve linearity of response.

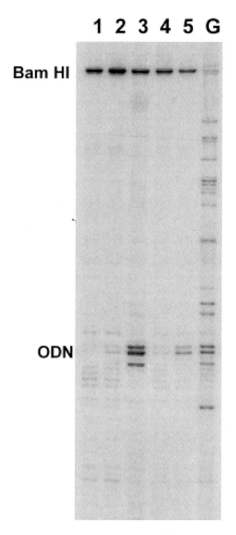

Fig. 2. RecA-mediated alkylation of the HLA DQβ1*0302 allele in human genomic DNA by chlorambucil–ODN$_R$ conjugates. An arbitrary site in the first intron of this single-copy gene was targeted using a RecA protein-coated, homologous 30-mer [5'-GAAGATACGAATTTC(U-chlmb)CCAGAGACACAGCA] or 50-mer [5'-GGTT ATTTTTGAAGATACGAATTTC(U-chlmb)CCAGAGACACAGCAGG ATTTGTCA]. After 6 h incubation, RecA protein was removed by phenol extraction, and the DNA was restricted with *Bam*HI. Quantitative LM-PCR was performed using the following primers (antisense strand): 5'-ATCCCCATCCTACAGGCT (primer 1), 5'-GCCTGGAAGAGAAGGAGAGAGGAG (primer 2), and 5'-^{32}P-GAGGAGACAA AGTGTACATTTACTACCAGTG (primer 3). Lane 1, no ODN or RecA protein; lane 2, 50-mer minus RecA protein; lane 3, 50-mer plus RecA protein; lane 4, 30-mer minus RecA protein; lane 5, 30-mer plus RecA protein; lane G, G-ladder.

References

1. Mueller, P. R. and Wold, B. (1989) In vivo footprinting of a muscle specific enhancer by ligation mediated PCR. *Science* **246**, 780–786.
2. Pfeifer, G. P., Steigerwald, S. D., Mueller, P. R., Wold, B., and Riggs, A. D. (1989) Genomic sequencing and methylation analysis by ligation mediated PCR. *Science* **246**, 810–813.
3. Kutyavin, I. V., Gamper, H. B., Gall, A. A., and Meyer, R. B. (1993) Efficient, specific interstrand cross-linking of double-stranded DNA by a chlorambucil-modified triplex-forming oligonucleotide. *J. Am. Chem. Soc.* **115**, 9303–9304.
4. Podyminogin, M. A., Meyer, R. B., and Gamper, H. B. (1996) RecA-catalyzed, sequence-specific alkylation of DNA by cross-linking oligonucleotides. Effects of length and nonhomologous base substitutions. *Biochemistry* **35**, 7267–7274.
5. Larhammar, D., Hyldig-Nielsen J. J., Servenius, B., Andersson, G., Rask, L., and Peterson, P. A. (1983) Exon–intron organization and complete nucleotide sequence of a human major histocompatibility antigen DC-beta gene. *Proc. Natl. Acad. Sci. USA* **80**, 7313–7317.
6. Gamper, H. B., Reed, M. W., Cox, T., Virosco, J. S., Adams, A. D., Gall, A. A., Scholler, J. K., and Meyer, R. B. (1993) Facile preparation of nuclease resistant 3'-modified oligodeoxynucleotides. *Nucleic Acids Res.* **21**, 145–150.
7. Tabone, J. C., Stamm, M. R., Gamper, H. B., and Meyer, R. B. (1994) Factors influencing the extent and regiospecificity of cross-link formation between single-stranded DNA and reactive complementary oligonucleotides. *Biochemistry* **33**, 375–383.
8. Cantor, C. R., Warshaw, M. M., and Shapiro, H. (1970) Oligonucleotide interactions. III. Circular dichroism studies of the conformation of deoxynucleotides. *Biopolymers* **9**, 1059–1077.
9. Pfeifer, G. P. and Riggs, A. D. (1993) Genomic footprinting by ligation mediated polymerase chain reaction. *Methods Mol. Biol.* **15**, 153–168.
10. Pfeifer, G. P., Singer-Sam, J., and Riggs, A. D. (1993) Analysis of methylation and chromatin structure. *Methods Enzymol.* **225**, 567–583.
11. Mueller, P. R., Garrity, P. A., and Wold, B. (1994) Ligation-mediated PCR for genomic sequencing and footprinting, in *Current Protocols in Molecular Biology*, vol. 2 (Ausubel, F. M., et al., eds.), John Wiley, New York, pp. 15.5.1–15.5.26.
12. Lee, J. S., Latimer, L. J. P., and Hampel, K. J. (1993) Coralyne binds tightly to both T·A·T- and C·G·C⁺-containing DNA triplexes. *Biochemistry* **32**, 5591–5597.
13. Praseuth, D., Francois, J.-C., and Helene, C. (1994) Triple helix-mediated antigene strategy. *Int. Antiviral News* **2**, 34–37.
14. Gamper, H. B., Kutyarin, I. V., Rhinehart, R. L., Lokhov, S. G., Reed, M. W., and Meyer, R. B. (1997) Modulation of C^m/T, G/A, and G/T triplex stability in the presence and absence of KCl. *Biochemistry* **36**, 14,816–14,826.
15. Freier, S. M., Kierzek, R., Jaeger, J. A., Sugimoto, N., Caruthers, M. H., Neilson, T., and Turner, D. H. (1986) Improved free-energy parameters for predictions of RNA duplex stability. *Proc. Natl. Acad. Sci. USA* **83**, 9373–9377.

15

Gene Targeting in Plants
via Site-Directed Mutagenesis

**Peter B. Kipp, Joyce M. Van Eck,
Peter R. Beetham, and Gregory D. May**

1. Introduction

Genetically engineered crops continue to arouse public controversy. One issue that causes much concern is the presence of antibiotic resistance genes in transgenic plants. These genes provide a means to select plant cells which have acquired the linked foreign gene that encodes a useful trait; selection genes are an unavoidable consequence of conventional transformation technologies. Reported herein are strategies to create, and select for, modifications to plant genes in vivo without the introduction of foreign DNA.

Several strategies have been developed to study the function of genes in plants. Two methods are commonly used to block the expression of a specific gene: introducing the gene of interest in a sense or antisense orientation *(1,2)*, and transposon tagging *(3)*. In addition, studies have been performed to develop strategies to direct insertion of foreign DNA into regions of interest; however, integration of DNA into plants generally occurs in a random fashion *(4)*. Attempts have been made to direct DNA to specific areas by introducing constructs that include homologous sequences from targeted regions, thus exploiting homologous recombination *(5,6)*. Although frequencies from homologous recombination are low, it is likely that these frequencies will increase once a standardized approach is established *(7,8)*. Ideally, a technology for directing site-specific alterations in genomic DNA would greatly advance the study of gene function in plants.

During the past few years, a technology for in vivo site-directed mutagenesis has been developed that holds promise for gene studies in plants. The tech-

From: *Methods in Molecular Biology, vol. 133: Gene Targeting Protocols*
Edited by: E. Kmiec © Humana Press Inc., Totowa, NJ

nology is based on the action of chimeric oligonucleotides (chimeraplasts) composed of DNA and 2'-O-methyl RNA, which can be used to direct single base changes at the site of interest (*9*; **Fig. 1**). Chimeraplasts are designed to pair to homologous sequences or target sites in genomic DNA, and thus can be used to introduce a change in known DNA sequences. The double-hairpin structure of the chimeraplast prevents its degradation by nucleases, which can destroy open-ended RNA/DNA duplex molecules.

Chimeraplasts have been demonstrated to introduce a site-specific change in mammalian cells (*10,11*). In one study, the chimeraplast technology was investigated as a possible treatment for metabolic liver disease, of which several result from single nucleotide mutations (*11*). A number of strategies have been employed for genetic modification of hepatic genes, but there are still major problems with these approaches (*12,13*). To determine the efficacy of chimeraplasts as a treatment for liver disease, a chimeraplast was designed to direct a change at a specific site in the alkaline phosphatase gene of HuH7 human hepatoma cells (*11*). It was demonstrated that a single base pair change can be introduced at a relatively high frequency. The important outcome of this and related mammalian studies is that chimeraplast technology provides an effective means of site-directed gene correction, or what is referred to as a conversion, in each system.

The authors are investigating the application of the chimeraplast technology in plants. Studies have focused on methods for delivery of chimeraplasts into plant cells, selection of target tissues, and the fate of chimeraplasts after introduction. There are various methods available for the introduction of DNA into plants, but the authors studies have focused on electroporation and biolistic methods for the introduction of chimeraplasts (*14,15*). To monitor the fate of the introduced chimeraplasts, the authors utilized fluorescently tagged chimeraplasts, in combination with fluorescence microscopy, to assess chimeraplast uptake and localization within plant cells.

Rhodamine-tagged chimeraplasts were electroporated into protoplasts isolated from tobacco NT-1 cells, and were then visualized using UV and confocal microscopy (**Fig. 2**). In biolistic studies, immediately after fluorescein-tagged chimeraplasts were introduced into intact onion epidermal cells (**Fig. 2**), chimeraplasts accumulated in the nucleus.

Once methods for the introduction of fluorescently tagged chimeraplasts into plant cells were determined, chimeraplasts were designed to direct a change in both an endogenous tobacco gene, acetolactate synthase (ALS), and a non-functional green fluorescent protein (GFP) transgene. ALS is the first dedicated step in branched-chain amino acid biosynthesis. A substitution at proline 196 in ALS confers resistance to sulfonylurea herbicides (*16*). Using chimeraplast technology, the authors created a mutation in the codon for proline 196. Chimeraplasts were designed for a native tobacco ALS gene, which contained a single base mismatch to the native sequence within the codon to proline 196.

The ALS chimeraplasts were introduced into 3-d-old cultures of a nonregenerable tobacco cell line (NT-1) via biolistics. Following a 3-d recovery period, the cells were plated onto selective medium containing 15–50 ppb chlorsulfuron, which would allow growth of only the converted cells. Putatively converted cells appeared as rapidly proliferating cell masses, which indicated resistance to chlorsulfuron (**Fig. 3**).

The fact that these herbicide-resistant cells are indeed caused by conversions within the codon, and are not a result of spontaneous mutations, was verified by nucleotide sequence analysis data. For analysis, DNA was purified from rapidly proliferating NT-1 cell masses, and PCR-derived ALS gene products were obtained and sequenced. Nucleotide sequence analysis of a region of the ALS gene from herbicide-resistant cells indicated that these cells (**Fig. 4**) harbor a base change specifically in the codon for proline 196.

The second approach using chimeraplast technology was to restore function of an introduced GFP transgene. GFPs are a unique class of proteins involved in the bioluminescence of many jellyfish. In plants, GFP has been extensively used as a reporter for gene expression in both transient and stable expression systems *(17)*. With the idea of using GFP as a model system to monitor conversion events in plant cells, the authors generated two mutant GFP expression vectors. These expression vectors contain either a point mutation that results in a premature stop codon in the mRNA or a single base pair deletion that results in a frame shift mutation, thus preventing translation of the protein.

Transgenic plants, expressing either wild-type or mutant GFP transcripts, were used for chimeraplast-directed conversion of the transgene *in planta*. Chimeraplasts designed to restore function to GFP were introduced by biolistics into callusing leaf tissues derived from GFP-mutant plants. Calli were initially surveyed 3 d after bombardment, and again at 5-d intervals, using fluorescence microscopy. Recovery of the GFP phenotype was observed (**Fig. 5**). Conversion events were scored on the basis of restoration of the GFP phenotype. Because both point mutations were at the same position within the codon, the same chimeraplast was used to restore functionality in the mutants.

The results from these preliminary studies demonstrate that chimeraplasts can efficiently direct site-specific mutations when introduced into plant cells. In addition, there is strong evidence that these molecules have the capacity to correct either deletion or substitution point mutations. Application of chimeraplast technology to plants should be viewed as a means to direct site-specific

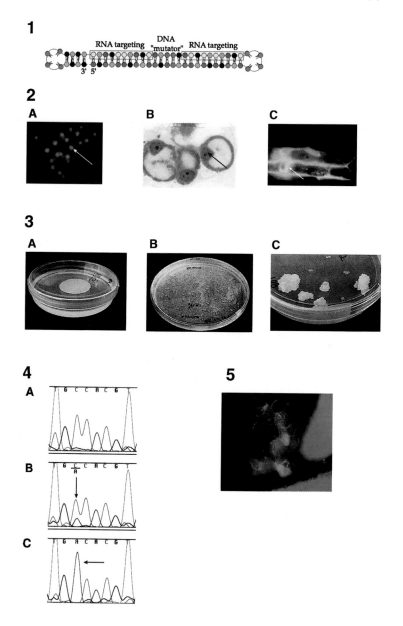

Fig. 1. Stylized chimeraplast with the following nucleotide representations: Green, A; Red, T; Black, G; Blue, C; Yellow, U.

Fig. 2. Efficient introduction of chimeraplasts. (**A**) UV photomicrograph depicting nuclear localization (indicated by arrow) of rhodamine-tagged chimeraplasts in the 2 min following electroporation into tobacco NT-1 cell protoplasts. (**B**) Confocal microscopy

mutagenesis *in planta*. The ability to target mutagenesis will provide a powerful tool for the investigation of gene function in plants.

2. Materials

2.1. Cell Suspension and Protoplast Culture Media

1. NT-1 cell suspension medium (CSM): Murashige and Skoog *(18)* salts (Gibco-BRL, Grand Island, NY), 500 mg/l MES, 1 mg/L thiamine, 100 mg/L myoinositol, 180 mg/L KH_2PO_4, 2.21 mg/L 2,4-diclorophenoxyacetic acid (2,4-D), 30 g/L sucrose. Adjust pH to 5.7 with 1 *M* KOH or HCl, and autoclave. For solidified medium, add 8g/L agar-agar (Sigma, St. Louis, MO) prior to autoclaving.
2. Plating-out medium (POM) for protoplasts: 80% (v/v) CSM, 0.3 *M* mannitol, 20% (v/v) conditioned medium (CM) (*see* **Note 1**).

2.2. Electroporation Media

1. Protoplast isolation medium (PIM): 0.25 *M* mannitol, 50 m*M* $CaCl_2 \cdot 2H_2O$, 10 m*M* NaOAc (anhydrous). Adjust to pH 5.8 or HCl, and filter-sterilize.

---

of fluorescence from a rhodamine-tagged chimeraplast localized in the nucleus (indicated by arrow) of NT-1 protoplasts. (**C**) UV photomicrograph depicting fluorescein-tagged chimeraplasts (indicated by arrow) introduced into intact onion epidermal cells.

Fig. 3. Generation and selection of chlorsulfuron resistant cells. From left to right: 3-d-old plate cultures of NT-1 cell suspension cultures used for biolistic delivery of an ALS chimeraplast; bombarded cultures maintained on 15 ppb chlorsulfuron for 2 wk; putatively converted NT-1 cell masses proliferating on medium containing 50 ppb chlorsulfuron.

Fig. 4. Automated nucleotide sequence analyses of gene-modification events. Electropherograms displaying the sequence of ALS-specific PCR products derived from DNA isolated from (**A**) NT-1 cells, and (**B**) herbicide-resistant NT-1 cells recovered as a result of an introduced chimeraplast, indicate an alteration in the native sequence for codon 196 (CCA). The conversion (C-to-A; arrow) in codon 196 (CCA) was detected (**B**), and is consistent with a targeted mutation induced by the chimeraplast. Because there are multiple copies of ALS alleles, modification of a single gene can confer herbicide resistance, but sequence analyses will indicate base-composition heterogeneity at the revised position. To characterize individual species from the heterogeneous population of the ALS-specific PCR products derived from the DNA of herbicide resistant cells, shown in (**B**), these products were cloned and sequenced. Sequence analysis of one of the 24 randomly selected clones, shown in (**C**), demonstrates the C-to-A conversion.

Fig. 5. Fluorescence photomicrograph of conversion to the GFP phenotype in leaf callus from a GFP mutant.

2. Cell suspension digestion medium: PIM with 0.3% cellulase (Karlan, Santa Rosa, CA) and 0.02% pectolyase Y23 (Karlan). Dissolve enzymes in PIM solution for 30 min, with constant stirring. Centrifuge for 10 min at 10,000*g* in 30 mL Corex tubes. Filter sterilize through a 0.2-μm filter. Store in 50-mL aliquots at –20°C.
3. Electroporation solution (POR): 200 m*M* mannitol, 120 m*M* KCl, 10 m*M* NaCl, 4 m*M* $CaCl_2 \cdot 2H_2O$, 10 m*M* HEPES (Sigma). Adjust to pH 7.2, then autoclave.

2.3. Materials for Biolistic Delivery

1. NT-1 cell suspension cultures that have been subcultured 3–5 d before bombardment.
2. A helium driven particle gun (Bio-Rad, Hercules, CA).
3. Microprojectiles: 1-μm gold particles (Bio-Rad).
4. Macroprojectiles and rupture disks (Rumsey-Loomis, Ithaca, NY) that have been soaked in 100% ethanol for several minutes, then allowed to dry.
5. Stopping screens (Rumsey-Loomis) that have been autoclaved.

3. Methods
3.1. Maintenance of NT-1 Cell Suspensions for Protoplasts

1. Transfer 4 mL of an established NT-1 cell culture into 40 mL CSM. The established cell suspension is maintained by weekly subcultures of 1 mL suspension into 49 mL CSM.

3.2. Isolation of Protoplasts from NT-1 Cell Suspensions

1. Use NT-1 cell suspensions 3–4 d after transfer to fresh CSM (*see* **Note 2**).
2. Centrifuge 10–20 mL cells at 112*g* (Allegra™ 6R centrifuge Beckman, Fullerton, CA) for 5 min at room temperature. Use these centrifugation conditions for all centrifugations in this protocol. Save the supernatant for CM in a 50-mL tube for use in POM near end of procedure.
3. After removing the supernatant, add an equal volume of PIM medium to the cells. Gently mix the cells by inversion, then centrifuge. Aspirate off supernatant.
4. Resuspend cells in an appropriate amount of enzyme solution. Use 30–35 mL PIM for 15–20 mL cells (pelleted volume). Distribute 20–25 mL of the mixture into individual Petri plates (100 × 20 mm). Incubate at 26°C in the dark on a gyratory shaker at 40 rpm for 3 h, then remove a small aliquot to a microscope slide, to determine that digestion is complete. Protoplasts will appear spherical (*see* **Note 3**).
5. Using a sterile, wide-bore pipet, carefully transfer the protoplast to a sterile, 50-mL centrifuge tube. Rinse Petri plates with 3 mL PIM to recover any remaining protoplasts. Centrifuge, then aspirate off the supernatant. Resuspend the pelleted protoplasts in a small, minimal volume of PIM, by inversion. Gently transfer the protoplasts to a sterile, 50-mL centrifuge tube, then rinse the previous centrifuge to recover any remaining protoplasts. Add PIM to the protoplasts, to bring to a final volume of 40 mL. Gently invert the tube several times to resuspend the protoplasts.

6. Centrifuge, then resuspend the protoplasts in 20–40 mL of PIM, depending on the initial volume of cell suspension used in **step 2**. For instance, if the initial volume was 10 mL, then add 20 mL PIM. Gently invert tube to resuspend the protoplasts.

7. Measure the protoplast density in an aliquot with a hemocytometer, and calculate the total number of protoplasts present in the tube.

8. Centrifuge, then resuspend the protoplasts in POR at a density of 2×10^6 protoplasts/mL.

9. Place protoplasts on ice for 10 min.

3.3. Electroporation of Protoplasts with Chimeraplasts

1. Aliquot 1 mL protoplasts into 0.4-mm electroporation cuvets. Add 0.5–5 μg of chimeraplast (Kimeragen, Newtown, PA) to each cuvet. Place cuvets on ice, invert to mix.

2. Apply one pulse, 250 V, capacitance 250 μF, and time constant 10–14 ms.

3. Place back on ice for 5 min. Transfer protoplasts to 7.5 mL POM in a Petri dish (100 × 20 mm).

4. Observe cells under a microscope.

3.4. Biolistic Delivery of Chimeraplasts

1. A special microprojectile-coating protocol was devised for chimeraplast delivery, which differs from the method used for delivery of plasmid DNA. The microprojectiles are first prepared for coating, then immediately coated with the chimeraplast. To prepare the microprojectiles, suspend 60 mg gold particles in 1 mL 100% ethanol (**see Note 4**). Sonicate the suspension for three 30-s bursts to disperse the particles. Centrifuge at 11,750*g* (Eppendorf 5415C microcentrifuge) for 30 s; discard supernatant. Add 1 mL 100% ethanol, vortex for 15 s, centrifuge at 11,750*g* for 5 min, then discard the supernatant. Resuspend the particles in water to a concentration of 60 mg/mL.

2. To coat the particles with chimeraplast: Transfer 35 μL particle suspension to a 1.5-mL microcentrifuge tube. Place tube on a vortex mixer. While vortexing, add the following in the order indicated: 40 μL chimeraplast (60 ng/μL water), 75 μL ice-cold 2.5 *M* CaCl$_2$, 75 μL ice-cold 0.1 *M* spermidine. Continue vortexing for 10 min at room temperature, then allow the particles to settle for 10 min. Centrifuge at 11,750*g* for 30 s; remove supernatant. Resuspend particles in 50 μL of 100% ethanol.

3. Dispense 10 μL resuspended particles onto each macroprojectile (flying disk). Allow to dry.

4. Plate out cultures 1 d prior to bombardment, and maintain under lights (16 h light + 8 h dark). Use NT-1 cell-suspension cultures that have been subcultured 3–5 d prior to preparing cultures for bombardment (*see Note 4*). Allow suspensions to settle, then dispense 0.6–1 mL settled cells onto each plate of solidified CSM.

5. Bombardment parameters: Bombard each plate once at 900 psi, with a gap distance (distance from power source to macroprojectile) of 1 cm and a target distance (distance from microprojectile launch site to target material) of 10 cm (*see Note 6*).

6. If applicable, transfer cultures to medium containing a selection agent (e.g., chorsulfuron 15 ppb) 2 d after bombardment (*see* **Note 7**).

4. Notes

1. Conditioned medium is the supernatant from the initial centrifugation of the NT-1 cell suspension prior to protoplast isolation.
2. It is advisable to check cell suspensions for contamination by microorganisms prior to protoplast isolation.
3. If there are a large number of undigested cell clumps, they can be removed by filtering through a 170-μm sieve (Sigma).
4. It is important to use a bottle of 100% ethanol that has not been opened for an long period of time.
5. Cell suspensions maintained for biolistic delivery were subcultured weekly by transferring 1 mL of an established suspension culture into 49 mL liquid CSM.
6. Alternative bombardment parameters are a pressure of 450 psi at a target distance of 6 cm.
7. For selection of chlorsulfuron resistant cells, cells were transferred from each bombarded plate to 15 mL tubes containing 5 mL liquid CSM 2 d after bombardment. The tubes were inverted several times to disperse cell clumps. The cells were then transferred to solidified CSM medium containing 15 ppb chorsulfuron (Dupont, Wilmington, DE). From approx 10–30 d, actively growing cells (raised, light-colored colonies) are periodically selected and transferred to solidified CSM containing 50 ppb chlorsulfuron. Three to four wk later, actively growing cells are selected, then transferred to solidified CSM containing 200 ppb chlorsulfuron. Cells that survive this treatment are then analyzed.

Acknowledgments

The authors would like to thank Ramesh Kumar, Eric Kmiec, and Keith Walker, as well as Naomi Thomson and Patricia Avissar of Kimeragen. In addition, the authors would like to recognize Xiaoping Zeng and Xenia Sawycky for their technical assistance, and Kenneth Palmer for reviewing the manuscript.

References

1. Sheehy, R. E., Kramer, M., and Hiatt, W. R. (1988) Reduction of polygalacturonase activity in tomato fruit by antisense RNA. *Proc. Natl. Acad. Sci. USA* **85,** 8805–8809.
2. Smith, C. J. S., Watson, C. F., Ray, J., Bird, C. R., Morris, P. C., Schuch, W., and Grierson, D. (1988) Antisense RNA inhibition of polygalacturonase gene expression in transgenic tomatoes. *Nature* **334,** 724–726.
3. Bensen, R. J., Johal, G. S., Crane, V. C., Tossberg, J. T., Schnable, P. S., Meeley, R. B., and Briggs, S. P. (1995) Cloning and characterization of the maize *An1* gene. *Plant Cell* **7,** 75–84.

4. Putcha, H. and Hohn, B. (1996) From centiMorgans to base pairs: homologous recombination in plants. *Trends Plant Sci.* **1(10)**, 340–348.
5. Paszkowski, J., Baur, M., Bogucki, A., and Potrykus, I. (1988) Gene targeting in plants. *EMBO J.* **7**, 4021–4026.
6. Thykjaer, T., Finnemann, J., Schauser, L., Christensen, L., Poulsen, C., and Stougaard, J. (1997) Gene targeting approaches using positive-negative selection and large flanking regions. *Plant Mol. Biol.* **35**, 523–530.
7. Kempin, S. A., Liljegren, S. J., Block, L. M., Rounsley, S. D., Yanofsky, M. F., and Lam, E. (1997) Targeted disruption in *Arabidopsis. Nature* **389**, 802–803.
8. Schaefer, D. G. and Zryd, J. P. (1997) Efficient gene targeting in the moss *Physcomitrella patens. Plant J.* **11**, 1195–1206.
9. Cole-Strauss, A., Nöe, A., and Kmiec, E. B. (1997) Recombinational repair of genetic mutations. *Antisense Nucleic Acid Drug Dev.* **7**, 211–216.
10. Cole-Strauss, A., Yoon, K., Xiang, Y., Byrne, B. C., Rice, M. C., Gryn, J., Holloman, W. K., and Kmiec, E. B. (1996) Correction of the mutations responsible for sickle cell anemia by an RNA-DNA oligonucleotide. *Science* **273**, 1386–1389.
11. Kren, B. T., Cole-Strauss, A., Kmiec, E. B., and Steer, C. J. (1997) Targeted nucleotide exchange in the alkaline phosphatase gene of HuH-7 cells mediated by chimeric RNA/DNA oligonucleotide. *Hepatology* **25**, 1462–1468.
12. Chang, A. G. Y. and Wu, G. Y. (1994) Gene therapy: applications to the treatment of gastrointestinal and liver diseases. *Gastroenterology* **106**, 1076–1084.
13. Strauss, M. (1994) Liver-directed gene therapy: prospects and problems. *Gene Ther.* **1**, 156–164.
14. Sanford, J. C., Smith, F. D., and Russell, J. A. (1993) Optimizing the biolistic process for different biological applications, in *Methods in Enzymology* (Abelson, J. N. and Simon, M. I., eds.), Academic Press, San Diego, pp. 483–509.
15. Potter, H. (1993) Application of electroporation in recombinant DNA technology, in *Methods in Enzymology* (Abelson, J. N. and Simon, M. I., eds.), Academic Press, San Diego, pp. 461–483.
16. Lee, K. Y., Townsend, J., Tepperman, J., Black, M., Chui, C. F., Mazur, B., Dunsmuir, P., and Bedbrook, J. (1988) Molecular basis of sulfonylurea herbicide resistance in tobacco. *EMBO J.* **7**, 1241–1248.
17. Chiu, W. L., Niwa, Y., Zeng, W., Hirano, T., Kobayashi, H., and Sheen, J. (1996) Engineered GFP as a vital reporter in plants. *Curr. Biol.* **6**, 325–330.
18. Murashige, T. and Skoog, F. (1962) Revised medium for rapid growth and bioassays with tobacco tissue cultures. *Plant. Phys.* **15**, 473–497.

16

Antisense Oligonucleotides as Modulators of Pre-mRNA Splicing

Halina Sierakowska, Sudhir Agrawal and Ryszard Kole

1. Introduction

Antisense oligonucleotides have been extensively used as downregulators of gene expression *(1)*, and as such are not only increasingly used in various fields as sequence-specific research tools *(2–4)*, but are also tested in clinical trials as antiviral and anticancer agents *(5–8)*.

The authors' recent work has shown that antisense oligonucleotides are not limited to downregulating gene expression, but can also restore the expression of genes inactivated by specific mutations *(9,10)*. This was accomplished by targeting antisense oligonucleotides to aberrant splice sites created by mutations that cause genetic diseases such as thalassemia or cystic fibrosis. Blocking these splice sites prevented aberrant splicing, and forced the spliceosomes to reform at correct splice sites, thus restoring the proper splicing pathway, and consequently the activity of the damaged gene. In this chapter, as an example of this novel application of antisense oligonucleotides, the methods leading to restoration of correct splicing in a thalassemic mutant, IVS2-654, will be described in detail.

In the IVS2-654 mutant of the human β-globin gene, a C-to-T mutation at position 654 of intron 2 creates an additional, aberrant 5' splice site at nucleotide 652, and activates a cryptic 3' splice site at nucleotide 579 of the β-globin pre-mRNA. During pre-mRNA splicing, a fragment of the intron contained between the newly activated splice sites is recognized by the splicing machinery as an exon, and is retained in the spliced mRNA. The aberrantly spliced mRNA appears to be relatively unstable, and, in addition, because of the presence of the stop codon in the retained fragment, leads to translation to a truncated β-globin polypeptide (**Fig. 1**). This molecular mechanism is responsible

From: *Methods in Molecular Biology, vol. 133: Gene Targeting Protocols*
Edited by: E. Kmiec © Humana Press Inc., Totowa, NJ

IVS2-654   IVS2-654 + oligo

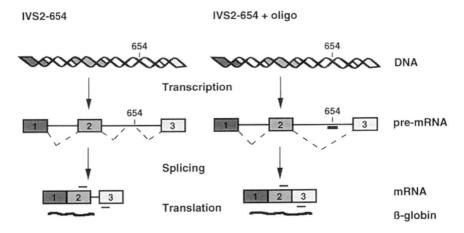

Fig. 1. Splicing of human β-globin IVS2-654 pre-mRNA in the presence of an antisense oligonucleotide. The human β-globin gene with a C-to-T IVS2-654 mutation is represented at the top of the figure (shaded areas, exons). In the absence of the antisense oligonucleotide (left panel), the transcribed pre-mRNA is spliced incorrectly. The oligonucleotide targeted to the aberrant 5' splice site created by the mutation (right panel) prevents aberrant, and restores correct, splicing of mRNA. As a result, full-length β-globin polypeptide is translated. Shaded boxes, exons; solid lines, introns; dashed lines indicate both correct and aberrant splicing pathways; the aberrant 5' splice site created by IVS2-654 mutation and the cryptic 3' splice site activated upstream are indicated; heavy bar, oligonucleotide antisense to the aberrant 5' splice site; light bars above and below exon sequences indicate primers used in the RT-PCR reaction; heavy line below mRNA represents β-globin polypeptide.

for the resulting β-globin deficiency, and manifests itself in affected individuals in a form of β-thalassemia, a blood disorder *(11)*. Note that aberrant splicing of IVS2-654 pre-mRNA takes place in the presence of unmodified, correct splice sites. Thus, one can anticipate that blocking of the aberrant splice sites by antisense oligonucleotides will direct the splicing machinery from the aberrant splice sites to the correct ones, modifying the splicing pathway. Indeed, the outcome of this approach is restoration of correct splicing of β-globin mRNA and its translation to β-globin protein (**Fig. 1**).

The modification of splicing can be obtained, in principle, by any antisense oligonucleotide that hybridizes strongly to the splice-site sequence, and does not promote cleavage of the RNA–oligonucleotide duplex by RNase H, an ubiquitous enzyme that cleaves RNA in RNA–DNA hybrids *(12)*. The latter property is essential, because, otherwise, the targeted pre-mRNA would have been degraded, leading to removal of the splicing substrate *(13)*. In the experiments described below, phosphorothioate 2'-O-methyl-oligoribonucleotides

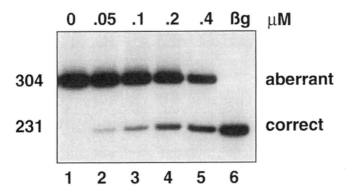

Fig. 2. Correction of splicing of IVS2-654 pre-mRNA in HeLa cells by antisense oligonucleotide targeted to the aberrant 5' splice site. Analysis of total RNA by RT-PCR. Lanes 1–5, IVS2-654 HeLa cells treated with increasing concentrations of the oligonucleotide (indicated in micromols at the top); βg (lane 6), RNA from human blood. The numbers on the left indicate the size, in nucleotides, of the RT-PCR products representing the aberrantly (304) and correctly (231) spliced RNAs.

have been used, because their duplexes with RNA do not constitute substrates for RNase H. Furthermore, these oligonucleotides are highly resistant to degradation by nucleases, resulting in their stability in cell culture environment *(14)* and in animal tissues *(15)*, and form duplexes with melting temperature (T_m) values higher than those of their ribo- or deoxyribo-congeners *(14)*.

The antisense oligonucleotide (**Fig. 1**) was targeted to the aberrant 5' splice site in the IVS2-654 β-globin pre-mRNA, which was constitutively expressed in a HeLa cell line stably transfected with the β-thalassemic globin gene cloned under immediate early cytomegalovirus (CMV) promoter. The cells were treated with a complex of cationic lipid, Lipofectamine *(16)*, and antisense 18-mer phosphorothioate 2'-O-methyl-oligoribonucleotide. The total RNA was isolated, and the spliced mRNAs were identified by reverse transcription polymerase chain reaction (RT-PCR) (**Fig. 2**). To ascertain that the protocol is suitable for quantitative analysis, the RT-PCR was carried out with α-^{32}P-dATP for no more than 18–20 cycles. Under these conditions, the amount of the PCR product is proportional to the amount of input RNA, as are the relative amounts of PCR products generated from aberrantly and correctly spliced RNAs *(10)*. Because the generated correctly spliced β-globin mRNA undergoes translation, the correction of splicing could be verified by detection of full-length β-globin polypeptide in the lysate of oligonucleotide treated cells. This was accomplished by immunoblots, using an antihemoglobin antibody *(10;* **Fig. 3**).

It is quite remarkable that oligonucleotides are effective in correcting aberrant splicing intracellularly, because their targets, the splice sites and adjacent

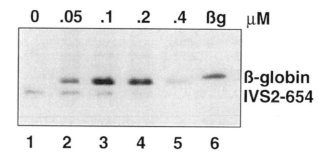

Fig. 3. Restoration of β-globin expression by antisense oligonucleotide in IVS2-654 HeLa cells. Immunoblot of total protein with antihuman hemoglobin antibody. Concentration of the oligonucleotide in micromols is indicated at the top (lanes 1–5); in lane 6, human globin (Sigma) was used as a marker. After treatment with oligonucleotides, the cells were treated with hemin preceding the isolation of proteins. The positions of human β-globin and the prematurely terminated β-globin IVS2-654 polypeptide are indicated.

regions such as the branch point, interact with a large splicing complex. Nonetheless, the results clearly indicate that the oligonucleotides were delivered into the cell and entered the nucleus, the site of splicing. There, in competition with the splicing factors, they hybridized to the aberrant splice site, preventing aberrant splicing and promoting the formation of the spliceosome and subsequent splicing at the correct splice sites. Apart from the potential clinical applications, this system provides an excellent general test for the efficacy of various antisense oligonucleotides. The correction of splicing may also serve as a measure of oligonucleotide uptake, their hybridization potential and/or other parameters involved in antisense activity. Because the action of the oligonucleotides generates a new product (either spliced mRNA or protein), even minor effects, difficult to discern when antisense oligonucleotides are used as downregulators of gene expression, are easily detectable.

2. Materials

2.1. Correction of Aberrant Splicing of Human β-Globin Pre-mRNA by Antisense Oligonucleotides

1. HeLa cell line stably expressing human β-globin thalassemic IVS2-654 pre-mRNA (provided by the authors on request). The RNA is transcribed from the human β-globin gene carrying the IVS2-654 mutation, and driven by the immediate early CMV promoter.
2. Phosphorothioate 2'-O-methyl-oligoribonucleotides, prepared and purified at Hybridon, Cambridge, MA, were dissolved in water under sterile conditions, and

stored at –20°C. The oligonucleotide, GCUAUUACCUUAACCCAG, was antisense to 5' splice site.

3. Minimum Essential Medium (S-MEM) (Life Technologies, Gibco-BRL, Gaithersburg, MD) was supplemented with 5% fetal calf and 5% horse sera, and 50 μg/mL gentamicin and 200 μg/mL kanamycin.
4. Trypsin-EDTA (TE), 1X (Life Technologies; Gibco-BRL).
5. OptiMEM I (Life Technologies; Gibco, BRL).
6. Lipofectamine, 2 mg/mL (Life Technologies, Gibco-BRL).
7. 20 mM NaOH, freshly prepared.
8. Hemin (Fluka). Dissolve 3.2 mg hemin in 5 mL 20 mM NaOH, and dilute 100-fold with S-MEM (without serum or antibiotics) at 37°C.

2.2. Isolation of Total RNA

1. 1X Hanks balanced salt solution (HBSS), low endotoxin, without calcium, magnesium or phenol red, pH 7.3.
2. (TRI) reagent, RNA/DNA/protein isolation reagent (Molecular Research Center, Cincinnati, OH).
3. Chloroform.
4. Glycogen for molecular biology, 20 mg/mL (Boehringer Mannheim).
5. Isopropanol.
6. 75% Ethanol.
7. Speed-Vac concentrator.

2.3. Analysis of RNA by Reverse Transcription-PCR and Gel Electrophoresis

1. GeneAmp Thermostable rTth Reverse Transcriptase RNA PCR Kit (Perkin-Elmer Cetus; Norwalk, CT).
2. 10 mM dATP, dCTP, dTTP, and dGTP (Perkin-Elmer Cetus).
3. Forward (5'), GGACCCAGAGGTTCTTTGAGTCC, and reverse (3'), GCACA-CAGACCAGCACGTTGCCC, primers spanning positions 21–43 of exon 2 and positions 6–28 of exon 3 of the human β-globin gene, respectively.
4. α-[^{32}P]-dATP aqueous solution, 10 μCi/mL, 6000 Ci/mmol (Amersham, Buckinghamshire, UK).
5. Mineral oil.
6. Perkin-Elmer Cetus DNA Thermal Cycler, and capped 0.5 mL polypropylene centrifuge tubes.
7. Hoefer 5E400 vertical slab electrophoresis apparatus (Amersham Pharmacia Biotech, Piscataway, NJ), with 16 × 18-cm glass plates and 1.5-mm thick spacers.
8. 0.5X tris-EDTA borate buffer (TEB), best prepared as 5X TEB, i.e., autoclaved aqueous 0.5 M Tris, 0.4 M boric acid, and 0.01 M EDTA.
9. 7.5% nondenaturing acrylamide gel stock (30:1, acrylamide: *bis*-acrylamide) in 0.5X TEB. Add 270 μL 10% ammonium persulfate and 27 μL (TEMED) to 40 mL gel stock immediately before pouring.

10. 10X loading dye: 0.42% bromophenol blue, 0.42% xylene cyanol F.F., and 25% Ficoll gel (Type 400, Pharmacia, Dublin, OH) in water.
11. Bio-Rad Gel Dryer (Hercules, CT) with an oil vacuum pump.
12. X-ray films.
13. Audioradiographic cassette with a Dupont Cronex Lightning intensifying screen.

2.4. Lysis of Cells and Electroblotting of Proteins.

1. Phosphate buffered saline (PBS).
2. Lysis buffer: to 6 mL 15% sodium dodecyl sulfate (SDS), 940 µL 2 M Tris-HCl, pH 6.8, 2 g sucrose and 150 µL 0.2M EDTA, pH 7.4; add distilled water to a final volume of 30 mL. Store at –20°C, adding the following proteolytic inhibitors immediately before use: phenylmethyl sulfonyl fluoride (PMSF) at 100 µM, leupeptin and aprotinin at 10 µg/mL each, and pepstatin A at 1 µg/mL.
3. Flat-tip sequencing gel loading pipet tips (Costar).
4. Becton Dickinson (Franklin Lakes, NJ) 0.5-cc insulin syringe with micro fine iv needle.
5. Gel electrophoresis apparatus and plates, as in **Subheading 2.3., step 7,** except for 0.75-mm thick spacers.
6. Gel buffer: 3 M Tris, 0.3% SDS, adjusted to pH 8.45 with HCl, stored at room temperature (RT), as in ref. *17*.
7. Gel stock: 48% acrylamide, 1.5% *bis*-acrylamide, w/v.
8. Separating gel: 3.05 mL gel stock, 5 mL gel buffer, 3.54 mL 50% aqueous glycerol, 3.41 mL distilled water; 50 µL 10% ammonium persulfate and 5 µL TEMED added immediately before pouring.
9. Stacking gel: 0.5 mL gel stock, 1.15 mL gel buffer, 4.2 mL distilled water; 50 µL 10% ammonium persulfate and 5 µL TEMED were added immediately before pouring.
10. Cathode buffer (–): 0.1 M Tris, 0.1 M Tricine (Sigma; St. Louis, MO), 0.1% SDS, pH 8.25, with no adjustment of pH necessary.
11. Anode buffer (+): 0.2 M Tris, adjusted to pH 8.9 with HCl.
12. Globin as immunoelectrophoretic marker: Dissolve, by heating to 100°C for 3 min, 1 mg globin (Sigma) in 0.5 mL lysis buffer with 50 µM dithiothreitol (DTT). Dilute sequentially with heating. Store diluted (40 ng/mL) solution at –20°C. Before use, thaw the solution by heating at 45°C for 15 min, and load 10–30 µL per lane.
13. Dilute 2 µL SDS-polycryamide gel electrophoresis (PAGE) low range mol wt standards (Bio-Rad) with 65 µL lysis buffer, 50 µM (DTT), heat at 100°C for 3 min and load 15 µL/lane.
14. Serva blue G or Brilliant blue G (Sigma).
15. Transfer buffer: 12.1 g Tris, 57.65 g glycine, 800 mL methanol, and distilled water to make 4 L. Store at room temperature.
16. Nitrocellulose, 0.2 µm (Schleicher and Schuell; Keene, NH).
17. Whatman 3 MM chromatographic paper.
18. Bio-Rad Trans-Blot Cell with a water cooling coil.

19. Ponceau S (Sigma) stock solution: 2 g Ponceau S, 30 g trichloroacetic acid, 30 g sulfosalicylic acid, and distilled water to 100 mL. For working solution, dilute 10-fold with distilled water.

2.5. Immunoblot Detection of β-Globin

1. Fisher clinical horizontal rotator.
2. 1% solution of Triton X-100 in PBS (PBST).
3. Blotto, 5% Carnation nonfat dry milk in PBST. Dissolve milk in PBS, filter, add Triton X-100 afterwards.
4. Tween-20.
5. Primary antibody: polyclonal affinity-purified chicken antihuman hemoglobin IgG (Accurate, Westbury, NY).
6. Secondary antibody: rabbit antichicken horseradish-peroxidase-conjugated IgG (Accurate).
7. Enhanced chemiluminescence (ECL) detection system (Amersham).

3. Methods

3.1. Correction of Aberrant Splicing of Human Thalassemic β-Globin pre-mRNA by Antisense Oligonucleotides

1. Culture HeLa cells (37°C, 5% CO_2) in monolayer on 75-cm^2 tissue culture plate in supplemented S-MEM to below 50% confluency. Treat the cells with 1 mL TE for 3–5 min, suspend at 10^5 cells/mL medium, and plate in 24-well plates (2 cm^2 well area) at 1 mL per well. Culture for 24 h before oligonucleotide treatment.
2. Prewarm 500 mL OptiMEM I in 37°C water bath and 50 mL vial of OptiMEM I in 26°C water bath. Work in tissue culture hood under sterile conditions.
3. Dilute 100 μM aqueous solution of the oligonucleotide to 5 μM with OptiMEM I at 26°C.
4. Aliquot 100 μL oligonucleotide solution (5 μM or appropriate dilutions) into individual Eppendorf tubes. Controls should contain no oligonucleotide.
5. Suspend 4 μL Lipofectamine in 100 μL OPTI-MEM I at 26°C, and mix thoroughly by inversion. For multiple samples, increase the reagent volumes as appropriate. Rapidly add 100 μL of this suspension to each Eppendorf tube containing the oligonucleotide and mix the contents by vigorous pipeting up and down. Incubate the tubes in 26°C water bath for 30 min, to form the Lipofectamine–oligonucleotide complex. Return the tubes under the hood, add 800 μL OptiMEM I at 26°C, mix by inverting 5×, and store at room temperature for up to 1 h.
6. Place the 24-well plate containing IVS2-654 HeLa cells under the hood, gently aspirate the medium, and wash the cells twice for 1 min with 1 mL OptiMEM I at 37°, to render them serum-free. Work with no more than six wells per plate, to prevent cooling of cells during the washes. Transfer 1 mL transfection complex from each Eppendorf tube to the appropriate well, and return the plate to the incubator for 10 h. Gently remove the transfection medium, add 1 mL supplemented medium at 37°C to each well, and incubate the cells for 36 h at 37°C.

7. For isolation of RNA, harvest the cells as in **Subheading 3.2.** For analysis of protein, pretreat the cells with hemin, which greatly facilitates detection of globin on immunoblots. Prerinse the cells twice with unsupplemented S-MEM at 37°C, incubate in hemin containing S-MEM for 4 h at 37°C and harvest as in **Subheading 3.4.**

3.2. Isolation of Total RNA

1. Gently aspirate the medium from the wells, and rinse them with 1 mL HBSS.
2. To each well, add 0.8 mL TRI reagent at RT for 5 min (*see* **Subheading 4.**). Pipet the lysate 5× up and down, transfer it to Eppendorf tubes, let sit for 3 min, invert the tubes several times, and touch spin. Use directly, or store at –80°C for up to a year.
3. Add 160 µL chloroform per tube, vortex vigorously for 30 s, and let sit for 3 min. Spin at 12,000g for 15 min at 4°C. Transfer 320 µL of the colorless upper aqueous phase to fresh Eppendorf tubes containing 2 µL glycogen. Vortex the tubes vigorously, and touch-spin. To each tube, add 400 µL isopropanol, vortex vigorously, invert twice, store on ice for 30 min, and centrifuge at 12,000g for 30 min at 4°C.
4. Pour off the supernatant and wash the pellet once with 1 mL 75% ethanol by vortexing and subsequent centrifugation at 12,000g for 10 min at 4°C. Carefully remove the supernatant without disturbing the pellet. Dry the pellet, avoiding overdrying, under the hood or in Speed-Vac.
5. Dissolve the RNA pellet in 60 µL autoclaved distilled water by incubating it for 30 min at 45–55°C with intermittent vortexing and touch-spins. The RNA solution can be stored at –20°C for at least 1 yr.

3.3. Analysis of RNA by RT-PCR and Gel Electrophoresis

1. Prepare the reverse transcription master mix (*see* **Subheading 4.**). Amounts are given for one sample: 6.4 µL autoclaved deionized water, 2 µL 10X rTth reverse transcription buffer, 2 µL 10 mM MnCl$_2$, 1.6 µL of a mixture of 2.5 mM dGTP, dATP, dTTP and dCTP, 1 µL (30 picomols) 3' primer, and 2 µL rTth DNA polymerase. For multiple samples, increase as appropriate. Vortex the master mix gently, prewarm to 37°C, and add 15 µL to each cycler tube containing 5 µL RNA (*from* **Subheading 3.2., step 5**) at RT, mixing the total with pipet tip. Overlay each sample with two drops of mineral oil.
2. Incubate the tubes in DNA Thermal Cycler at 70°C for 15 min, followed by soak at 4°C.
3. Prepare the PCR master mix. The amounts are given for one sample: 65 µL autoclaved deionized water, 8 µL 10X chelating buffer, 8 µL 10 mM MgCl$_2$, 1 µL (32 pmols) 5' primer, and 2.5 µCi α-^{32}P dATP. For multiple samples, increase as appropriate. Vortex.
4. Dispense 80 µL PCR master mix to each reverse transcription reaction tube, centrifuge at 12,000g for 30 s, and subject to PCR programmed for 3 linked files as follows:
   a. Step cycle: 3 min at 95°C for 1 cycle.
   b. Step cycle: 1 min at 95°C and 1 min at 65°C for 18 cycles.
   c. Soak: 4°C.

5. Pour a vertical 1.5 mm thick polyacrylamide slab gel (*see* **Subheading 2.3., step 9**). Use 0.5X TEB buffer as running buffer.
6. Withdraw 20 µL of the amplified material from under the mineral oil, combine with 4 µL 10X Ficoll loading dye, vortex, spin, and load onto the gel. Store the remaining samples at –20°C for up to 1 wk.
7. Electrophorese at RT for a total of 900 V × h, until xylene cyanol dye leaves the gel. Keep the voltage for the initial 45 min below 150 V, and, throughout electrophoresis within 45 to 250 V.
8. Dry the gel in gel dryer at 80°C, and autoradiograph using an X-ray film and a cassette with an intensifying screen.

3.4. Lysis of Cells and Electroblotting of Proteins

1. Wash the hemin-treated cells twice in HBSS, once with PBS, and lyse them for 15 min at RT in 75 µL lysis buffer. Scrape the wells with flat-tip sequencing-gel-loading pipet tips, and transfer the lysate with 0.5-mL insulin syringe with 28G½ needle into Eppendorf tubes. Homogenize the lysate by passing it 5× through the syringe. Use the lysate directly, as in **Subheading 3.4., steps 3** and **4**, or store at –80°C.
2. Pour 0.75-mm-thick vertical Tricine-SDS-polyacrylamide slab gel, as in ref. *17*, as follows: the separating gel, up to 2 cm, from the bottom of the comb, and overlay with water. Upon polymerization, remove the water, add stacking gel solution to fill up the plates, and insert the comb.
3. Add to each tube of cell lysate 4.5 µL 1 *M* DTT and 6 µL 0.1% aqueous Serva blue dye, heat at 100°C for 5 min, and load 40 µL/lane. As markers, use globin and low-range mol wt standards.
4. Electrophorese the gel with anode buffer in the lower chamber and cathode buffer in the upper one for 1 h at 30 V, and subsequently for 5 h at 150 V, until the dye reaches 1 cm from gel bottom.
5. Always handle nitrocellulose and blots with gloves and flat tip filter forceps (Gelman Sciences, Ann Arbor, MI). Wet nitrocellulose in distilled water, and equilibrate in transfer buffer for 5 min. On the transfer holder, place buffer soaked sponge, 3MM filter paper, and the gel, and cover it with nitrocellulose, preventing formation of air bubbles. Cover the nitrocellulose with buffer-soaked 3MM filter paper and sponge, and place the loaded holder in Trans-Blot Cell containing transfer buffer and a water-cooling coil. Electrotransfer at 60 V overnight at room temperature. Mark the protein side of the membrane. If desired, stain it with a working solution of Ponceau S for 5–10 min at RT, wash with several changes of distilled water, and mark the positions of protein standards.
6. Proceed with immunodetection of β-globin, or store the air-dried blot wrapped in Saran Wrap in the refrigerator.

3.5. Immunoblot Detection of β-Globin

1. Perform all immunoreactions and rinses with agitation on a clinical rotator at RT. Rinse blot in PBST for 15 min.

2. Block with Blotto for 2 h.
3. Incubate with primary antibody diluted 1000-fold with Blotto, for 20 min.
4. Wash in Blotto, 3× for 10 min each, and with PBST twice, for 10 min each.
5. Incubate with the secondary antibody diluted 2000-fold with Blotto, for 1 h.
6. Wash for 10 min each: twice with Blotto, 3× with PBST containing 0.02% Tween-20, and twice with PBST.
7. Mix equal volumes of ECL detection solution 1 with detection solution 2, to obtain a final volume of 0.125 mL/cm^2 membrane.
8. Drain excess buffer from the washed blot, and place it in a flat-bottomed plastic dish, protein-side-up. Add the detection reagent to the protein side of the blot, so that the solution is held by surface tension on blot surface. Do not allow the surface of the blot to dry. Incubate for precisely 1 min at RT without agitation.
9. Remove the blot by holding it vertically and touching its edge to filter paper, to drain excess reagent. Place the blot protein-side-down on Saran Wrap, avoiding air pockets. Close the Saran Wrap to form an envelope, without pressure on the blot.
10. Quickly place the blot envelope, protein-side-up, in a film cassette, and immediately take it to the dark room. Place an X-ray film on the blot and expose it for 30 s. Remove the film and replace it with a fresh one. Immediately develop the first film, and, on the basis of signal strength, estimate the desired length of exposure of subsequent film(s), which may vary from 2 min to over 2 h. Note that the intensity of luminescence signal diminishes rapidly with time.

4. Note

1. The procedures described for isolation of RNA (**Subheading 3.2.**) and its analysis by RT-PCR (**Subheading 3.3.**) are as recommended by the manufacturers of TRI reagent and the reverse transcriptase RNA-PCR kit, respectively. The Tricine-SDS-PAGE system is as described in **ref. *17***.

References

1. Crooke, S. T. and Bennett, CF. (1996) Progress in antisense oligonucleotide therapeutics. *Ann. Rev. Pharm.Tox.* **36,** 107–129.
2. Pasternak, G. W. and Standifer, K. M. (1995) Mapping of opioid receptors using antisense oligodeoxynucleotides: correlating their molecular biology and pharmacology. *Trends Pharmacol. Sci.* **16,** 344–350.
3. Niggli, E., Schwaller, B., and Lipp, P. (1996) Antisense oligodeoxynucleotides directed against the Na–Ca exchanger mRNA. Promising tools for studies on the cellular and molecular level. *Ann. NY Acad. Sci.* **779,** 93–102.
4. Ramchandani, S., MacLeod, R. A., Pinard, M., von Hoffe, E., and Szyf, M. (1997) Inhibition of tumorigenesis by a cytosine-DNA, methyltransferase, antisense oligodeoxynucleotide. *Proc. Natl. Acad. Sci. USA* **94,** 684–689.
5. Zhang, R., Y. J., Shahinian, H., Amin, G., Lu, Z., Liu, T., Saag, M.S., Temsamani, Y., and Martin, R. R. (1995) Pharmacokinetics of an anti-human immunodeficiency virus antisense oligodeoxynucleotide phosphorothioate (GEM 91) in HIV-infected subjects. *Clin. Pharm. Ther.* **58,** 44–53.

6. Bishop, M. R., Iversen, P. L., Bayever, E., Shar, J. G., Greiner, T. C., Copple, et al. (1995) Phase I trial of an antisense oligonucleotide OL(1)p53 in hematologic malignancies. *J. Clin. Oncol.* **14,** 1320–1326.
7. Agrawal, S (1996) Antisense oligonucleotides: towards clinical trials. *Trends Biotech.* **14,** 376–378.
8. Tonkinson, J. L. and Stein, C. A. (1996) Antisense oligonucleotides as clinical therapeutic agents. *Cancer Invest.* **14,** 64–65.
9. Dominski, Z. and Kole, R. (1993) Restoration of correct splicing in thalassemic pre-mRNA by antisense oligonucleotides. *Proc. Natl. Acad. Sci. USA* **90,** 8673–8677.
10. Sierakowska, H., Sambade, M. J., Agrawal, S., and Kole, R. (1996) Repair of thalassemic human β-globin mRNA in mammalian cells by antisense oligonucleotides. *Proc. Natl. Acad. Sci. USA.* **93,** 12840–12844.
11. Weatherall, D. J. (1994) Thalassemias, in *The Molecular Basis of Blood Diseases* (Stamatoyannopoulos, G., et al., eds.), W.B. Saunders, Philadelphia, pp. 157–205.
12. Mirabelli, C. K., and Crooke, S. T. (1993) Antisense oligonucleotides in the context of modern molecular drug discovery and development, in *Antisense Research and Applications* (Crooke, S. T. and Lebleu, B., eds.), CRC, Boca Raton, FL, pp. 7–35.
13. Furdon, P. F., Dominski, Z., and Kole, R. (1989) RNase H cleavage of RNA hybridized to oligonucleotides containing methylphosphonate, phosphorothioate and phosphodiester bonds. *Nucleic Acids Res.* **17,** 9193–9204.
14. Sproat, B. S. and Lamond, A. I. (1993) 2'-O-alkyloligoribonucleotides, in *Antisense Research and Applications* (Crooke, S. T. and Lebleu, B., eds.), CRC, Boca Raton, FL, pp. 351–363.
15. Zhang, R., Lu, Z., Zhao, H., Zhang, X., Diasio, R. B., Habus, I., et al. (1995) In vivo stability, disposition and metabolism of a "hybrid"oligonucleotide phosphorothioate in rats. *Biochem. Pharm.* **50,** 545–556.
16. Hawley-Nelson, P., Ciccarone, V., Gebeyehu, G., Jessee, J., and Felgner, P. L. (1993) Lipofectamine reagent: a new, higher efficiency polycationic liposome transfection reagent. *Focus* **15,** 73–79.
17. Schagger, H. and von Jagov, G. (1987) Tricine-sodium dodecyl sulfate-polyacrylamide gel electrophoresis for the separation of proteins in the range from 1 to 100 kDa. *Anal. Biochem.* **166,** 368–379.

Index